# Advanced Technique of Endoscopic Cervical and Thoracic Spine Surgery

Hyeun Sung Kim • Dong Hwa Heo
Kangtaek Lim • Cheol Woong Park
Chun-Kun Park
Editors

# Advanced Technique of Endoscopic Cervical and Thoracic Spine Surgery

Springer

*Editors*
Hyeun Sung Kim
Department of Neurosurgery
Gangnam Nanoori Hospital
Seoul, Korea (Republic of)

Dong Hwa Heo
Department of Neurosurgery
Champodo Spine Hospital
Seoul, Korea (Republic of)

Kangtaek Lim
Department of Neurosurgery
Seoul Segyero Hospital
Seoul, Korea (Republic of)

Cheol Woong Park
Department of Neurosurgery
Daejeon Woori Hospital
Daejeon, Korea (Republic of)

Chun-Kun Park
Department of Neurosurgery
The Catholic University of Korea
Seoul, Korea (Republic of)

ISBN 978-981-99-1132-5 ISBN 978-981-99-1133-2 (eBook)
https://doi.org/10.1007/978-981-99-1133-2



This Springer imprint is published by the registered company Springer Nature Singapore Pte Ltd.
The registered company address is: 152 Beach Road, #21-01/04 Gateway East, Singapore 189721, Singapore

# Preface by Chun-Kun Park

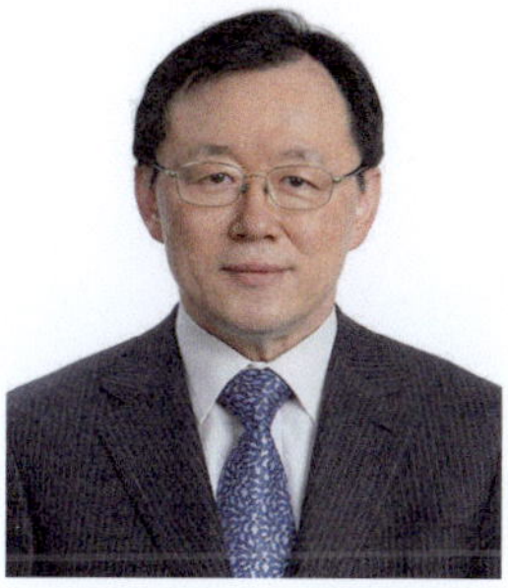

First of all, it would be congratulatory to the current and former presidents of Korean Research Society of Endoscopic Spine Surgery (KOSESS), the editorial staffs and all the authors that are publishing a contemporary book of endoscopic spine surgery (ESS). What impressed us the most was that the youngest spine group in Korea, KOSESS inaugurated only less than 3 years ago, made the textbook of spinal endoscopy. Nowadays, the development of ESS is so rapid that a traditional textbook cannot contain the newest issue in a specific clinical field. It takes more than 2 years to complete a traditional textbook. In this regard, a contemporary textbook could be a solution and medium to keep a reader updated with the qualified new subjects of ESS.

As a strong supporter during Dr. G Choi's inauguration preparation of KOSESS, it must be proud that publishing the contemporary textbook of ESS was done by such so young-aged group. In the Korean Minimally Invasive Spine Surgery Society (KOMISS), particularly in KOSESS, there are many globally leading personalities in the frontier spirit, by whom KOSESS could make the current textbook without significant difficulty in such a short period. The book would be made smaller in size than an ordinary textbook for a user to carry in a pocket, perhaps as a matter of efficiency. Hopefully, this would become a handbook of ESS for beginners and trainees of ESS, and also any endoscopic spine surgeon who needs to be updated and feeding their ESS procedure into the text. It would be recommendable for all the readers not to understand the handbook as a low-quality one. The editor should have wanted the book to be useful for a surgeon practically at the front line.

Finally, it should be our hope that the contemporary textbook must be published annually in line with the role of this book although the contents are a fewer than this textbook to keep the surgeons not to drop out of line.

Seoul, Korea (Republic of) Chun-Kun Park, MD, PhD

# Preface by Cheol Woong Park

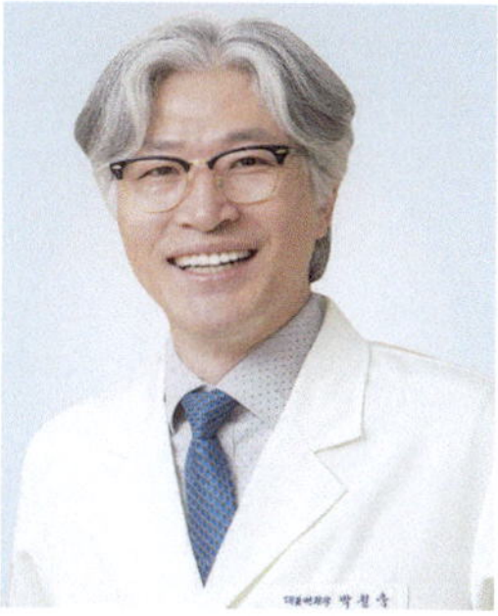

Throughout history, science has developed by breaking down the pre-existing knowledge, ideas, prejudices, and beliefs of that period of time. It has always faced strong objections, attacks, and skepticism from the majority of the community whenever someone tries to go further. But with someone who believes in his findings based on nothing but scientific studies and keeps working on them till others can see and agree with them.

There was skepticism about endoscopic spine surgery (ESS): its safety, efficacy, effectiveness, practicality, and so on. But there have been changes in recent years, ESS is gaining more attention and approval among spine surgeons. This wouldn't have been possible without those great pioneers who had the vision and contributed to the continuous development of ESS from their own experiences. We have come a long way, and it is not the end of our journey. For this, it is beyond my words how honored and proud I am to be part of this project.

This book is the second edition of the Endoscopic Spine Surgery textbook, published by Korean Research Society of Endoscopic Spine Surgery (KOSESS) shortly after the first edition was published. This book has wider applications and techniques of ESS as it has been evolving significantly over the past few years, such as its applications to the cervical and thoracic spine, and inter-body fusion. This, in my humble opinion, helps both young and experienced spine surgeons stay up-to-date in ESS scene.

This cannot be done without those surgeons who share their experiences and knowledge with colleagues to broaden our horizons. There will be more new findings, technologies, and instruments to come, and it makes me thrilled. This project could not be completed without those authors who are masters of ESS in their own right. I cannot thank them enough for their efforts and remarkable work in making this art. With these people, there is a bright future for ESS where it will be treated as the gold standard treatment of choice in the future.

Daejeon, Korea (Republic of) Cheol Woong Park, MD, PhD

# Preface by Dong Hwa Heo

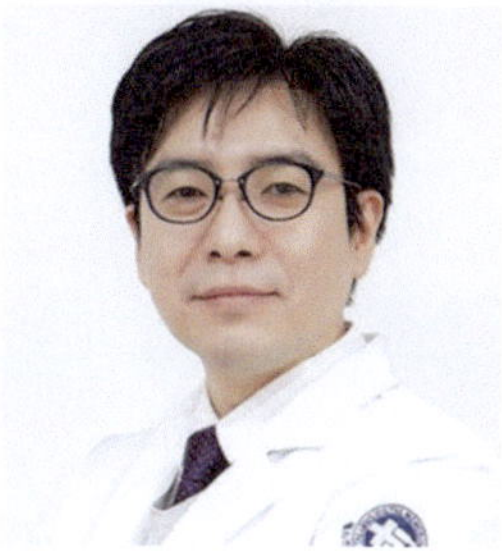

In recent years, spinal endoscopic surgeries have advanced and developed dramatically. Indications for spinal endoscopic surgery were extended from the lumbar to cervical and thoracic lesions.

Spinal endoscopic surgeries have been performed for the treatment of various spinal diseases, and various spinal diseases are being treated with spinal endoscopic surgery instead of conventional spine surgeries.

Through this textbook of spinal endoscopic surgery, I would like to introduce advanced surgical techniques of endoscopic spine approaches. This textbook contains many figures, surgical images, and video clips. Therefore, I believe that it will be of great help in learning cervical and thoracic endoscopic surgery.

Although cervical and thoracic spine endoscopic surgeries have many advantages, they also have risks and complications. Before starting endoscopic surgery for cervical and thoracic spine, you must have sufficient experience in lumbar spine endoscopic surgery and microsurgery.

Many thanks to the many authors and springer nature who contributed to this textbook.

Seoul, Korea (Republic of) — Dong Hwa Heo, MD, PhD

# Preface by Hyeun Sung Kim

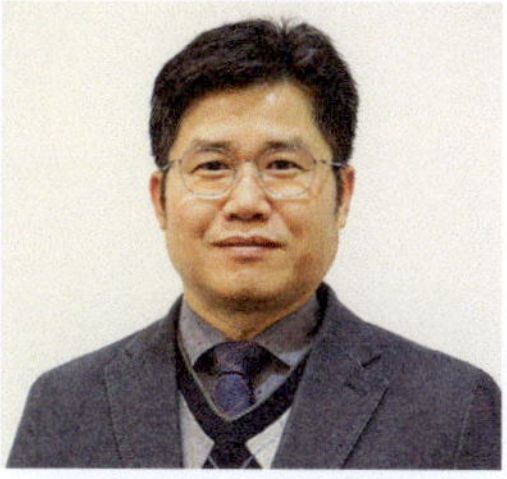

**Things that seemed to last forever change suddenly one day!!**

The development of industry is changing many patterns of society, and the development of medicine also undergoes many changes and developments.

With the development of spinal endoscopy drills and radiofrequency ablation system for spinal endoscopy, the development of uniportal endoscopic surgery techniques, and the development of biportal endoscopic endoscopic surgery, we believe that endoscopic spinal surgery and treatment will now lead the spine surgery and treatment. And, it is believed that these will be done with the development of endoscopic spinal fusion surgery, endoscopic spine surgery (ESS) of the cervical and thoracic spine.

In that sense, the second endoscopic spine surgery textbook of Korean Research Society of Endoscopic Spine Surgery (KOSESS) can be said to be very meaningful in the history of endoscopic spinal surgery and treatment.

Things that seemed to last forever change suddenly one day. If we do not prepare in advance, we will not be able to join the new era, but those who prepare will be given more opportunities.

Seoul, Korea (Republic of)  
20, Feb 2022

Hyeun Sung Kim, MD, PhD

# Preface by Kangtaek Lim

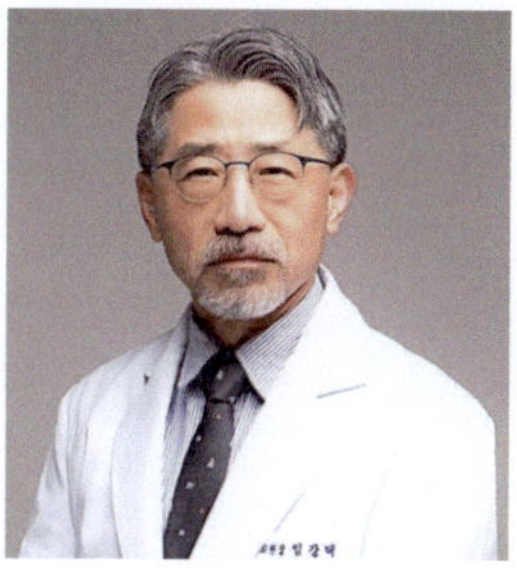

A year ago, KOSESS (Korean Research Society of Endoscopic Spine Surgery) published its first textbook about endoscopic surgery for lumbar spine, which drew significant attention from the readers. A year later, the second textbook about cervical, thorax spine was published.

As the technology and the approach of endoscopic spine surgery (ESS) continues to develop, endoscopic surgery extended its limit from just solving lumbar spine pathology to solving the cervical and thoracic spine such as decompression and fusion.

Much has changed in cervical and thoracic spine surgery since the endoscopic procedures came out, but the ultimate goal of surgery has not. That is, by using endoscopic procedures introduced here, surgeons will be able to avoid the damage of normal anatomical structures which can result in decrease of postoperative complications, reduced postoperative pain, shortened hospital stay, and expedited recovery.

In this textbook, step-by-step guidance from a highly experienced expert will provide a detailed description, which includes the utilization of endoscopic instruments, image-guided approach, methods for preoperative planning, complication avoidance strategies, and postoperative care.

KOSESS has one of the world's most advanced spinal endoscopic surgical technology. We publish our textbook to introduce our latest understanding about theoretical and technical methods of endoscopic surgery. It is our desire that sharing our understanding with the world will elicit more novel and innovative ideas.

We hope this textbook serves as a valuable resource to a spine surgeon who wants to advance their understanding in ESS.

Seoul, Korea (Republic of) Kangtaek Lim

# Acknowledgment

This textbook was produced with the support of the Korean Minimally Invasive Spine Surgery Society (KOMISS) and the Korea Research Society of Endoscopic Spine Surgery (KOSESS).

# Contents

# Part I

# Cervical - Introduction

# Anatomical Consideration of Posterior Cervical Endoscopic Approaches

Dong Hwa Heo, Jae Won Jang,
and Don Young Park

**Abstract**

Recently, endoscopic spine approaches using uniportal or biportal endoscopy have been performed for cervical radiculopathy or myelopathy. Posterior cervical approaches were the most common endoscopic approaches and compared to the anterior cervical endoscopic approach, posterior cervical endoscopic surgery is safer. Compared to microscopic approaches, the surgical field of endoscopic approach is narrow. Therefore, surgical landmarks and anatomical orientation are important for complete decompression in cervical endoscopic approaches. The radiological anatomy of preoperative computed tomography (CT) and magnetic resonance imaging (MRI) is also important. In addition, a portal for endoscopic surgery is made while looking at the C-arm fluoroscopy. Therefore, it is also important to understand the C-arm fluoroscopic images.

**Keywords**

Endoscopy · Cervical · Anatomy · Posterior

## 1 Radiological Anatomy for Cervical Endoscopic Posterior Approach

### 1.1 Simple X-Ray and C-Arm Fluoroscopic Anatomy

Two portals for biportal endoscopic procedures are made over pedicle line in anteroposterior (AP) view (Fig. 1a). Intraoperatively, an X-ray AP view is usually checked to make the portals of endoscopy. In patients with a short neck, lower levels of the cervical spine such as C 6–7 and C7-T1 cannot be demonstrated on lateral X-ray view due to shoulder obstruction (Fig. 1b). In these cases, the exact level of marking of the lower C6–7 and C7-T1 using C-arm lateral X-ray view was difficult. C-arm AP X-ray view was very helpful in confirming the operation level in the lower cervical level (Fig. 1a). The first thoracic vertebrae had the first rib, and it can give information to confirm the operating lesion on cervicothoracic junction. However, we always check the possibility of C7 rib using a preoperative cervical CT scan.

D. H. Heo (✉)
Neurosurgery, Endoscopic Spine Surgery Center, Champodonamu Spine Hospital, Seoul, South Korea

J. W. Jang
Neurosurgery, Spine Center, Leon Wiltse Memorial Hospital, Suwon, South Korea

D. Y. Park
Orthopedics, David Geffen School of Medicine, UCLA, Los Angeles, CA, USA
e-mail: DYPark@mednet.ucla.edu



H. S. Kim et al. (eds.), *Advanced Technique of Endoscopic Cervical and Thoracic Spine Surgery*,
https://doi.org/10.1007/978-981-99-1133-2_1

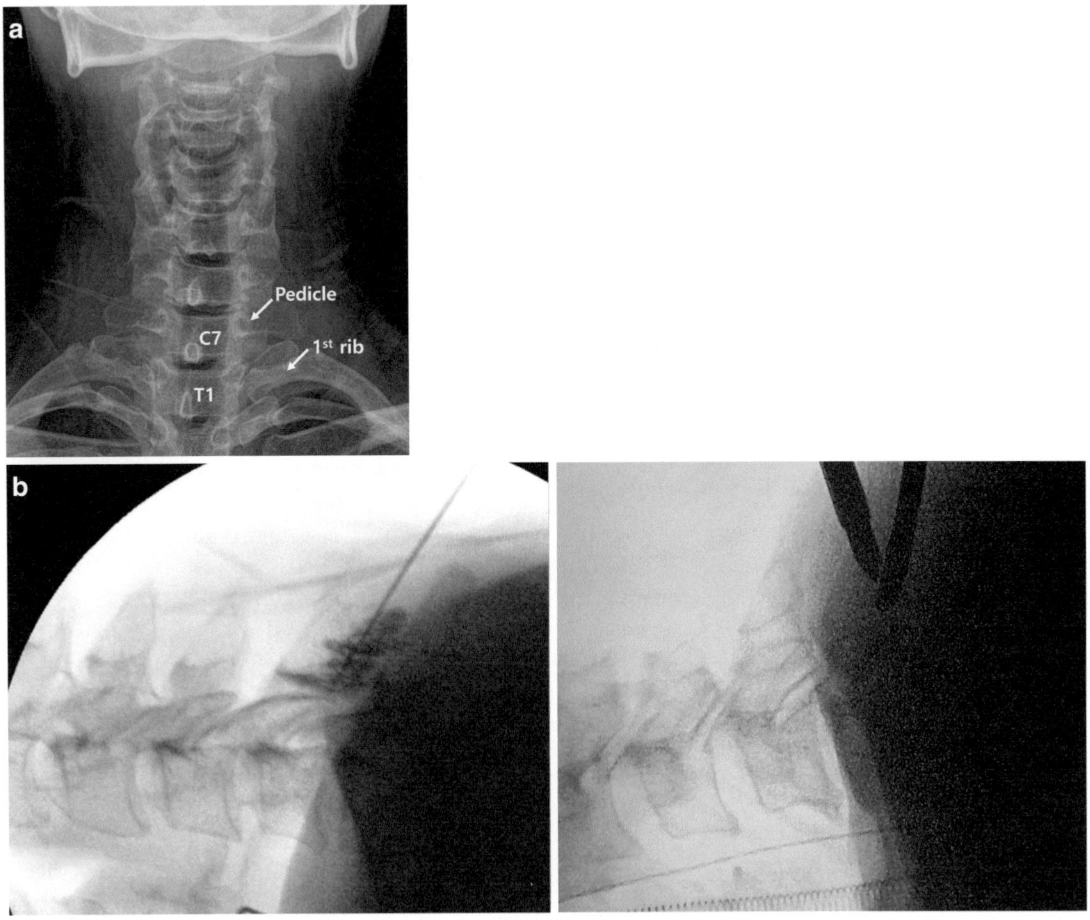


**Fig. 1** (**a**) Anteroposterior X-ray views of cervical spine. The first rib-attached T1 vertebra is an important point for intraoperative level marking. A pedicle is also an important radiological marking of making endoscopic corridor. (**b**) Cervicothoracic junction is often invisible due to shoulder joint

## 1.2 Computed Tomography Anatomy

We recommend taking preoperative cervical computed tomography (CT) scan, including three-dimensional (3D) reconstruction (Fig. 2a). Cervical CT and its 3D reconstruction images are important and useful in making decisions on the cervical endoscopic approach and surgical plan. A cervical CT scan can demonstrate osteophyte, ossification of posterior longitudinal ligament, disc calcification, pedicle orientation, and rib more accurately than a magnetic resonance imaging (MRI) (Fig. 2b). Especially, 3D reconstruction CT image can show the operation-level V point. The actual appearance of the V point can be predicted through the 3D CT image. Also, the first rib and first rib-attached T1 vertebra should be checked on CT scan because there is a possibility of C7 rib [1] (Fig. 2c).

## 1.3 Magnetic Resonance Imaging Anatomy

MRI reveals muscular anatomy (myoarchitecture), location of the vertebral artery, and pathological lesions such as central stenosis with

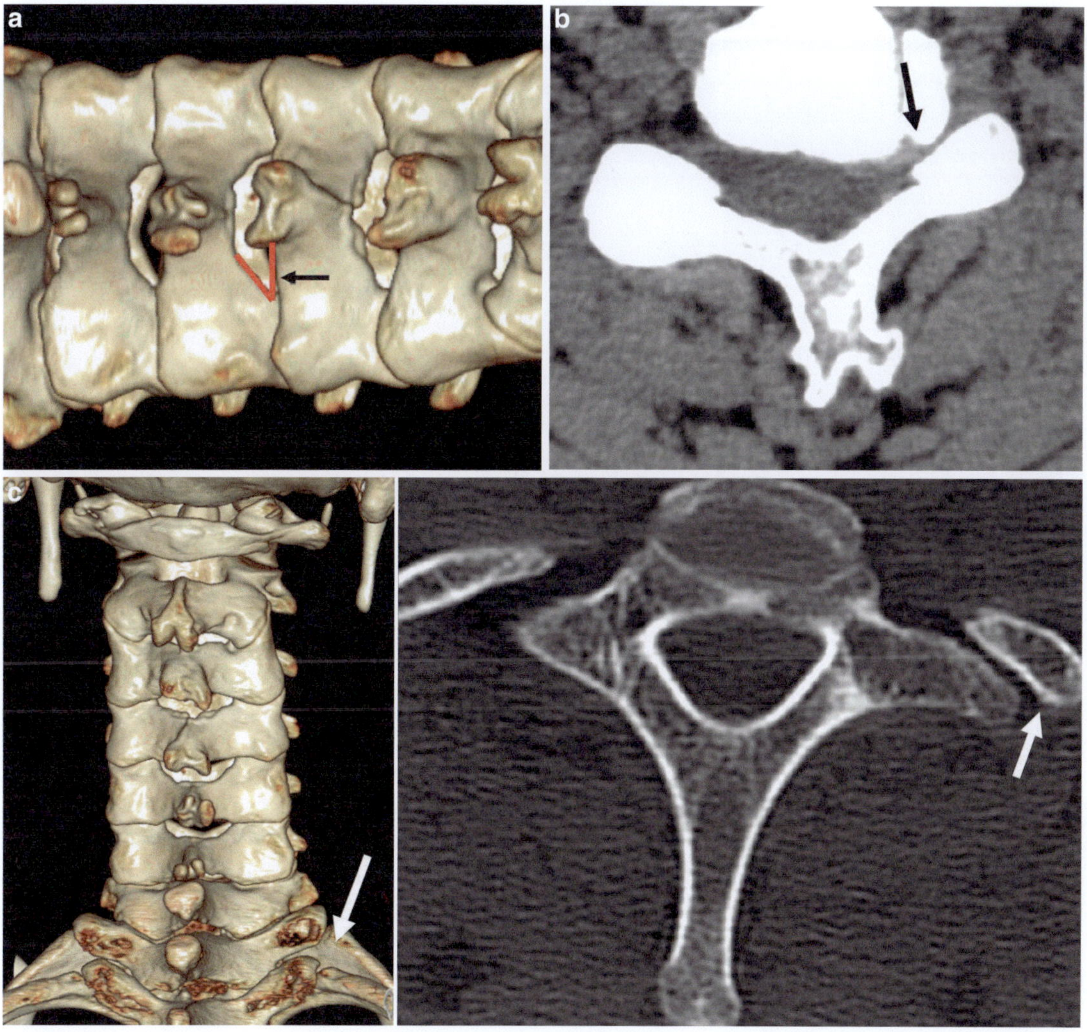


**Fig. 2** A cervical CT scan with a 3D demonstration is important in making a decision on a surgical plan. (**a**) 3D reconstruction image of cervical CT demonstrates the bony surface anatomy and V point for posterior cervical endoscopic approach (red line and black arrow). (**b**) Cervical CT axial image reveals osteophyte and foraminal stenosis (black arrow). (**c**) The rib and its attached vertebral should be checked using cervical CT images

hypertrophy of ligamentum flavum, foraminal ruptured disc, foraminal stenosis, or existence of myelopathy. Preoperative MRI was important for making decisions on the endoscopic posterior cervical approach. If an imaginary line is drawn on both lateral borders of the myelon (spinal cord) and most of the lesion is located inside the imaginary line, that is, in the myelon region, it is difficult to remove it with a posterior endoscopic approach (Fig. 3a). The pathological lesion outside the lateral borders of the spinal cord was suitable for posterior cervical foraminotomy (Fig. 3b).

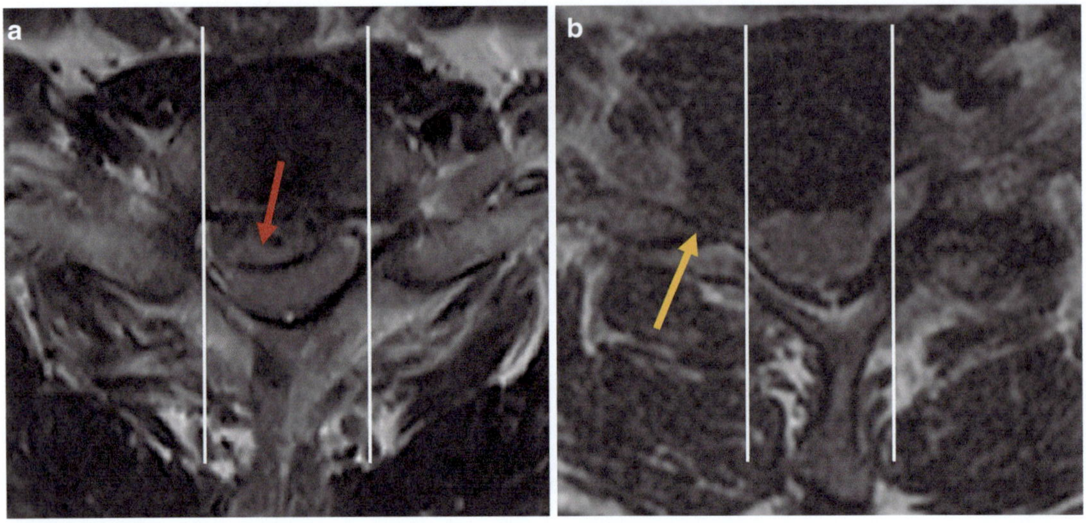


**Fig. 3** We draw two lines on both lateral borders of the (spinal cord), and if most of the lesion is located inside the two lines, the posterior endoscopic approach is not suitable (**a**) If the pathological lesion is located outside the two lines, it means cervical foraminal lesion (**b**) and it is suitable for posterior cervical endoscopic foraminotomy or lamino-foraminotomy

## 2 Endoscopic Anatomy

### 2.1 Bony Surface Anatomy

- V point: The V point is the first landmark of the bony surface anatomy in endoscopic posterior cervical foraminotomy (Fig. 4a) [2]. The V point consists of the lower margin of the upper lamina, and upper margin of the lower lamina and facet joint (Fig. 4b). Cervical lamino-foraminotomy starts at the V point. The V point of intraoperative bone anatomy should be exposed first using a radiofrequency or dissectors in uniportal or biportal endoscopic cervical posterior approaches. After finding the V point and cleanly exposing it, bone work must be started with the correct anatomical orientation.

### 2.2 Cervical Ligamentum Flavum

The ligamentum flavum covered dura and nerve roots like lumbar area (Fig. 5). The ligamentum flavum was easily exposed after partial hemi-laminotomy. The medial part of the ligament above the dura is usually thick, and the lateral part of the ligamentum flavum above the root is thinned by the dura. The ligamentum flavum should be partially removed to find the dura and nerve root (Fig. 5).

### 2.3 Peridural Membrane

Spine endoscopy can clearly demonstrate the peridural membrane over the dura and nerve root (Fig. 6 a and b). A peridural membrane is sometimes observed located between the dura and the ligamentum flavum [3]. If the ligamentum flavum is removed but the dura and nerve root are not clearly visible, the peridural membrane should be evaluated and removed (Fig. 6a). Care must be taken as the peridural membrane can look like dura. Cervical nerve root was clearly exposed after removal of the peridural membrane (Fig. 6c). The peridural membrane contains vessels; hence, to prevent bleeding, the vessels must be coagulated prior to removal.

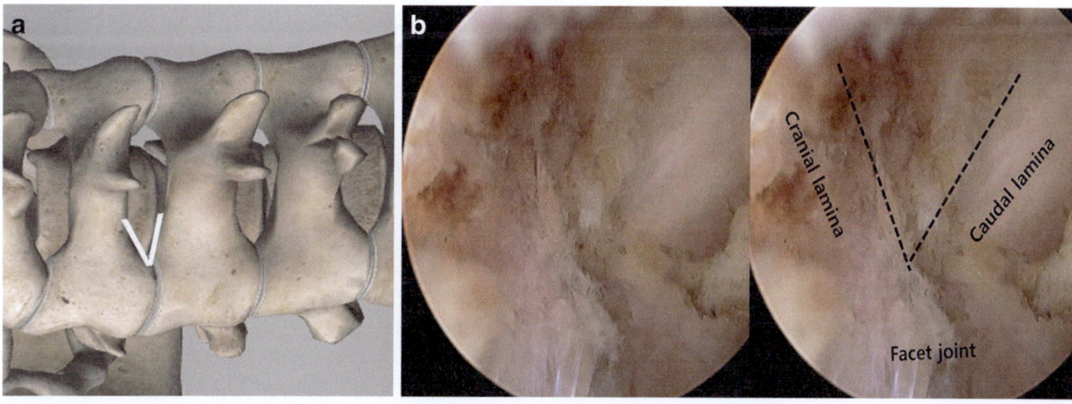


**Fig. 4** The V point consists of the cervical upper lamina, lower lamina, and facet joint (**a**). For clear dissection of the V point, soft tissue over the lamina should be removed using a radiofrequency probe or pituitary forceps (**b**)

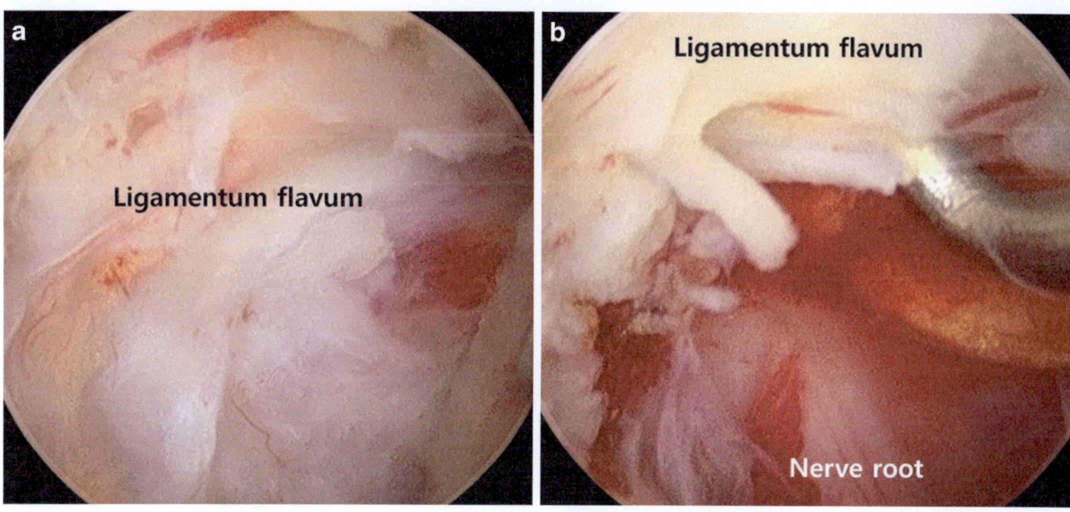


**Fig. 5** Cervical ligamentum flavum. Ligamentum flavum covered dura and nerve root (**a**). After partial removal of the ligamentum flavum, the dura and nerve root were visible (**b**)

## 2.4 Cervical Dura and Nerve Root

- Nerve root anatomy: Dual nerve roots were frequently seen [4]. A motor nerve root was placed beneath a sensory nerve root (Fig. 7). There was a possibility of cervical motor nerve root injury during discectomy or axillar dissection. Moreover, motor nerve root may be mistaken for ruptured disc particle or protruded disc during the learning curve period. In order to accurately expose the nerve root during surgery, it is necessary to expose it from the central dura and find the proximal part of the nerve root.

## 2.5 Axillar and Pedicle Area

Axillar area of the cervical nerve root consisted of the dura lateral margin, nerve root, and pedicle (Fig. 8). The pedicle should be dissected and

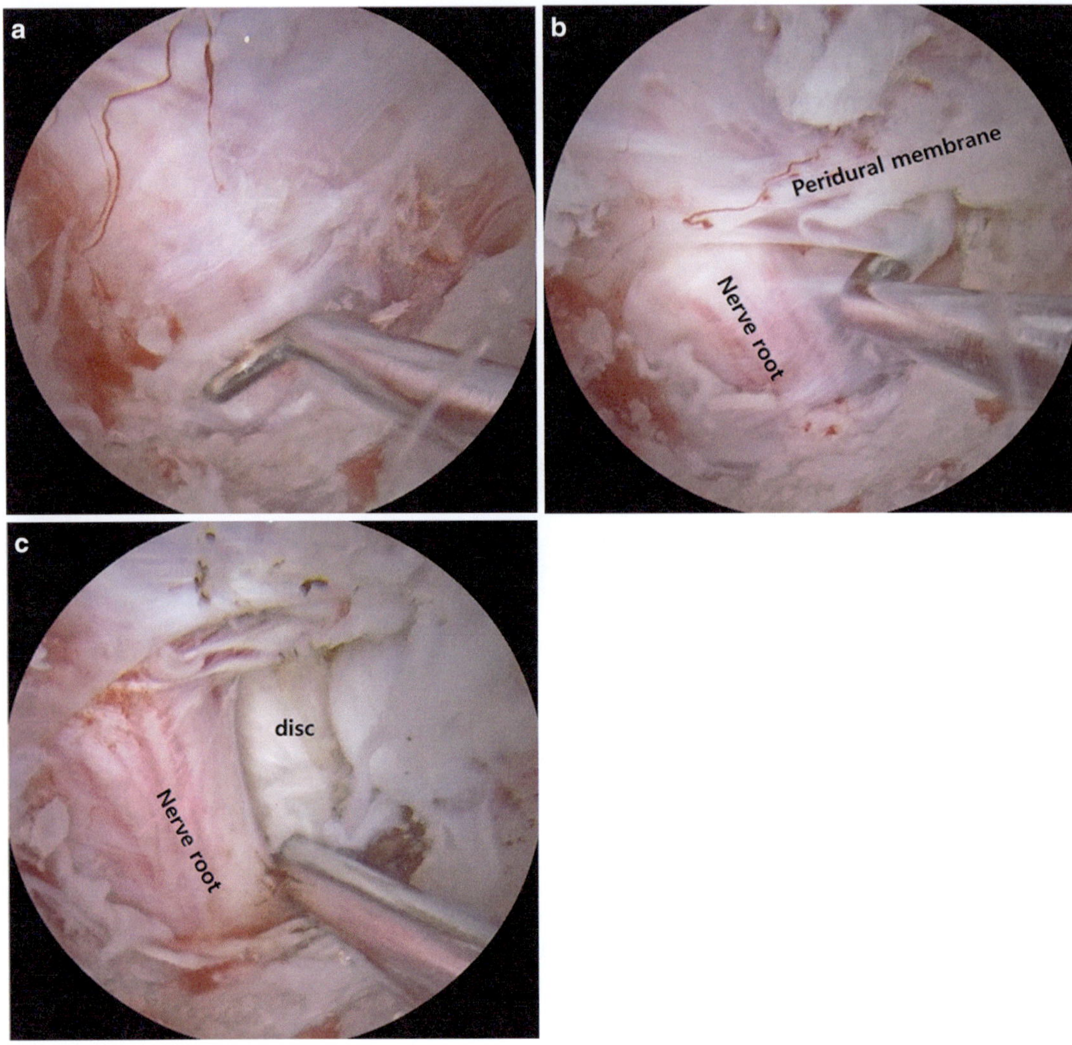


**Fig. 6** Peridural membrane-covered dura and nerve root (**a**, **b**). After removal of the membrane, the nerve root was clearly exposed (**c**)

exposed (Fig. 8). In case with a narrow space of axillar area, the pedicle should be partially removed to remove ruptured disc particles with minimal nerve root retraction. Endoscopic decompression from pedicle to pedicle was performed for full decompression of the cervical nerve root. The lower margin of the upper pedicle and upper margin of the lower pedicle were checked using a hook or a dissector before the end of the endoscopic surgery.

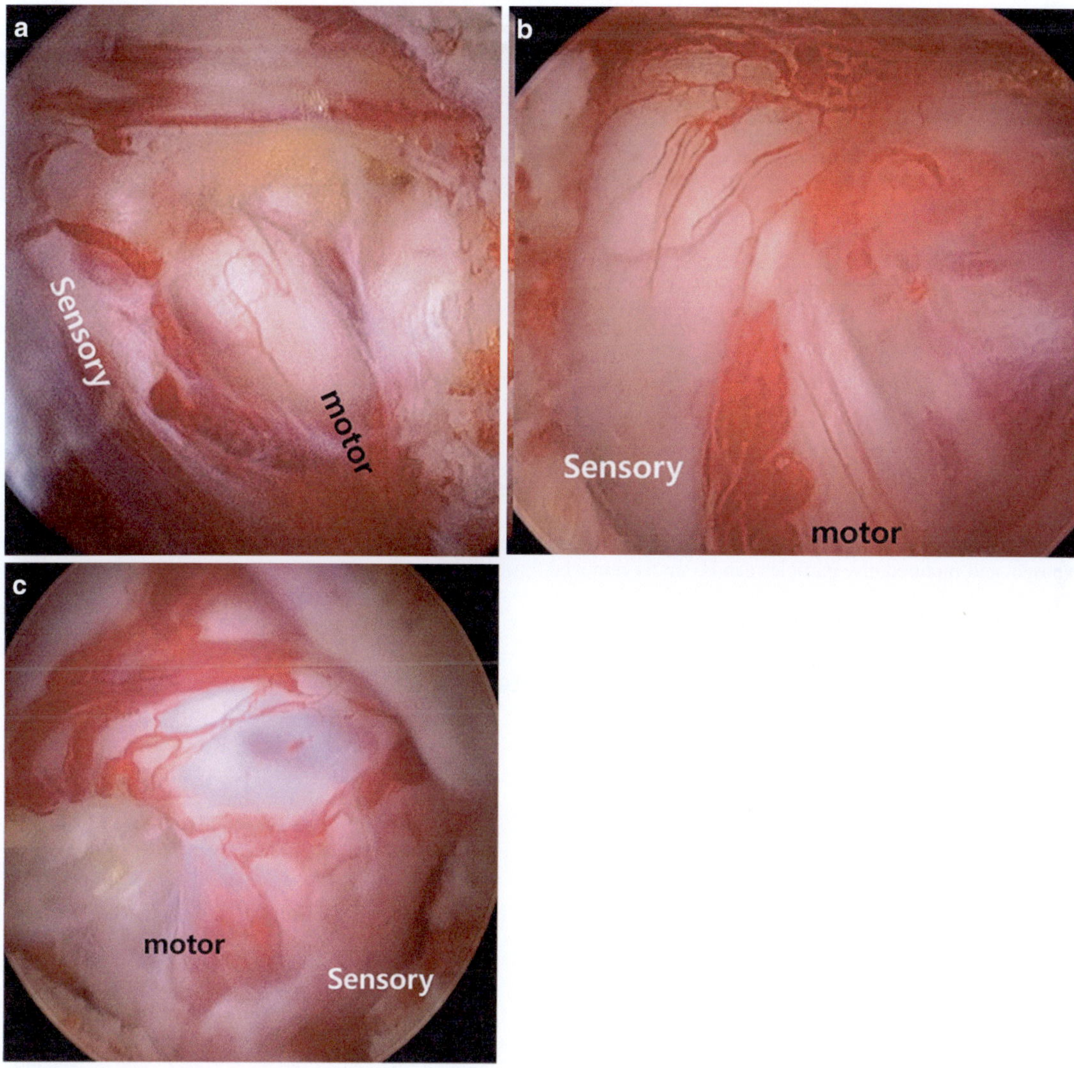


**Fig. 7** Dual cervical nerve root. A motor nerve root was beneath a sensory nerve root. Left posterior cervical approach (**a**, **b**) and right posterior cervical approach (**c**)

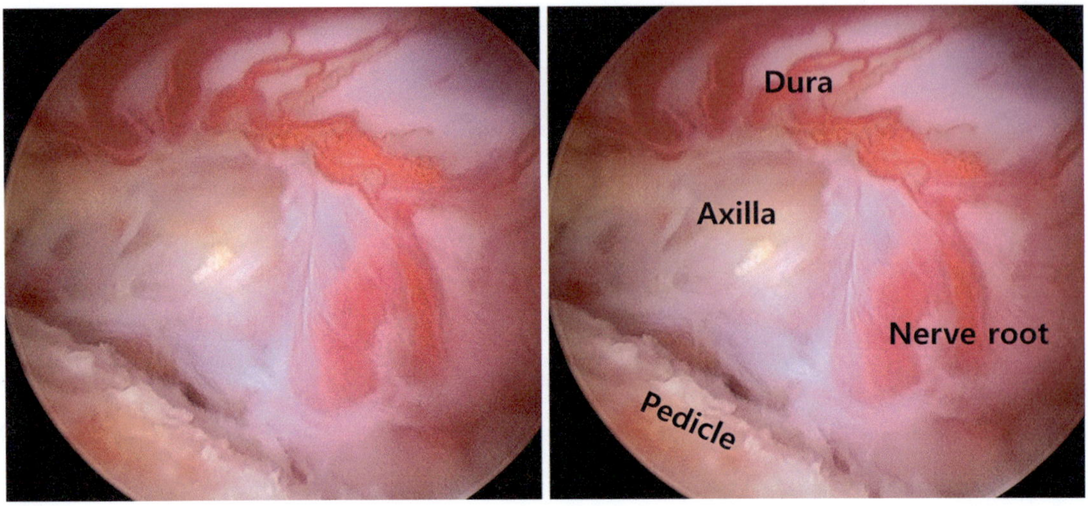


**Fig. 8** Axillar area of the cervical dura and nerve root. If the pedicle is partially removed, the axillar can be clearly exposed, and ruptured disc particles can be safely removed through the axillar

## 3 Conclusion

Cervical endoscopic approaches, including uniportal or biportal endoscopy, provide a magnified and accurate surgical view, but have a disadvantage in that the field of view is narrow compared to microsurgery [5]. Therefore, an accurate understanding of the spinal endoscopy anatomy is essential for safe surgery. The image matching between endoscopic field view and preoperative radiological exams, including CT scan and MIR, should be trained. The surgeon must try to find and understand the anatomical differences of individual patient in preoperative CT and MRI scans to prevent complications and wrong-level surgery.

## References

1. Guttentag AR, Salwen JK. Keep your eyes on the ribs: the spectrum of normal variants and diseases that involve the ribs. Radiographics. 1999;19(5):1125–42.
2. Kim JY, Kim DH, Lee YJ, Jeon JB, Choi SY, Kim HS, et al. Anatomical importance between neural structure and bony landmark: clinical importance for posterior endoscopic cervical Foraminotomy. Neurospine. 2021;18(1):139–46.
3. Bosscher HA, Grozdanov PN, Warraich II, MacDonald CC, Day MR. The anatomy of the peridural membrane of the human spine. Anat Rec (Hoboken). 2021;304(4):677–91.
4. Kitamura K, Yamamoto M, Hirota Y, Sato N, Machida T, Ishikawa N, et al. Cervical nerve roots and the dural sheath: a histological study using human fetuses near term. Anat Cell Biol. 2020;53(4):451–9.
5. Kim JY, Hong HJ, Lee DC, Kim TH, Hwang JS, Park CK. Comparative analysis of three types of minimally invasive posterior cervical foraminotomy for foraminal stenosis, uniportal endoscopy, biportal endoscopy, and microsurgery: radiologic and mid-term clinical outcomes. Neurospine. 2022;19:603.

# Prevention of Complications

Hee Seok Yang and Jeong Yoon Park

**Abstract**

With the development of spinal endoscopic surgery, cervical decompression and discectomy has become the major endoscopic cervical spine surgery. The lack of clear anatomical landmarks and hindered visualization of anatomical structures due to narrow operating view are significant limitations in the endoscopic approach to the spine. Complications during the learning curve period of endoscopic spine surgery usually occur due to unfamiliarity with endoscopic image orientation and inappropriate approach to the surgical target. This can result in injury to neural structures, incomplete decompression, dural tear, wrong-level procedures, and excessive removal of facet joint in the initial series of patients. The learning curve is steep because endoscopic drilling is performed close to neural structures. To avoid complications associated with endoscopic spine surgery, various factors should be considered. The important step for obtaining a good surgical outcome after endoscopic spine surgery is an ideal entry point and trajectory during the surgical approach. To prevent insufficient decompression, the widest decompression as possible is often required. However, excessive facet joint removal and surgically induced instability could lead to persistent symptoms, recurrent disc herniation, and progressive neck pain. Prevention of postoperative dysesthesia is also an important factor for successful cervical endoscopic decompression. The surgeon is responsible for optimal outcomes, which could affect the frequency and severity of adverse events. Endoscopic cervical spine surgery should be performed carefully using an appropriate surgical technique with sufficient experience.

**Keywords**

Anterior endoscopic cervical discectomy
Posterior endoscopic cervical foraminotomy
Posterior endoscopic cervical discectomy
Unilateral biportal endoscope · Cervical complication

**Supplementary Information** The online version contains supplementary material available at https://doi.org/10.1007/978-981-99-1133-2_2.

H. S. Yang
Department of Neurosurgery, Seoul Barunsesang Hospital, Seoul, South Korea

J. Y. Park (✉)
The Spine and Spinal Cord Institute, Department of Neurosurgery, Gangnam Severance Hospital, Yonsei University College of Medicine, Seoul, South Korea
e-mail: spinepjy@yuhs.ac


H. S. Kim et al. (eds.), *Advanced Technique of Endoscopic Cervical and Thoracic Spine Surgery*, https://doi.org/10.1007/978-981-99-1133-2_2

# 1 Introduction

## 1.1 Cervical Endoscopic Decompression and Discectomy

Cervical radiculopathy is a common cervical spine condition leading to significant disability from nerve root dysfunction [1, 2]. Conservative therapy is recommended for at least 6 weeks in the treatment of cervical radiculopathy without myelopathy. However, a significant proportion of patients remain symptomatic despite being compliant with conservative management, and such patients might need surgical treatment.

Anterior cervical discectomy and fusion (ACDF) or artificial disc replacement has been popular as the gold standard treatment [3, 4]. Morbidity attributed to anterior cervical surgery ranges from 13.2% to 19.3%, with pseudoarthrosis and adjacent segment disease being the most common postoperative complications [3, 5, 6]. Anterior and posterior cervical decompression and discectomy have gained popularity as an alternative to ACDF, sparing patients from problems associated with fusion and surgical instrumentations with equally good clinical results with the added advantage of motion preservation [2, 7–9].

With the development of spinal endoscopic surgery, cervical decompression and discectomy has become the major endoscopic cervical spine surgery. Anterior endoscopic cervical discectomy (AECD) is performed with one-portal full endoscope. Posterior cervical foraminotomy has recently been performed with one-portal full endoscope or unilateral biportal endoscope (UBE), and posterior endoscopic cervical foraminotomy (PECF) and discectomy (PECD) have become the main endoscopic cervical spine surgeries [1, 2, 7, 10–13].

## 1.2 Anatomical Landmarks

The lack of clear anatomical landmarks and hindered visualization of anatomical structures due to narrow operating view are significant limitations in the endoscopic approach to the spine. Complications during the learning curve period of endoscopic spine surgery usually occur due to unfamiliarity with endoscopic image orientation and inappropriate approach to the surgical target. This can result in injury to neural structures, dural tear, wrong-level procedures, and excessive removal of facet joint in the initial series of patients. The most important step for obtaining good surgical outcome after endoscopic spine surgery is an ideal entry point and trajectory during the surgical approach [14].

## 1.3 Learning Curve

An initial learning curve is essential in endoscopic spine surgery because the use of long instruments is inevitable, and the surgical field of view is narrow. The learning curve is steep because endoscopic drilling is performed close to neural structures. Competence in using endoscopic instruments can be achieved with experience. Depending on surgical experience, different types and frequencies of endoscopic spine surgery-specific complications can occur [14, 15].

# 2 Anterior Endoscopic Cervical Discectomy

Anterior endoscopic cervical discectomy (AECD) is an endoscopic cervical spine surgery with a one-portal full endoscope in which the trocar is inserted into the midline of the disc while pushing the trachea in front of the cervical vertebrae (Fig. 1). The route of surgical approach to the cervical spine is generally determined using magnetic resonance imaging (MRI), and the lesion should be approached diagonally, from the opposite side of the disc rupture site. In AECD, the most dangerous and important aspect is to safely place the needle or trocar inside the disc; once the trocar is placed inside the disc, the working sleeve and endoscope insertions are relatively safe procedures.

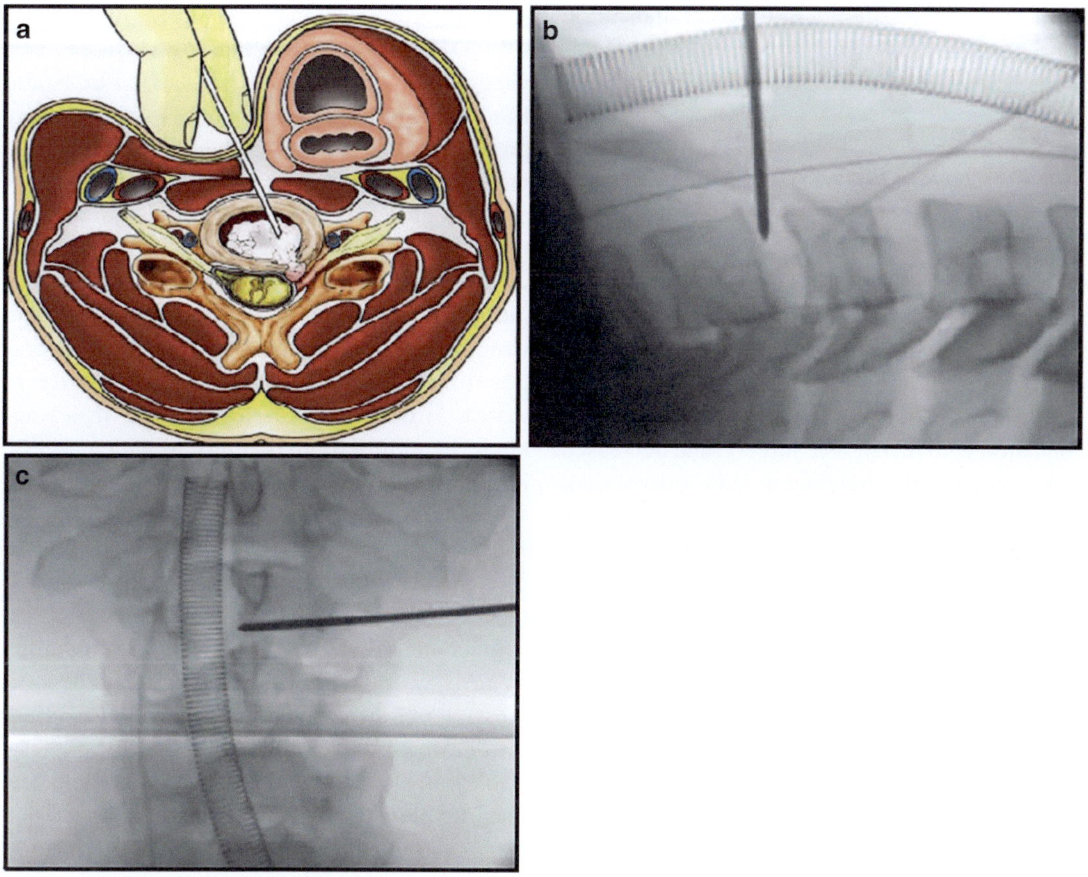


**Fig. 1** In AECD, the needle or trocar is inserted into the midline of the disc while pushing the trachea in front of the cervical vertebrae (**a**) and should be approached from the opposite side of the disc rupture site. Lateral (**b**) and anteroposterior (**c**) X-ray images during trocar insertion. The intubation tube is pushed laterally

## 2.1 Anatomical Consideration before AECD

In the anterior cervical approach, safe and precise targeting is the most essential factor for effective discectomy. The surgeon should identify the carotid pulse and push their fingertips down into the space between the carotid artery and trachea to identify the anterior surface of the vertebral body [1, 16, 17]. (Fig. 1a) If anterior neck surgery, such as thyroid surgery, has previously been performed, the carotid artery and trachea should not be pushed due to soft-tissue adhesion. Thus, AECD is contraindicated because damage to vascular structures (carotid artery, jugular vein) or trachea could be a life-threatening complication.

In patients with a narrow disc space and advanced spondylosis with osteophytes, the AECD is contraindicated. The AECD can only be performed when the working sleeve is accurately positioned near the lesion. If the disc prolapses, mounting the working sleeve to the desired area and changing the position of the working sleeve might be hindered, and the ruptured disc cannot be removed properly. The purpose of AECD is to remove a ruptured disc without enlarging the foramen. Because disc prolapse patients frequently have foraminal stenosis, AECD is contraindicated. Due to the difficulty of proper positioning of the working sleeve, ACDF or posterior foraminotomy is recommended. A significant migrated disc herniation not located at the precise disc level could be a contraindication because the up and down movement of the endoscope is limited.

## 2.2 Prevention of Disc Height Reduction

AECD requires penetrating and removing a normal disc from the anterior portion to access the posterior laterally ruptured disc. Because the range of disc removal is wide, a high possibility exists that disc height after surgery will decrease compared with that before surgery, and decreased and prolapsed disc height can lead to foraminal stenosis, which is associated with unsatisfactory surgical outcome. To avoid height reduction, the amount of normal disc removal should be minimized, or a transcorporeal route might be advantageous. In addition, due to the very narrow surgical field through the vertebral body, the use of an endoscope with a high visual angle might be ideal [1, 11, 12].

## 2.3 AECD-Specific Instruments Are Required

Because the AECD has to be approached through the disc, the diameter of the endoscope (4 mm) is thinner than in other cervical endoscopic surgeries. Because the instruments have to be inserted through the working channel, thin and long instruments are necessary, which require a longer procedure time and learning curve. Therefore, use of a laser is necessary during AECD. The laser can effectively remove the disc and ligaments in a narrow space and minimize the amount of normal disc removal. Thus, the decrease in disc height after AECD is reduced and the operation time shortened.

# 3 Posterior Endoscopic Cervical Foraminotomy and Discectomy

Posterior endoscopic cervical foraminotomy (PECF) has recently been performed with one-portal full endoscope or UBE, and PECF and posterior endoscopic cervical discectomy (PECD) has become the major endoscopic cervical spine surgery [2, 7, 11–13]. PECF and PECD are preferred over AECD because they provide direct access to the foraminal lesion without extensive discectomy. The posterior cervical procedure has other benefits, including good visualization and an extended field of vision, less muscle and soft-tissue trauma, low rate of complications (bleeding, infection, wound healing), and cost-effectiveness (operation time, hospital stay, recovery, capacity to work). However, the procedure has disadvantages, including limited ability to widen access, less ability to perform an endoscopic dural suture, and limited intradiscal accessibility [2, 7–10, 15].

Generally accepted indications are persistent or intolerable radicular pain and/or neurological deficits due to cervical disc herniation, foraminal stenosis, zygapophyseal joint cysts with compression of the nerve root, and anterior foraminal residual pathologies following anterior surgery. Neck pain alone, medial disc herniation with cervical myelopathy or central nervous symptoms, bony central spinal canal stenosis, and deformity or instability requiring correction are considered contraindications [2, 7].

## 3.1 Incomplete Decompression

The factors associated with increased risk of failure after PECF and PECD are spondylosis, residual medial disc protrusion, and persistent radicular pain due to insufficient decompression [7, 15]. To prevent failure, the widest decompression as possible is often required; however, overly aggressive resection of a facet joint leading to instability should be considered. The surgeon is responsible for optimal outcomes, which could greatly affect the frequency and severity of reported adverse events. The main limitation of PECF and PECD is centrally located lesions. Because cervical cord retraction is not possible using the endoscope working tube, the endoscope cannot gain access to a centrally located lesion, and the possibility of incomplete decompression increases.

## 3.2 Dural Injury

Attention is focused on the attachment between the ligamentum flavum (LF) and the dural sac during foraminotomy and discectomy to avoid dural injury. After the dural sac is identified, coagulation of the epidural venous plexus is performed using radiofrequency to maintain a clear visual field and accurately identify the nerve roots. The relationships between the intervertebral disc and nerve root between segments differ; thus, surgeons should be knowledgeable concerning the anatomical relationships of the cervical vertebrae to achieve accurate decompression and avoid damage to the nerve roots and spinal cord. The nerve root pathway could be winding due to cervical spondylosis and bony spurs, and risk of dural injury could be increased [18]. Because dural tears mainly occur during dissection of the root, sufficient medial pediculectomy is performed to secure sufficient space, and if adhesion is present, it should be delicately peeled off (Video 1). A dural tear could also occur during pediculectomy or foraminotomy, and the risk of dural tear can be decreased using a diamond drill burr. A dural tear can be disastrous and should be covered with the patch-blocking repair technique or gluing for small incidental tears [19, 20] (Video 1). In more extensive injury, the dura should be directly repaired after changing to an open procedure.

## 3.3 Postoperative Dysesthesia and Injuries to Nerve Roots or the Spinal Cord

Nerve root injury could lead to postoperative dysesthesia, a specific complication in PECF and PECD. Even if the nerve root has been successfully decompressed, postoperative dysesthesia inhibits a quick recovery and delays the return to daily life. Therefore, prevention of postoperative dysesthesia is the most important factor for successful cervical endoscopic decompression [2, 7, 9, 10].

The nerve root is considered the key landmark before decompression, and minimal retraction is allowed at the nerve root. Ossification of the posterior longitudinal ligament (OPLL) and myelopathy due to central disc herniation are contraindications for PECF and PECD. Due to continuous intraoperative high water pressure, there is a potential risk of injury to the spinal cord in myelopathy. In myelopathy patients, input pressure and smooth drainage should be secured to ensure excessive increase in saline pressure, and a working cannula is recommended in UBE. Spinal cord retraction should never be performed to prevent catastrophic neurological sequelae. Spinal cord injury can occur even in patients with appropriate indications for PECF and PECD and can cause irreversible and fatal complications (Fig. 2). If disc removal is difficult, medial pediculectomy should be performed rather than retracting the spinal cord.

## 3.4 Hematoma

Bleeding obstructs the intraoperative view. Subtle hemostasis should be ensured during preparation using the radiofrequency electrode. Intraspinal venous plexus hemorrhage is an important consideration in cervical spinal surgery. The posterior venous plexus is located in the anterior epidural fat of the vertebral arch and LF. The plexus is irregular, and numerous lateral anastomoses are present. In decompression of the neural foramen, the line of circumference of the intervertebral disc space should be considered to avoid excessive preparation in an anterior direction and contact with the vertebral artery. Hemostasis should be performed before removal of the endoscope, and a drain should be inserted [2, 9, 11]. If neurological symptoms are not present and the hematoma is small, surgical treatment might not be necessary; however, if neurological symptoms occur, surgical treatment should be considered immediately (Fig. 3).

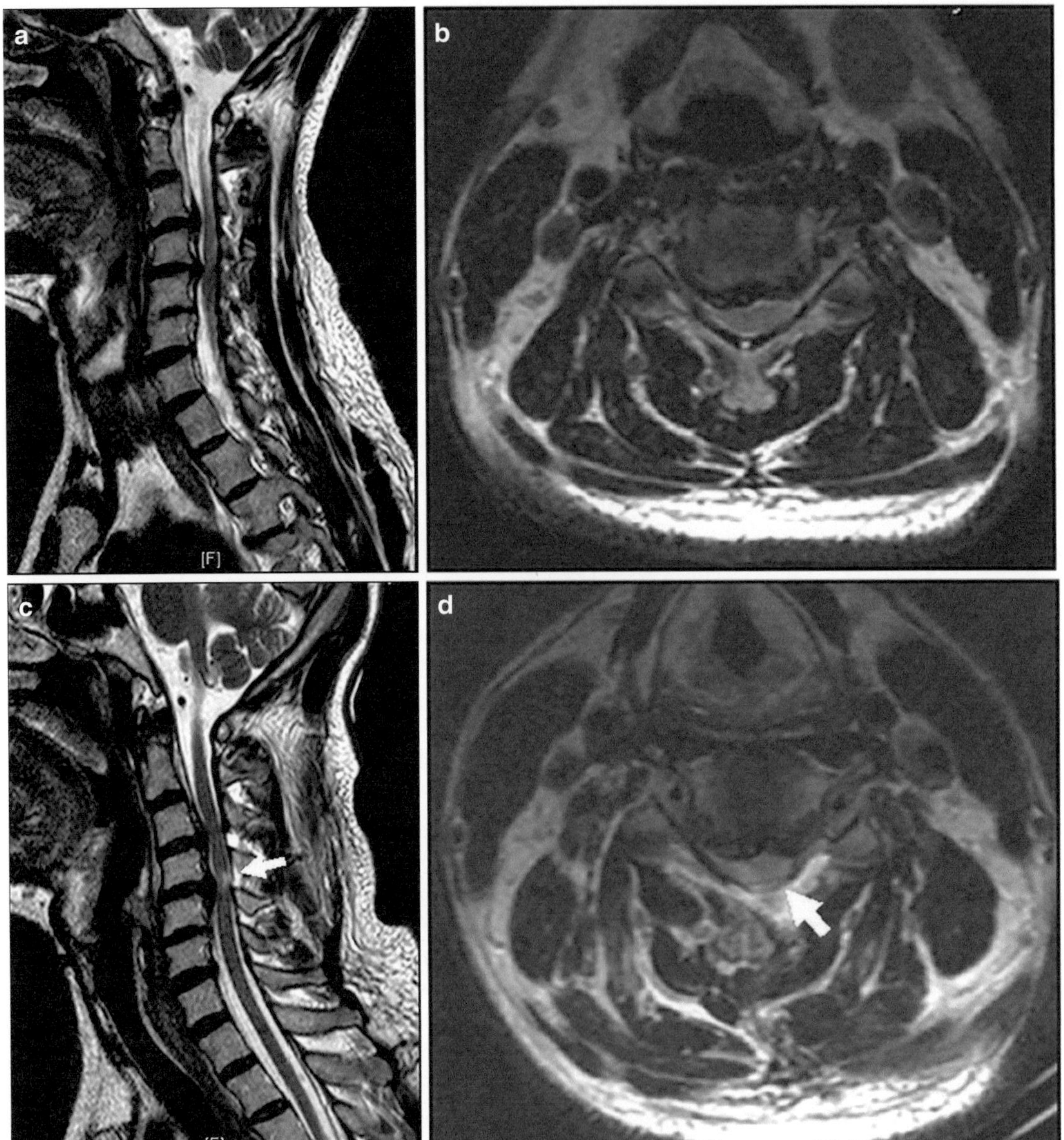


**Fig. 2** A 52-year-old male with spinal cord injury that occurred after PECF with a biportal endoscope. Preoperative sagittal (**a**) and axial MRI images at C4/5 (**b**), postoperative sagittal (**c**) and axial MRI images, (**d**) and postoperative 3D computed tomography (CT) (**e**). Postoperative MRI shows spinal cord injury (**c** and **d**, white arrow), and CT shows foraminotomy site (**e**, white arrow)

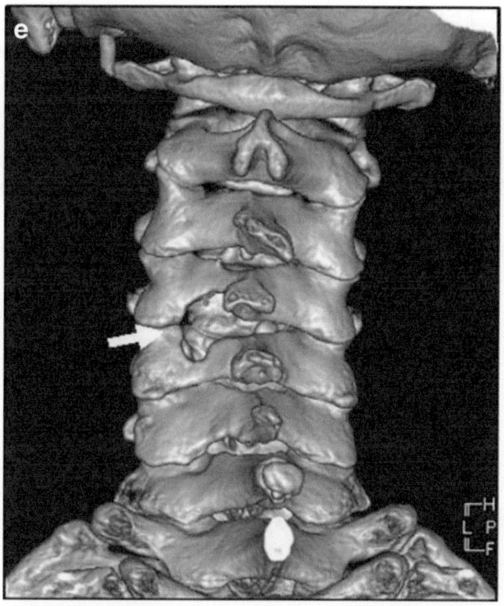


**Fig. 2** (continued)

## 3.5 Persistent Neck Pain and Surgically Induced Instability

When the nerve root is compressed to the lateral side, parts of the articular processes need to be removed to achieve sufficient decompression. If the extent of the facet joint excision is less than 50%, the stability of the cervical spine can be preserved, and successful decompression can be achieved [21]. Excessive facet joint removal and surgically induced instability (Fig. 4) could lead to persistent symptoms, recurrent disc herniation, and progressive neck pain. Therefore, preserving as much facet as possible with sufficient nerve root decompression is important to preserve stability of the cervical spinal column. Because the endoscope lens is positioned at the distal tip of the endoscope, inclined facetectomy and partial pediculectomy without excessive facet joint removal are possible [8, 9, 11, 13].

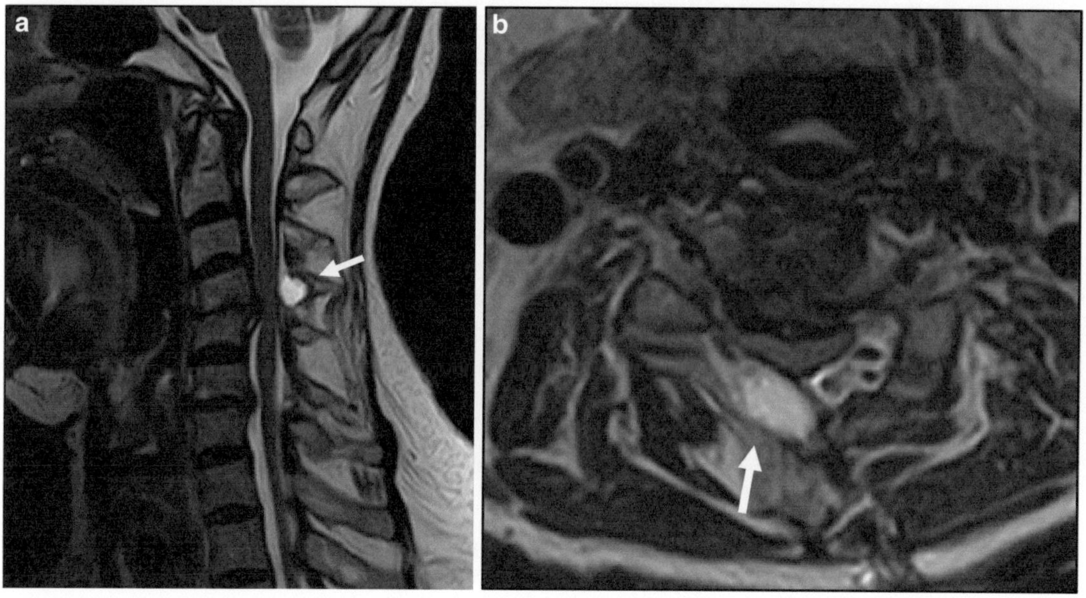


**Fig. 3** Postoperative epidural hematoma after PECF. Neurological symptoms were not present and the hematoma was small; thus, surgical treatment was not performed. Postoperative sagittal (**a**) and axial MRI images (**b**)

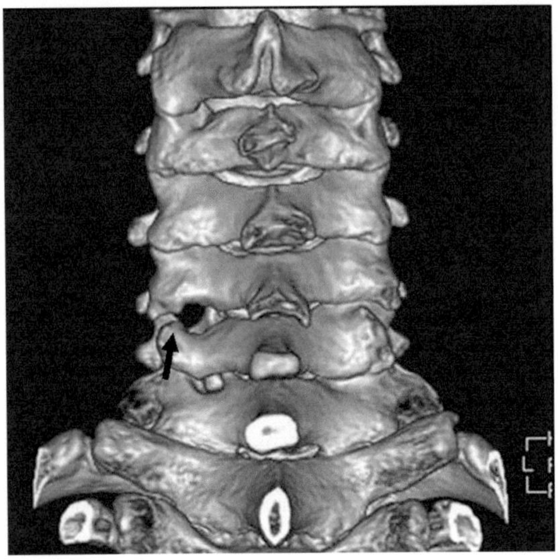

**Fig. 4** Greater than 50% facet joint removal can lead to surgically induced instability

## 4 How to Avoid Complications in Endoscopic Spine Surgery

To avoid complications associated with endoscopic spine surgery, various factors should be considered.

1. The surgeon should be familiar with spinal endoscopic techniques and undergo strict training in minimally invasive surgery.
2. Foraminal anatomy should be evaluated using preoperative MRI and CT scans.
3. Fluoroscopic visualization is essential during endoscope placement with level confirmation, and the endoscopic depth must be validated via lateral fluoroscopy.
4. The nerve root and spinal cord should be manipulated carefully to prevent injury.
5. If general anesthesia is used, nerve electrophysiology monitoring might reduce the incidence of nerve root or spinal cord injury.
6. A dural tear could be disastrous; if an incidental small dural tear occurs, it should be covered with a dural patch or glued. In cases of more extensive dural tears, it is recommended to change an open procedure and directly repair the tear.
7. The facet and lamina must be removed layer by layer until the cortical bone is visible.
8. After the interlaminar windows are enlarged, the LF is resected. If the LF is resected early, the working sheath and burr of the endoscope can slide into the interlaminar space and cause spinal cord injury.
9. Endoscopic cervical spine surgery should be attempted only if the surgeon has sufficient experience. The safety of endoscopic spine surgery for myelopathy is uncertain. After sufficient experience and numerous considerations, the surgeons should proceed carefully.

## 5 Conclusion

During the last decade, endoscopic technologies have significantly advanced, and the surgical indications have expanded to spinal stenosis. Currently, most soft disc herniation and some spinal stenosis can be treated with endoscopic spine surgery. However, the learning curve associated with endoscopic cervical decompression and discectomy is steep. Understanding which endoscopic cervical surgery technique offers the best clinical long-term success and lowest complication rate is important, and the surgeon is responsible for the outcome of endoscopic spine surgery. To prevent complications, endoscopic cervical spine surgery should be performed using an appropriate surgical technique to obtain the desired outcome.

## References

1. Lee JH, Lee SH. Clinical and radiographic changes after percutaneous endoscopic cervical discectomy: a long-term follow-up. Photomed Laser Surg. 2014;32(12):663–8.
2. Ruetten S, Komp M, Merk H, Godolias G. A new full-endoscopic technique for cervical posterior foraminotomy in the treatment of lateral disc herniations using 6.9-mm endoscopes: prospective 2-year results of 87 patients. Minim Invasive Neurosurg. 2007;50(4):219–26.
3. Epstein NE. A review of complication rates for anterior cervical Diskectomy and fusion (ACDF). Surg Neurol Int. 2019;10:100.

4. Maharaj MM, Mobbs RJ, Hogan J, Zhao DF, Rao PJ, Phan K. Anterior cervical disc arthroplasty (ACDA) versus anterior cervical discectomy and fusion (ACDF): a systematic review and meta-analysis. J Spine Surg. 2015;1(1):72–85.
5. Lubelski D, Healy AT, Silverstein MP, Abdullah KG, Thompson NR, Riew KD, et al. Reoperation rates after anterior cervical discectomy and fusion versus posterior cervical foraminotomy: a propensity-matched analysis. Spine J. 2015;15(6):1277–83.
6. Choi D, Petrik V, Fox S, Parkinson J, Timothy J, Gullan R. Motion preservation and clinical outcome of porous coated motion cervical disk arthroplasty. Neurosurgery. 2012;71(1):30–7.
7. Ruetten S, Komp M, Merk H, Godolias G. Full-endoscopic cervical posterior foraminotomy for the operation of lateral disc herniations using 5.9-mm endoscopes: a prospective, randomized, controlled study. Spine (Phila Pa 1976). 2008;33(9):940–8.
8. Won S, Kim CH, Chung CK, Choi Y, Park SB, Moon JH, et al. Comparison of cervical sagittal alignment and kinematics after posterior full-endoscopic cervical Foraminotomy and discectomy according to preoperative cervical alignment. Pain Physician. 2017;20(2):77–87.
9. Kim HS, Wu PH, Lee YJ, Kim DH, Kim JY, Lee JH, et al. Safe route for cervical approach: partial Pediculotomy, partial Vertebrotomy approach for posterior endoscopic cervical Foraminotomy and discectomy. World Neurosurg. 2020;140:e273–e82.
10. Bucknall V, Gibson JA. Cervical endoscopic spinal surgery: a review of the current literature. J Orthop Surg (Hong Kong). 2018;26(1):2309499018758520.
11. Komp M, Oezdemir S, Hahn P, Ruetten S. Full-endoscopic posterior foraminotomy surgery for cervical disc herniations. Oper Orthop Traumatol. 2018;30(1):13–24.
12. Park Jae H, Jun SG, Jung Je T, Lee SJ. Posterior percutaneous endoscopic cervical Foraminotomy and Diskectomy with unilateral Biportal endoscopy. Orthopedics. 2017;40(5):e779–e83.
13. Song KS, Lee CW. The Biportal endoscopic posterior cervical inclinatory Foraminotomy for cervical radiculopathy: technical report and preliminary results. Neurospine. 2020;17(Suppl 1):S145–s53.
14. Sclafani JA, Kim CW. Complications associated with the initial learning curve of minimally invasive spine surgery: a systematic review. Clin Orthop Relat Res. 2014;472(6):1711–7.
15. McAnany SJ, Kim JS, Overley SC, Baird EO, Anderson PA, Qureshi SA. A meta-analysis of cervical foraminotomy: open versus minimally-invasive techniques. Spine J. 2015;15(5):849–56.
16. Lee S-H, Lee JH, Choi W-C, Jung B, Mehta R. Anterior minimally invasive approaches for the cervical spine. Orthop Clin N Am. 2007;38(3):327–37.
17. Ahn Y. Endoscopic spine discectomy: indications and outcomes. Int Orthop. 2019;43(4):909–16.
18. Haviarová Z, Matejčík V, Kuruc R, Halgaš F. Extradural and intradural characteristics of the cervical nerve root anomalies. J Clin Neurosci. 2020;73:259–63.
19. Kim HS, Raorane HD, Wu PH, Heo DH, Sharma SB, Jang IT. Incidental Durotomy during endoscopic stenosis lumbar decompression: incidence, classification, and proposed management strategies. World Neurosurg. 2020;139:e13–22.
20. Kim J-E, Choi D-J, Park EJ. Risk factors and options of Management for an Incidental Dural Tear in Biportal endoscopic spine surgery. Asian Spine J. 2020;14(6):790–800.
21. Jonas R, Demmelmaier R, Wilke HJ. Influences of functional structures on the kinematic behavior of the cervical spine. Spine J. 2020;20(12):2014–24.

# Part II

# Cervical - Uniportal

# Uniportal Cervical Posterior Foraminotomy and Discectomy

Chul-Woo Lee, Dong-Chan Lee, and Tae-Hyun Kim

**Abstract**

The radicular symptoms of arm pain are usually caused by lateral disc herniation or osteophyte in the foramen and vertebrae that originate from cervical degenerative changes. Various surgical options are available to treat the pathologies that cause cervical radiculopathy. Anterior cervical approach, including anterior cervical discectomy and fusion (ACDF) and cervical artificial disc replacement (ADR), has been considered the gold standard treatment for degenerative cervical diseases. However, unfavorable postoperative complications of the anterior cervical approach such as instrument failure, pseudoarthrosis, and adjacent segment disease have been reported (13.2–19.3%) and criticized by those limitations. Posterior cervical foraminotomy (PCF) gained popularity as an alternative to ACDF by sparing problems associated with fusion and surgical instrumentations. Despite these advantages, postoperative neck pain was the most common complication to be overcome in posterior cervical. Several authors reported relative advantages of posterior endoscopic cervical discectomy and foraminotomy to minimize iatrogenic injury of the posterior cervical structures and achieve similar goals of conventional posterior cervical foraminotomy without significant complications. In this chapter, surgical procedure and practical tips and pearls for endoscopic posterior cervical approach are described in detail.

**Supplementary Information** The online version contains supplementary material available at https://doi.org/10.1007/978-981-99-1133-2_3.

C.-W. Lee
Department of Neurosurgery, Saehim Hospital, Seoul, Republic of Korea

D.-C. Lee (✉) · T.-H. Kim
Department of Neurosurgery, Anyang Wiltse Memorial Hospital, Anyang-Si, Kyeonggi-Do, Republic of Korea


H. S. Kim et al. (eds.), *Advanced Technique of Endoscopic Cervical and Thoracic Spine Surgery*,
https://doi.org/10.1007/978-981-99-1133-2_3

**Keywords**

Endoscopic · Posterior cervical · Cervical approach

## 1 Advantages of this Approach

Compared to the anterior cervical approach, the posterior cervical approach technique has significant advantages, such as no vital organ damage in the anterior neck, preservation of a cervical range of motion, and no complications caused by a bone graft or implant [1–3]. Most common complication of posterior cervical surgery is the postoperative axial neck pain [4–6]. So, most of all, the preservation of the posterior neck muscles and ligamentous structures would be the most valuable advantage that is crucial to prevent postoperative instability and axial neck pain. Posterior endoscopic cervical foraminotomy and discectomy have many merits such as less postoperative pain, short duration of hospital stay, and early return to normal life due to their minimal invasiveness. The endoscopic posterior cervical approach follows the same anatomical principle of the traditional posterior cervical approach that provides thorough decompression of the whole length of exiting nerve root from the upper pedicle to the lower pedicle. However, minimal invasiveness of endoscope surgery goes on to have a more favorable outcome than the traditional approach [7–13]. The posterior endoscopic cervical approach has certain challenges like the feasibility of approaches, limitation in maneuvering the instruments, and achieving adequate decompression [14–18]. However, more delicate handling of instruments is possible with an endoscope that provides a magnified, clear operative view in an endoscopic posterior cervical approach. Drilling with an endoscope, which can be rotated, tilted, and permits various operative angles, can be more helpful to preserve the integrity of facet joint compared to the traditional posterior cervical approach. In what follows, surgical procedure and practical tips and pearls for endoscopic posterior cervical approach will be described in detail.

## 2 Indications and Contraindications

**Indications**

1. Foraminal or lateral cervical disc herniation in which the main part of the disc is located lateral to the lateral edge of the spinal cord on MRI and CT scan.
2. Unilateral cervical radiculopathy.
3. Craniocaudal disc migration as long as the lateral localization was maintained.
4. Concomitant foraminal stenosis.
5. Unsuccessful conservative therapy.

**Relative contraindications**

1. Intra-canal stenosis.
2. Medial localization of the disc herniation.

**Contraindications**

1. Definitive segmental instability.
2. Cervical deformities.
3. Neurological or vascular pathologies mimicking a herniated disc.

## 3 Anesthesia and Position

1. The operation is performed under general anesthesia with the patient in a prone position using three-point pin fixation devices with a table-mounted holder (Mayfield system, Intergra, Painsboro, JN) (Fig. 1a).
2. The patient's head also could be fixed without cervical fixation device. The head is fixed and both shoulders were pulled by plasters. A gel-type facial pad should be used to protect the face and eyeballs from direct high-contact pressure. The neck is flexed and upper back is slanted down for good venous return in order to reduce the chance of intraoperative bleeding (Fig. 1b).
3. The abdomen is relaxed using an H-shape pillow in order to avoid increasing abdominal pressure.

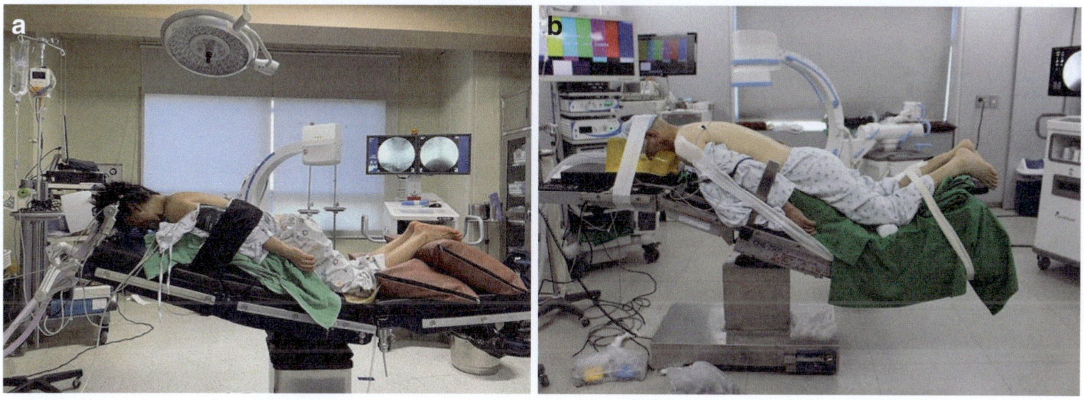

**Fig. 1** Operative position and set-up in the operating room: (**a**) operative position with Mayfield system; (**b**) operative position with facial pad and plaster

## 4 Special Instruments (Fig. 2)

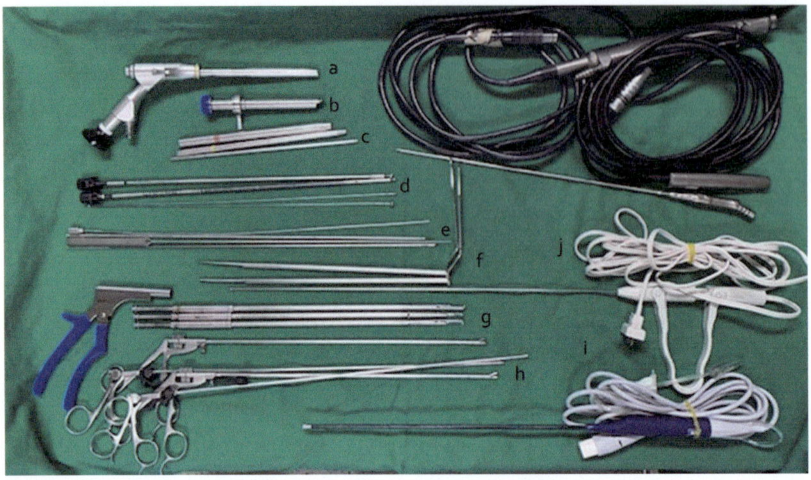


**Fig. 2** Instruments for posterior endoscopic cervical approach. (**a**) Endoscopy (whole length: 125 mm; outer diameter: 10 mm; working channel diameter: 6 mm). (**b**) Working cannula (outer diameter: 11.5 mm). (**c**) Serial dilators (3,7,10 mm). (**d**) Endoscopic burrs and drills -RPM 16,000–20,000, burr diameter 2.5–5.0 mm, cutting and diamond types. (**e**) Endoscopic hooks and flexible dissector probe. (**f**) Nerve root retractor. (**g**) Kerrison punches (variable sizes). (**h**) Endoscopic forceps and cutter. (**i**) Radiofrequency probe. (**j**) Ellman RF coagulator

# 5 Procedures

## 5.1 Preoperative Targeting By Needle and Skin Incision

1. Preoperative targeting is performed by needle under fluoroscopy to check the operative level and plan the working trajectory.
2. Target is the junction of the lower margin of target disc space and uncovertebral joint line. The tip of the needle should be located at the upper margin of lower vertebral body in lateral X-ray image and uncovertebral joint line on AP (anteroposterior) X-ray (Fig. 3b–d).
3. A 1 cm vertical skin incision on the symptomatic side is made at more medial to uncovertebral joint line (0.5–1 cm lateral from the midline), which provides a trajectory angle of 5–15 degrees (Fig. 3a).

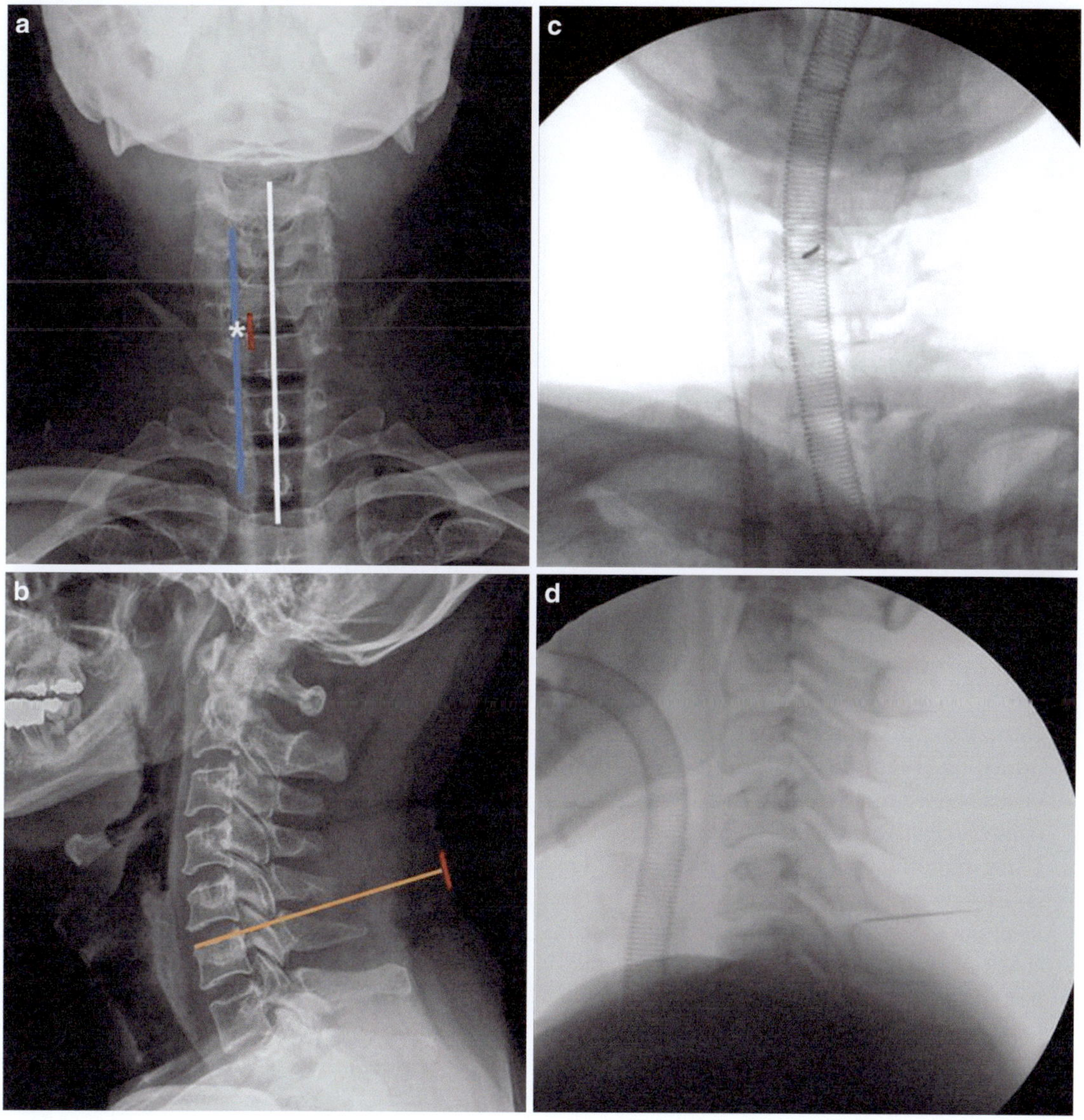


**Fig. 3** Preoperative needle targeting point and skin incision site in X-ray. (**a**, **b**) Needle trajectory (brown line) is parallel to the lower margin of target disc space in X-ray lateral images. Skin incision (red line) is made on more medial area to the target in X-ray AP image. (**c**, **d**) The tip of the needle was placed at the initial target (asterisk) in c-arm AP and lateral images. White line: midline; blue line: uncovertebral joint line; asterisk: target at the junction of the lower margin of target disc space and uncovertebral joint line

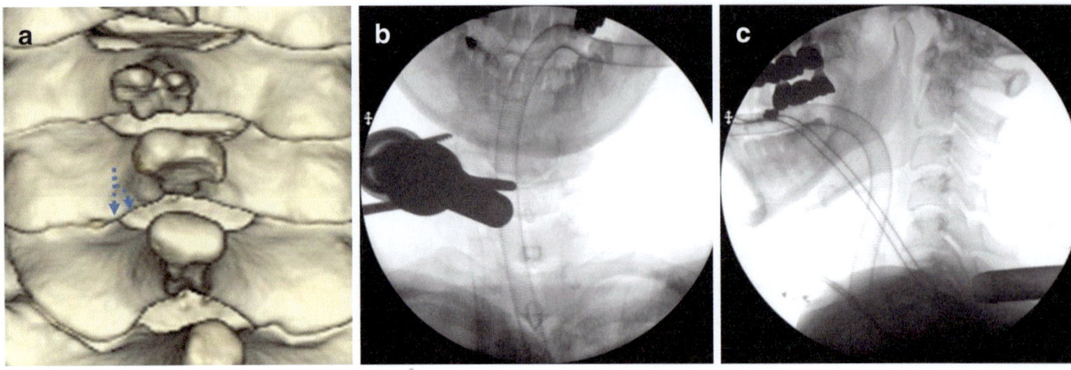


**Fig. 4** (**a**) Inferior margin of the upper lamina is palpated by the initial first dilator with scraping maneuver (blue dotted arrows). (**b**, **c**) Final position of the working cannula in C-arm AP and lat images

## 5.2 Sequential Dilation and Working Cannula Insertion (Fig. 4)

1. The upper lamina is palpated by the first dilator and then the dilator slides down to search the inferior margin of the lamina, taking care to avoid entering the spinal canal (Fig. 4a).
2. Aggressive scraping or dissection around facet joint should be avoided in order to prevent undue active bleeding from the branch of radicular artery.

## 5.3 Confirmation of Anatomical Landmark (V Point) (Fig. 5)

1. Once the working cannula position is confirmed on C-arm images, endoscopy is introduced under irrigation system with water pump (irrigative pressure 35–50 mmHg)
2. Using radiofrequency (RF) probe, soft tissue is dissected to expose the medial part of the facet joint (V point), inferior articular process (IAP) of the upper vertebrae, and the medial part of the superior articular process (SAP) of lower vertebrae

## 5.4 Circumferential Decompression

Bony decompression is performed in a circumferential fashion by endoscopic drill, including a part of the upper and lower lamina, IAP of upper vertebrae, and cranial tip of SAP is removed under direct endoscopic vision (Fig. 6a).

* Anatomical landmarks for decompressive boundary.

Cranial: origin of the ligament flavum (LF).
Lateral: cranial tip of SAP.
Caudal: insertion of LF

## 5.5 The Removal of a Lateral Part of LF, Soft-Tissue Dissection, and Adhesiolysis Around the Exiting Root

A part of ligament flavum is detached from the decompressed bone margin and removed in order to expose the lateral margin of dural sac and the exiting root (ER) (Fig. 6b). The soft tissue around ER is dissected and adhesiolysis is performed.

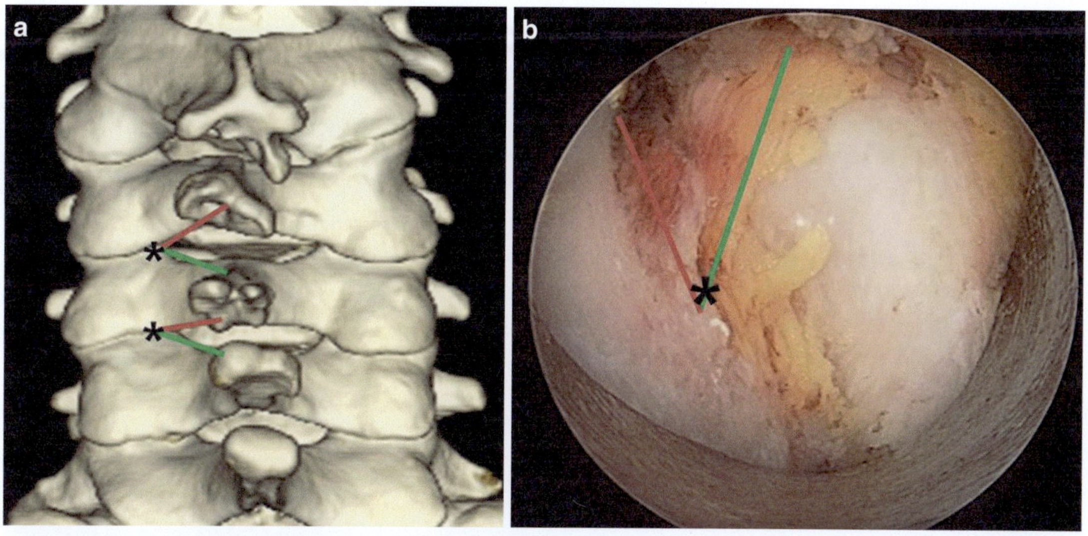


**Fig. 5** (**a**) V point (asterisk): junction of the lower margin of the upper lamina (brown line) and the upper margin of the lower lamina (green line). (**b**) V point in endoscopic view

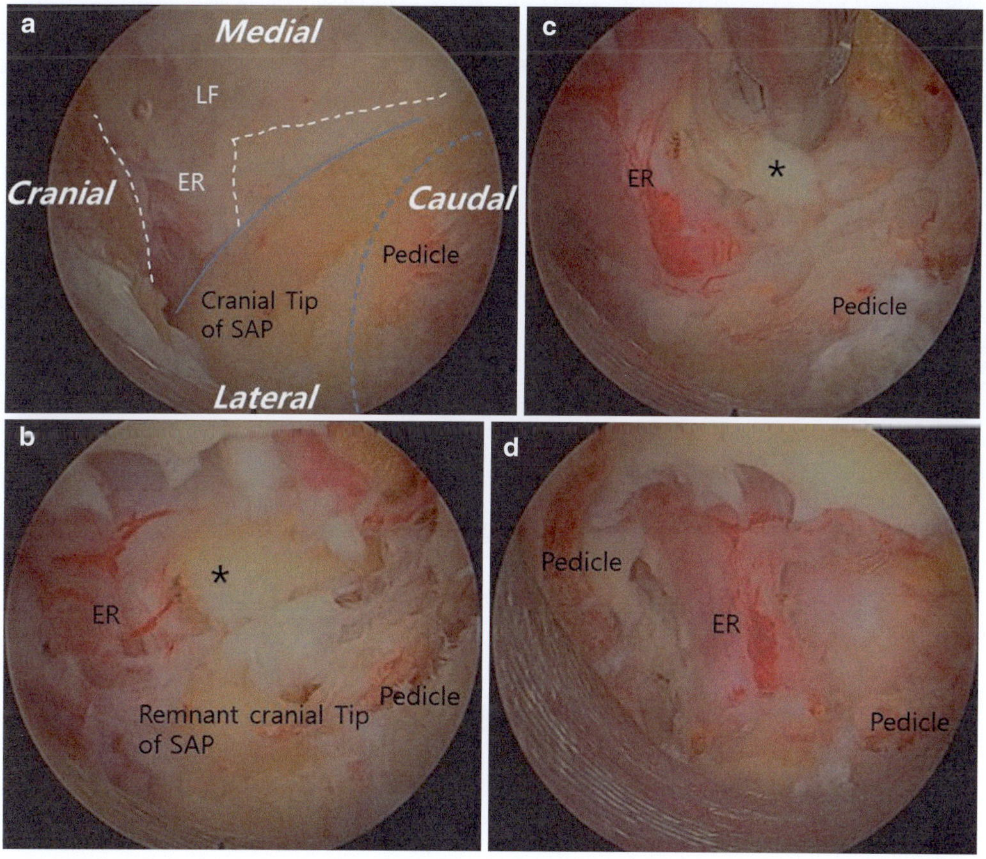


**Fig. 6** (**a**) Initial circumferential drilling was performed; (**b**) the removal of partial LF and thinned cortical bone of lower lamina and SAP revealed ER. Protruded disc was found in the axilla area of ER. (**c**) Protruded disc was removed by endoscopic forcep. (**d**) Fully decompressed exiting root was exposed from pedicle to pedicle. LF: ligament flavum; ER: exiting root. Asterisk: protruded disc

### 5.6 Additional Decompression (Discectomy, Foraminotomy, or Pediculotomy) and Confirmation of the Decompressed Exiting Root

Protruded or redundant disc material, remnant bony structure, and LF that are compressing ER in the shoulder area of the exiting root are removed. If required, pediculotomy should be done. Bony spur of lower vertebral body and remnant disc under the exiting root also should be decompressed (Fig. 6c). The decompression of entire length of ER should be confirmed from the axilla area of the exiting root to the distal foraminal area and from the upper pedicle to the lower pedicle (Fig. 6d). Further foraminotomy is performed until the footplate of a 2-mm Kerrison rongeur could be easily passed into the foramen. Once the foramen is deemed decompressed, a nerve hook is passed to palpate the foramen, as well as the medial and lateral walls of the pedicle to ensure adequate foraminal decompression.

### 5.7 Hemostasis and Closure

Complete hemostasis should be achieved. Drain insertion in all cases followed by closure (Fig. 7)

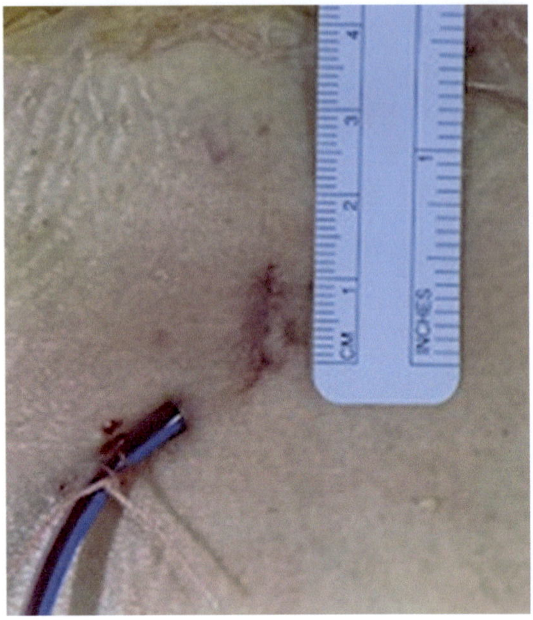


**Fig. 7** Skin closure and drain

## 6 Illustrated Cases

### 6.1 Case 1: Paracentral Disc Herniation

A 58-year-old male patient presented with left-side arm pain of 20 days duration with inability to sleep at night due to severe pain. On examination, the VAS scores of 5 and 8 for neck and arm, respectively, with elbow flexion weakness of grade 3 on the left side were noted. Routine X-ray revealed no evidence of instability, and MRI showed left paracentral disc compressing spinal cord and exiting nerve root on the C5–6 level (Fig. 8a, b). The patient underwent spinal decompression with discectomy via uniportal endoscopic posterior cervical approach (Video 1). Intraoperatively, pediculotomy was needed in order to acquire enough space to dissect to axilla area of the exiting root and lateral margin of the dural sac (Fig. 8e–g). The protruded disc in the paracentral region was not revealed until the dural sac was gently retracted by the tip of the working cannula (Fig. 8h). The protruded disc herniation that was located in the paracentral area was removed using various endoscopic instruments such as curved ball probe and angled forcep (Fig. 8i, j). Postoperatively the patient had

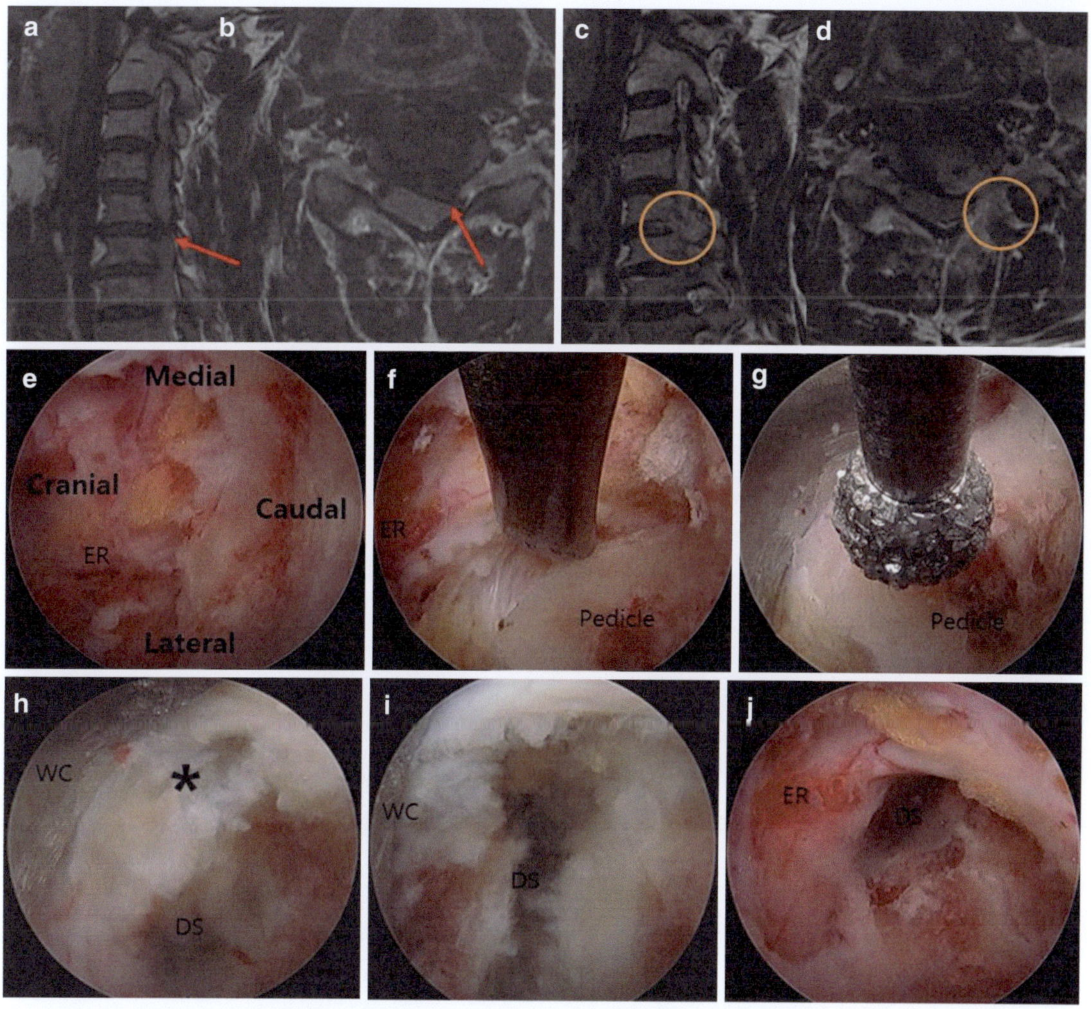


**Fig. 8** (**a**, **b**) Preoperative MRI T2 sagittal and axial images demonstrated paracentral disc herniation compressing spinal cord and exiting nerve root (red arrows). (**c**, **d**) Postoperative MRI images showed laminoforaminotomy state with decompressed spinal cord and exiting nerve by the removal of herniated disc (orange-colored circles). (**e**) Dural sac and a proximal exiting root were exposed after the removal of IAP, SAP, and lateral part of the ligament flavum. (**f**, **g**) After the dissection of axilla of the exiting root from superolateral margin of the pedicle, pediculotomy was performed with protection of neural structure by working cannula. (**h**, **i**) Paracentral ruptured disc was exposed by retraction of dural sac and removed. (**j**) Intraoperative endoscopic view at final stage showed a fully decompressed exiting root. Asterisk: ruptured disc material; ER: exiting nerve root, DS: disc space

resolution of arm pain with no features of immediate postoperative complications. Postoperative MRI revealed a successful result with the removal of herniated disc and decompressed nerve root (Fig. 8c, d).

## 6.2 Case 2: Foraminal Stenosis

A 63-year-old man presented with 9 months history of posterior neck pain, right arm pain, and numbness over the forearm, thumb, and index finger. He had failed conservative management, including analgesic, nonsteroidal anti-inflammatory medications, and nerve block. X-ray showed degenerative changes at multiple levels with no features of instability. Preoperative MRI and CT showed narrowed right-side foramen with compressed root at the C5–6 level (Fig. 9a–c). The patient underwent uniportal endoscopic decompression surgery (Fig. 9g, h, and i) Cervical nerve root was com-

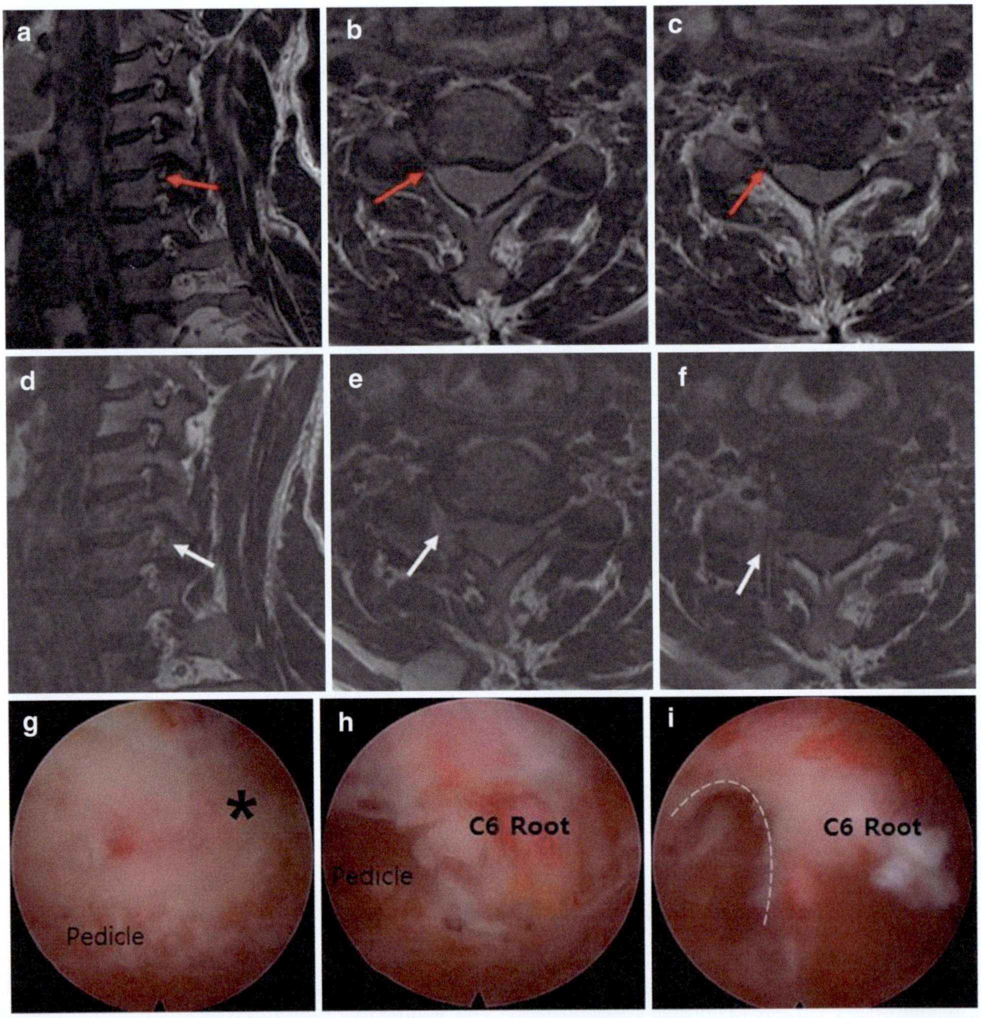


**Fig. 9** (**a–c**) MRI T2 oblique and axial images showed compressed root at C5–6 right foramen with severe degenerative changes (red arrows). (**d–f**) Postoperative axial and sagittal T2 MRI images showed decompressed foramen on the right side at C5–6 level by partial lamino-foraminotomy and pediculotomy (white arrows). (**g**) Intraoperative image showed the cranial tip of SAP (asterisk) and medial part of a pedicle after drilling of a part of IAP and SAP. (**h**) Further bony work and removal of a part of the ligament flavum exposed exiting nerve root along the superomedial margin of the pedicle. (**i**) Full decompressed exiting nerve root was shown after pediculotomy. Asterisk: cranial tip of SAP; dotted curve line: pediculotomy site

pletely decompressed by endoscopic foraminotomy (Video 2). The patient's symptoms were improved with a reduction in VAS score of neck and arm pain from 7 and 8 preoperatively to 2 and 2 after the operation, respectively, with no neurological deficits. Postoperative X-ray showed no evidence of any immediate instability with MRI and CT suggestive satisfactory decompression of neural foramen at C5–6 (Fig. 9d–f).

### 6.3 Case 3: Bilevel Foraminal Decompression

A 64-year-old man presented with severe posterior neck pain and left upper-limb radicular pain for 6 months with VAS score of 4 and 8 for neck and arm pain, respectively, on examination. X-ray of the cervical spine revealed slightly reduced disc space height at C-5-6-7, with no evidence of instability on dynamic X-rays. Preoperative MRI showed foraminal stenosis on the right side of C5–6 and C6–7, both two levels combined with foraminal disc herniation on the C5–6 level (Fig. 10a–c). The patient underwent selective diagnostic root block with time interval to confirm the pain generator, which offered temporary relief at both levels. Initial foraminal decompression was performed at the C67 level. Removal of protruded disc and decompressive foraminotomy for the C6–7 level was followed by a sliding technique without further skin incision (Video 3). C6 and 7 nerve roots were fully decompressed (Fig. 10g, h, and i). The patient was ambulated at 6 hours after the surgery with a reduction in VAS scores of 3 and 2 for neck and arm pain, respectively, and discharged on the first postoperative day. Postoperative images showed no immediate postoperative instability and well-decompressed left foraminal area of C5–6 and C6–7 levels (Fig. 10d–f, j).

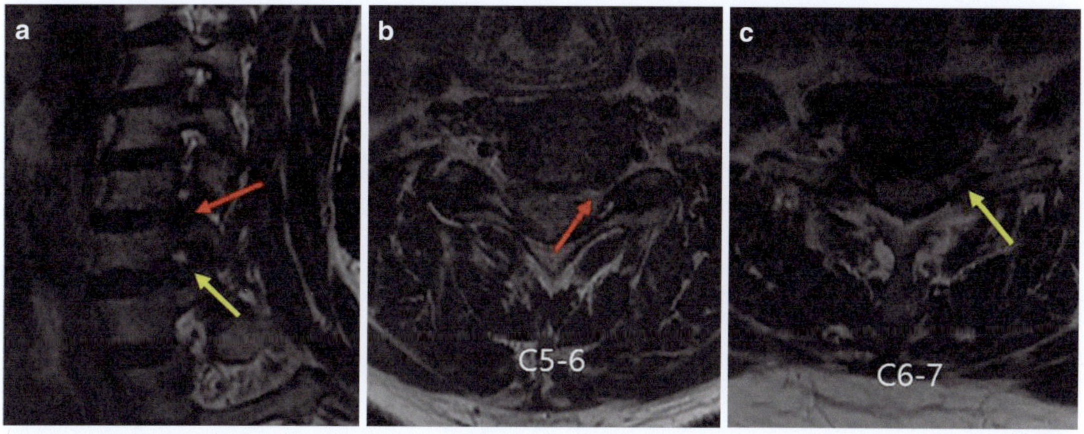


**Fig. 10** (**a–c**) Preoperative T2 oblique and axial MRI showed foraminal stenosis combined with focal foraminal disc on the left side at the C5–6 level (red arrows) and foraminal stenosis at the C6–7 level (yellow arrows). (**d–f**) Postoperative oblique and sagittal T2 MRI images showed decompressed foraminal area at the left side of C5–6 and C6–7 bilevels (white arrows). (**g**) Decompression at the axilla area of C7 root was confirmed by retraction with probe. (**h**) Protruded focal disc herniation (asterisk) was revealed around the axilla area of C6 root by retraction of the working cannula after bony work. (**i**) Fully decompressed C6 root was shown after partial pediculotomy and discectomy. (**j**) Postoperative 3D reconstruction CT image showed keyhole-shaped laminoforaminotomy site at C5–6 and C6–7 bilevels (orange circle)

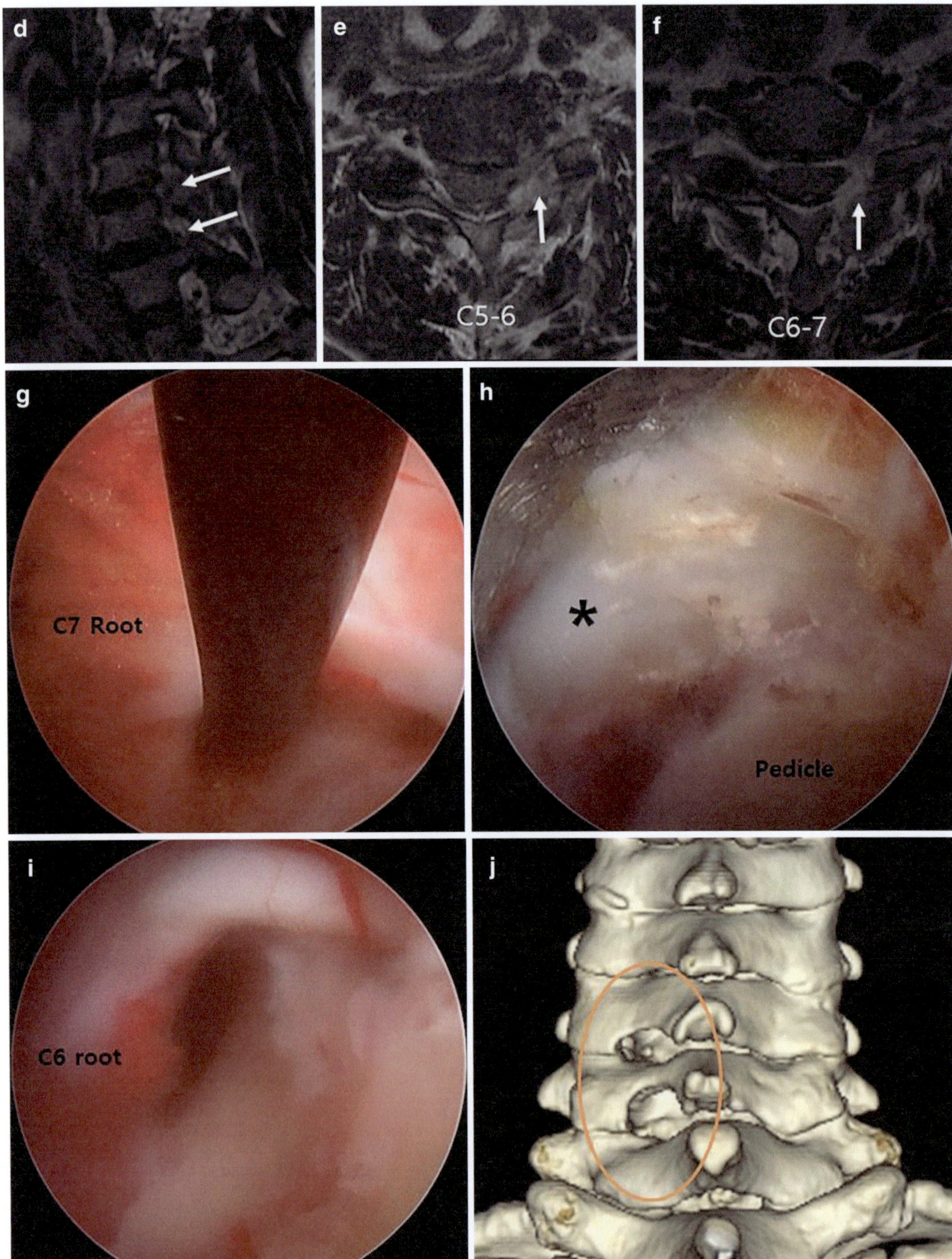


**Fig. 10** (continued)

## 7 Prevention and Management of Complications

1. Neurological complications.
   - These complications can manifest in the form of dysthesia and motor weakness caused by excessive manipulation of the exiting root or inappropriate usage of RF probe.
   - The operation for the C4–5 level should be performed with more caution for the prevention of C5 palsy.
   - Measures to avoid neural injury include delicate manipulation of ER after acquisition of enough space around the ER by initial decompression (such as discectomy and bony unroofing of ER) and separation of ER from around the perineural structure by adhesiolysis. The use of sharp instruments should be prohibited.
   - RF should be used at adequate voltage in pinpoint fashion (soft-tissue ablation and bone bleeding control: 250 Watts, but around the neural structures: below 90 Watts) and in proper direction, posterior end of RF probe should be directed against nerve root so that discharge RF current is away from the neural structure not directly on it.
2. Incomplete decompression.
   - Incomplete decompression can lead to persistence of preoperative symptoms.
   - Target points of decompression should be determined by preoperative investigation (patients' neurological symptom and radiological images).
   - The structures that can compress ER and evoke patients' symptom should be thoroughly decompressed and confirmed decompressed status for a successful postoperative outcome.
     (a) Redundant disc.
     (b) IAP compressing the shoulder of ER.
     (c) Cranial tip of SAP compressing distal portion of ER.
     (d) Adhesive band-like structures entrapping ER.
     (e) Pedicle that pushes up the axilla of the exiting root craniomedially: pediculotomy needed.
   - Free space in the foraminal area along the distal pathway of ER should be checked by a ball tip probe for the confirmation of complete decompression of ER.
3. Excessive facet violation.
   - Facet joint plays an important role in maintaining stability, but in certain cases, resection of the facet joint is inevitable for adequate decompression.
   - To avoid such complications, after initial exposure to ER, tailored, limited removal of the bony structure along just the ER pathway in direct endoscopic view is recommended.
   - The intraoperative modification of medial to lateral operative angle is also helpful to obliquely undercut SAP, preserve the facet joint by more than 50%, and prevent iatrogenic instability.
4. Intraoperative bleeding and postoperative hematoma
   - Intraoperative bleeding is usually from venous plexus around ER. An unexpected bleeding can be troublesome, leading to longer operative time interrupting the operative flow.
   - Tips to control bleeding include beforehand coagulation and dissection at the area where it is easy to meet bleeding along the course of the exiting root. Temporary elevation of the irrigation fluid pressure may be helpful to find bleeding focus in blurred operative view.
   - The application of hemostatic agents (Floseal®) and "wait and see" strategy is useful to manage uncontrollable bleeding from an unknown origin.
   - The insertion of Hemo-vac drain after the operation is recommended for the prevention of postoperative hematoma.
5. Dura tear
   - Dura tear is not uncommon in posterior endoscopic cervical approach.
   - It often occurs during drilling the cranial tip of SAP, adhesiolysis, and vigorous retraction of ER.

- Making a thin bony shell at the margin of the ligament flavum and medial border of SAP by drilling and removal of the bony shell by punch or curette can be a useful method to protect dura and avoid root injury during drilling.
- During the removal of adhesive membranous tissues from dura and ER, meticulous and careful surgical attitude is important to prevent dura tear.
- ER should be retracted after adequate release of ER from adhesed perineural structures.

## 8 Discussion (Surgical Tips and Pitfalls)

1. Importance of preoperative diagnosis for endoscopic simple foraminal decompression.
    - Symptoms and sign: history and neurological examination.
    - Identify the pathological origin and rule out other causes.
    - Imaging: target pathology, rule out candidates for other kinds of operation (ACDF, wide posterior cervical foraminotomy and fusion, other endoscopic approaches).
    - Diagnostic selective nerve root block.
2. Anatomical landmarks.
    - Initial operative trajectory should be determined parallel to the lower end plate of disc space.
    - "V point" is the initial landmark to provide the endoscopic surgical orientation and point to start drilling.
    - The boundary of the primary bony resection is determined by the origin and insertion of LF, cranial tip of SAP, and superomedial border of the pedicle of the lower vertebra.
3. Complete decompression.
    - The most common cause of unfavorable outcome is incomplete decompression.
    - Based on preoperative planning, adequate decompression of key structure must be ensured.
    - Protruded or redundant disc that is verified at shoulder and axilla area should be removed or shrunk appropriately.
    - The removal of cranial tip of SAP and partial pedicle is sometimes needed for complete decompression of ER.
    - Pulsatility and enough free space at the distal area of ER always should be checked at the final stage of the procedure. Those are the important signs of adequate decompression.
4. Facet joint preservation.
    - Biomechanically facet joint limits movement of the spinal motion segment but excessive bone resection that can occur during unroofing the ER for complete decompression could lead to postoperative instability and postoperative chronic neck pain.
    - More medial skin entry, bony decompression in medial to lateral direction with rotation, and tilting of endoscope enable oblique undercutting of facet joint. It could be advantageous to minimize the violation of facet joint and preserve the segmental stability.
5. Intraoperative bleeding.
    - Most of the intraoperative bleeding during posterior endoscopic cervical approach is from internal venous plexus and bone matrix.
    - Beforehand coagulation of vessel with RF bipolar is essential for a bloodless endoscopic view and to prevent any postoperative hematoma and maintain stable operation without ceasement.
    - Temporary elevation of irrigative water pressure and intermittent compression by the blunt tip of RF coagulator in a blind fashion are practical tips to help the surgeon to find bleeding focus and control it in blurred operative view from bleeding. The time and amount of pressure elevation should be as short and less as possible (< 30 sec, < 50 mmHg).
    - The resected bone margin and muscle outside of the working cannula can be the ori-

gin of unknown bleeding. When the operator encounter blurred operative view by unknown origin, such origins should be checked with slight withdrawal of endoscope and examination.

6. Neural injury.
   - To avoid neural injury such as postoperative motor weakness or dysthesia.
   - Initial adequate bony decompression and adhesiolysis from around soft tissues should precede the manipulation of root. Aggressive manipulation of root should be avoided. Mobilized root that is partially decompressed and freed from around structures should be dealt with in a careful and delicate manner.
   - The RF bipolar should be used with much caution. The surgeon should adhere to adequate power and direction when using RF.

## References


1. Tasiou A, Giannis T, Brotis AG, Siasios I, Georgiadis I, Gatos H, et al. Anterior cervical spine surgery-associated complications in a retrospective case-control study. J spine Surg (Hong Kong) [Internet]. 2017 Sep [cited 2022 Jan 17];3(3):444–59. Available from: https://pubmed.ncbi.nlm.nih.gov/29057356/
2. Bertalanffy H, Eggert HR. Complications of anterior cervical discectomy without fusion in 450 consecutive patients. Acta Neurochir (Wien) [Internet]. 1989 Mar [cited 2022 Jan 17];99(1–2):41–50. Available from: https://pubmed.ncbi.nlm.nih.gov/2667284/
3. Epstein NE. A review of complication rates for anterior cervical Diskectomy and fusion (ACDF). Surg Neurol Int [Internet] 2019 [cited 2022 Jan 17];10. Available from: https://pubmed.ncbi.nlm.nih.gov/31528438/
4. Jagannathan J, Sherman JH, Szabo T, Shaffrey CI, Jane JA. The posterior cervical foraminotomy in the treatment of cervical disc/osteophyte disease: a single-surgeon experience with a minimum of 5 years' clinical and radiographic follow-up - clinical article. J Neurosurg Spine 2009 Apr;10(4):347–356.
5. Fehlings MG, Gray RJ. Posterior cervical foraminotomy for the treatment of cervical radiculopathy. J Neurosurg Spine 2009 Apr;10(4):343–344.
6. Grieve JP, Kitchen ND, Moore AJ, Marsh HT. Results of posterior cervical foraminotomy for treatment of cervical spondylitic radiculopathy. Br J Neurosurg [Internet] 2000 [cited 2022 Jan 17];14(1):40–43. Available from: https://pubmed.ncbi.nlm.nih.gov/10884883/
7. Wen H, Wang X, Liao W, Kong W, Qin J, Chen X, et al. Response to: Comment on "effective Range of Percutaneous Posterior Full-Endoscopic Paramedian Cervical Disc Herniation Discectomy and Indications for Patient Selection." Biomed Res Int 2020;2020.
8. Ji-jun H, Hui-hui S, Zeng-wu S, Liang Z, Qing L, Heng-zhu Z. Posterior full-endoscopic cervical discectomy in cervical radiculopathy: a prospective cohort study. Clin Neurol Neurosurg [Internet]. 2020;195(98):105948. https://doi.org/10.1016/j.clineuro.2020.105948.
9. Yao S, Ouyang B, Lu T, Chen Q, Luo C, Dora Z. Treatment of cervical spondylotic radiculopathy with posterior percutaneous endoscopic cervical discectomy: Short-Term outcomes of 24 cases. Med (United States). 2020;99(20):3–9.
10. Gu BS, Park JH, Seong HY, Jung SK, Roh SW. Feasibility of posterior cervical Foraminotomy in cervical Foraminal stenosis. Spine (Phila Pa 1976). 2017;42(5):E267–71.
11. Kim CH, Kim KT, Chung CK, Park SB, Yang SH, Kim SM, et al. Minimally invasive cervical foraminotomy and diskectomy for laterally located soft disk herniation. Eur Spine J. 2015;24(12):3005–12.
12. Ruetten S, Komp M, Merk H, Godolias G. Full-endoscopic cervical posterior foraminotomy for the operation of lateral disc herniations using 5.9-mm endoscopes: a prospective, randomized, controlled study. Spine (Phila Pa 1976). 2008;33(9):940–8.
13. Wan Q, Zhang D, Li S, Liu W, Wu X, Ji Z, et al. Posterior percutaneous full-endoscopic cervical discectomy under local anesthesia for cervical radiculopathy due to soft-disc herniation: a preliminary clinical study. J Neurosurg Spine. 2018;29(4):351–7.
14. Vaishnav AS, Louie P, Gang CH, Iyer S, McAnany S, Albert T, et al. Technique, time demand, radiation exposure, and outcomes of skin-anchored intraoperative 3D navigation in minimally invasive posterior cervical laminoforaminotomy. Clin Spine Surg A Spine Publ. 2021;00:1–7.
15. Zhang Y, Ouyang Z, Wang W. Percutaneous endoscopic cervical foraminotomy as a new treatment for cervical radiculopathy: a systematic review and meta-analysis. Medicine (Baltimore). 2020;99(45):e22744.
16. Yu KX, Chu L, Chen L, Shi L, Deng ZL. A novel posterior trench approach involving percutaneous endoscopic cervical discectomy for central cervical intervertebral disc herniation. Clin Spine Surg. 2019;32(1):10–7.
17. Zheng C, Huang X, Yu J, Ye X. Posterior percutaneous endoscopic cervical Diskectomy: a single-center experience of 252 cases. World Neurosurg [Internet]. 2018;120:e63–7. https://doi.org/10.1016/j.wneu.2018.07.141.
18. Song KS, Lee CW. The biportal endoscopic posterior cervical inclinatory foraminotomy for cervical radiculopathy: technical report and preliminary results. Neurospine. 2020;17(Suppl 1):S145–53.

# Cervical Multilevel Foraminotomy Using Single Incision

Han Ga Wi Nam, Chun-Kun Park, and Kangtaek Lim

**Abstract**

Endoscopic spine surgery for the treatment of degenerative spinal diseases from the lumbar to the cervical spine has accelerated over the past two decades. Posterior cervical foraminotomy is an effective surgical treatment method for relieving radicular symptoms that result from cervical nerve root compression. Minimally invasive techniques and tubular retractor systems are available to minimize tissue retraction, but minimally invasive approaches can carry with them the surgical challenge of trying to pass instruments through a long narrow retractor that is also the port for visualizing the surgical pathology. We describe a surgical technique for a fully endoscopic multilevel posterior cervical foraminotomy performed through a 8-mm incision using a 8.4-cm working channel high-definition endoscope with a 5.7-mm working channel.

**Keywords**

Endoscopic spine surgery · Minimally invasive · Cervical foraminotomy · Cervical radiculopathy · Stenoscope

## 1 Advantages of this Approach (Introduction)

Traditional posterior cervical foraminotomy is performed without additional stabilization and thus preserves the mobility of the segment. However, there is potential significant perioperative morbidity from neck pain and wound issues in conventional open cervical foraminotomy that limits the enthusiasm for this treatment option [1]. Unlike open surgery, the blunt insertion of a dilator and a working tube onto the facet joint makes the incision of posterior endoscopic cervical decompression by foraminotomy and/or discectomy (PECD) only less than 1 cm, without extensive subperiosteal stripping of the paraspinal musculature [2]. It has the advantage of being a minimally invasive technique that conserves soft tissue, while achieving cervical foraminal decompression and discectomy for prolapsed intervertebral disc and foraminal stenosis [3]. It may avoid excessive resection of facet that can

**Supplementary Information** The online version contains supplementary material available at https://doi.org/10.1007/978-981-99-1133-2_4.

H. G. W. Nam
Department of Neurosurgery, Suncheon Chuck Hospital, Suncheon, South Korea

C.-K. Park
Department of Neurosurgery, Seoul St. Mary's Hospital, The Catholic University of Korea, Seoul, South Korea

K. Lim (✉)
Department of Neurosurgery, Seoul Sagyero Hospital, Hanam, South Korea



H. S. Kim et al. (eds.), *Advanced Technique of Endoscopic Cervical and Thoracic Spine Surgery*, https://doi.org/10.1007/978-981-99-1133-2_4

lead to instability of cervical spine. Moreover, with the high-definition endoscope and underwater infusion, a clear field of surgery can be achieved by inhibition of the bleeding. With the minimally invasive approach, morbidity is reduced and recovery and hospital stay are shortened [4]. Furthermore, the author can be sure that the aforementioned benefits can be maximized if multilevel cervical pathology is treated using a single skin incision.

## 2 Indications and Contraindications

- The possible indications for the procedure include.
  1. Cervical radiculopathy at one or more levels caused by disk herniation and/or foraminal stenosis by osteophyte formation.
- The possible contraindications include.
  1. Cervical myelopathy.
  2. Midline disk herniation.
  3. Vertebral body pathology.
  4. Cervical instability at the pathologic level.

## 3 Anesthesia and Position

- Before surgery, magnetic resonance imaging should be carefully reviewed to assess the position of herniated disc and degree of foraminal stenosis. Computed tomography (CT) scan is performed for a detailed analysis of foraminal zone such as the degree of stenosis and the degree of calcification in the herniated disc. In addition, the shape of the lamina and the thickness and deviation of the spinous process should be checked through a CT scan. This provides a reference of inserting the endoscopic position and the size of bone resection of facet joint while preserving segmental stability.
- The patient was positioned prone on hip and chest bolsters on the operating room table with the table flexed under general anesthesia. The arms were positioned caudal on the body and immobilized with adhesive tape (Fig. 1).
- The cervical spine was delordosated and the head should be on foam supporting head frame to avoid any direct pressure to the eye. (It is not necessary to use a skull clamp; Fig. 2).

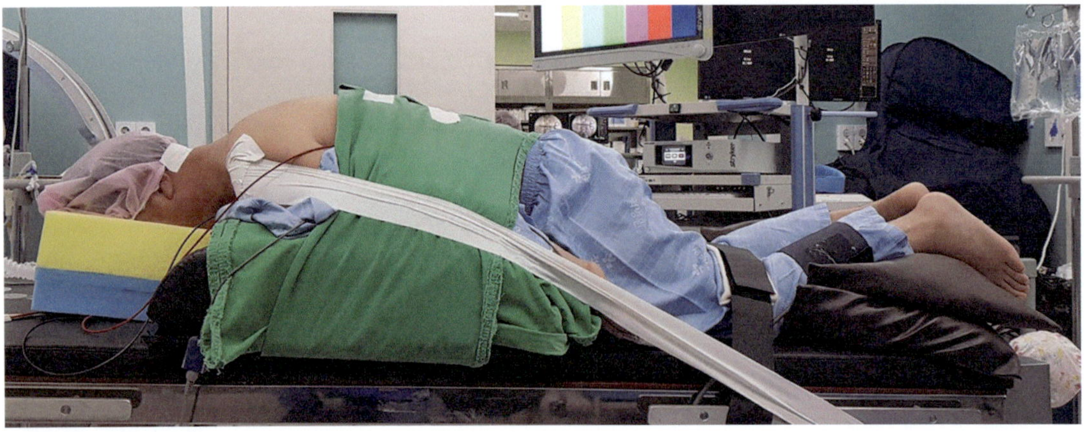

**Fig. 1** Patient positioning

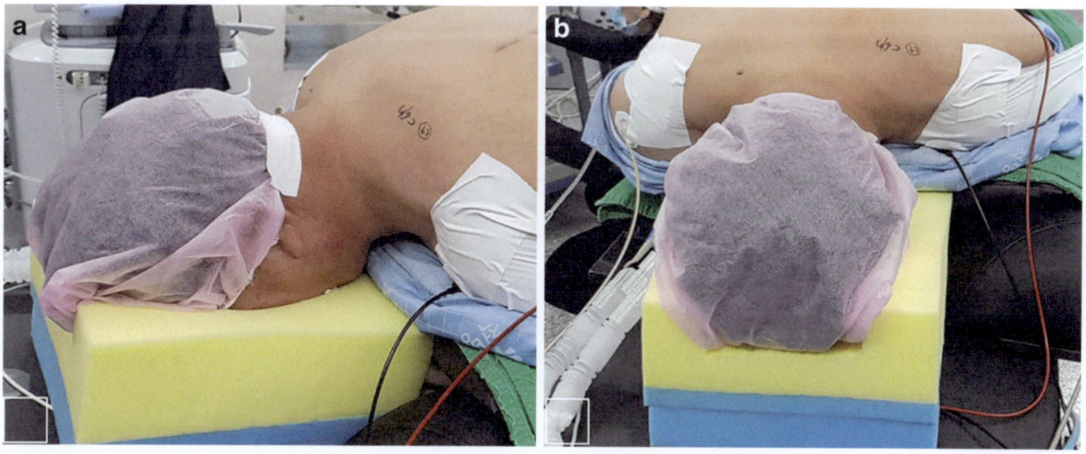


**Fig. 2** The images of the head position and the head frame (**a**, **b**)

## 4 Special Instrument

- All operative procedures were performed with a complete uniportal endoscopic instrument system: Techcord Endoscopic System (Techcord, Daejeon, Korea) (Fig. 3). Uniportal endoscopes are used in a different fashion as an operating microscope employed for open spinal surgery in aspects of 360 degree operating field rotation.
- Surgical instruments can be categorized into four groups (Fig. 4):

1. Mechanical instruments: Kerrison punches, long pituitary forceps (small/middle/large), dissectors (small/large), blunt-angled probe, ball-tipped probe.
2. Special instruments: obturator, working sleeve, endoscopic customized root retractor.
3. Electrosurgical instruments: bipolar radiofrequency electro-coagulator (OK MedinetKorea, Seoul, Korea), DELPHI radiofrequency electrode (C&S Medical, Pocheon, Korea).
4. Motorized instruments: LDRON endoscopic drill system (SAESHIN, Daegu, Korea).

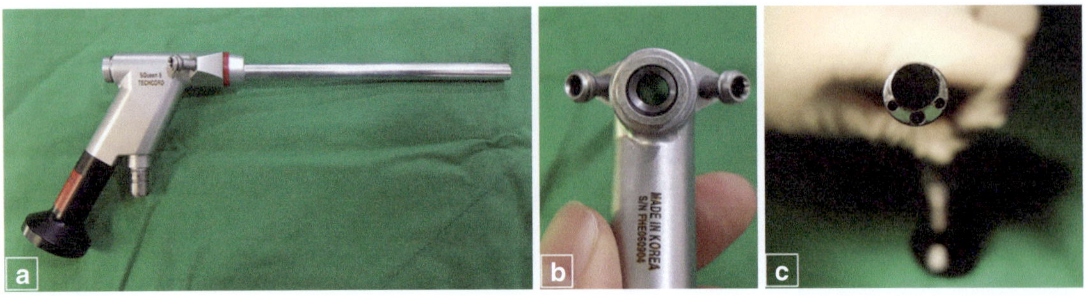


**Fig. 3** Techcord Endoscopic System (8.4-mm outer diameter, 5.7-mm working channel, and 12 degree direction of view, 80 degree field of view). (**a**) Side view; (**b**) working channel and irrigation channels; (**c**) working channel and lens

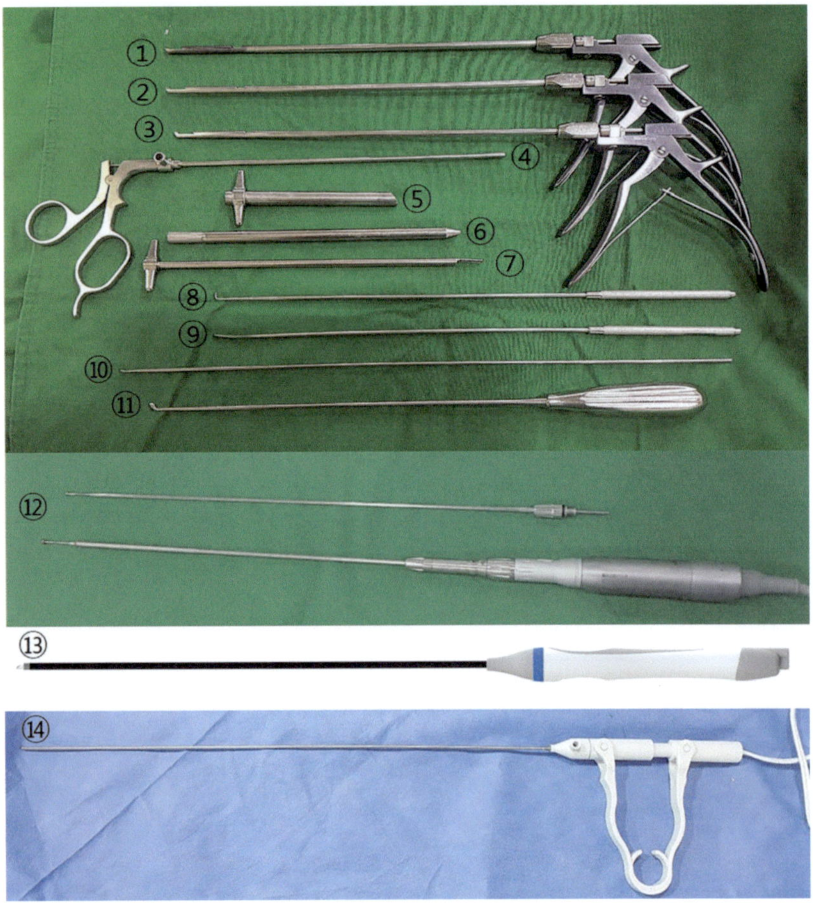


**Fig. 4** Essential unit for uniportal endoscopic decompression: (1–3) Kerrison punches, (4) pituitary forcep (large), (5) working sleeve, (6) obturator, (7) endoscopic customized root retractor, (8) ball-tipped probe, (9–10) dissectors (small/large), (11) up-angled curette, (12) LDRON endoscopic drill system (3 mm, 4-mm-sized burr) (SAESHIN, Daegu, Korea), (13) DELPHI radiofrequency electrode, and (14) bipolar radiofrequency electro-coagulator

## 5 Procedures

- Step 1: skin entry point.
  1. Midline drawing: The midline is drawn after the midline is identified through the C-arm (Fig. 5).
  2. V-point line drawing: The V-point (the "V" point is due to the V-shaped appearance on the margin of the superior laminar, inferior laminar, and medial point of the facet joint) line is drawn after the V-point is identified through the C-arm (Fig. 6). The average distance from the midline to the V-point is about 1–1.5 cm away from the midline of the cervical spine. The distance from the midline to the V-point can be confirmed in advance with a preoperative CT scan (Fig. 7).
  3. Confirmation of trajectory site: A less than 1-cm skin incision is made vertically toward the V-point based on the angulation of disc space with lateral C-arm images (Figs. 8 and 9).
- Step 2: dilation and endoscope insertion (Videos 1 and 2).
  1. With a one-step dilatation, the working sleeve, endoscope, and instruments are directly placed over the surface of the facet joint place through the skin incision.
  2. The 9.5-mm working sleeve was inserted via the dilator before the dilator was removed (Fig. 10). A guidewire or sharp dilator should be avoided for iatrogenic spinal cord injuries via the interlaminar space.

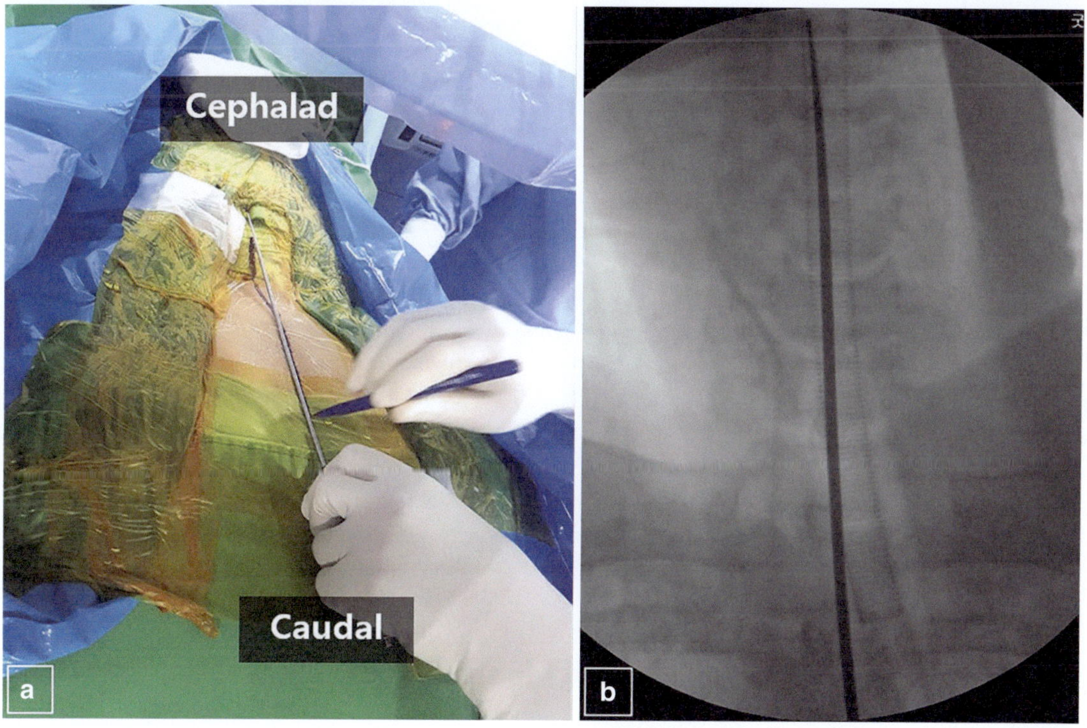


**Fig. 5** (**a**) Midline drawing image. (**b**) The midline is identified through the C-arm

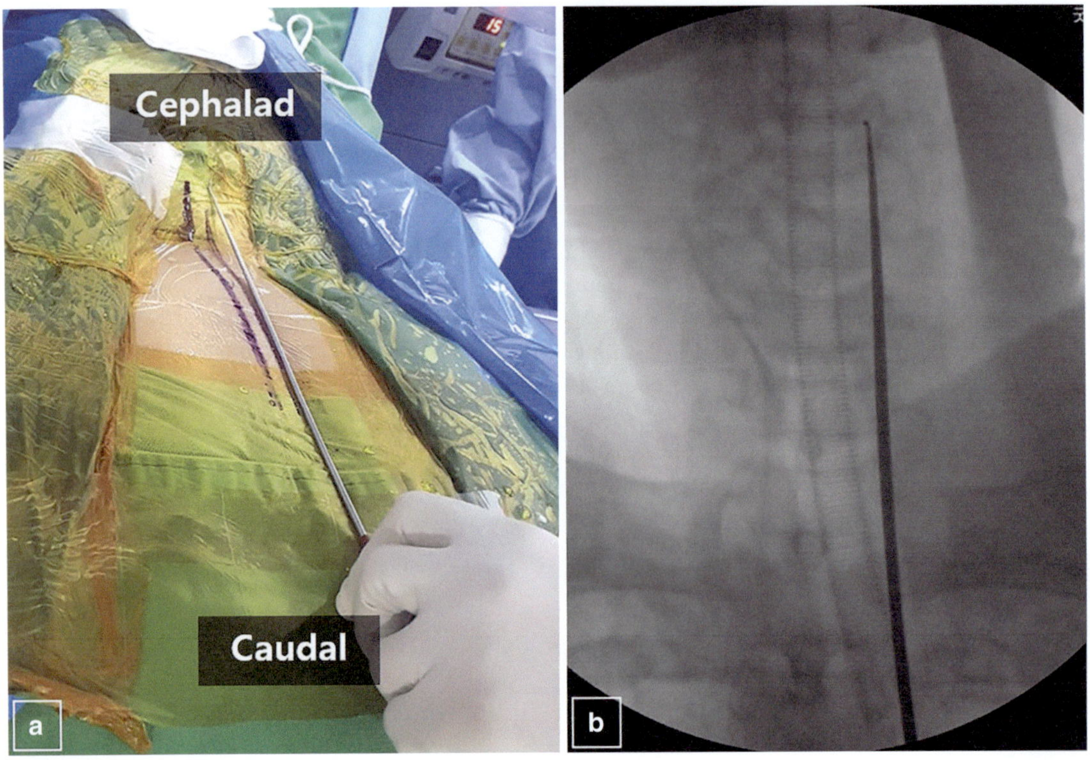


**Fig. 6** (**a**) V-point line drawing image. (**b**) The V-point is identified through the C-arm

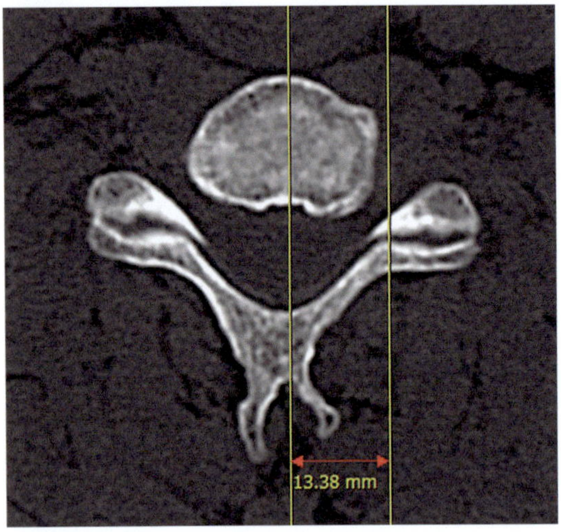


**Fig. 7** Image of the distance from the midline to the V-point on a CT scan

- Step 3: cervical foraminotomy and discectomy (Video 3).
  1. After insertion of the 8.4-mm endoscope, further operation is performed under visual control and continuous irrigation. The endoscopic procedure is performed with below 30 mmHg of irrigation fluid pressure. The pressure of the fluid should be adjusted to provide optimal clarity of endoscopic view but no more than 30 mmHg.
  2. After cleaning the soft tissue on the joint with a bipolar radiofrequency coagulation or radiofrequency electrode, the V-point was identified. A keyhole foraminotomy was performed at the lamina–facet junction using a 4-mm diamond burr and a 1-mm-sized Kerrison punch.

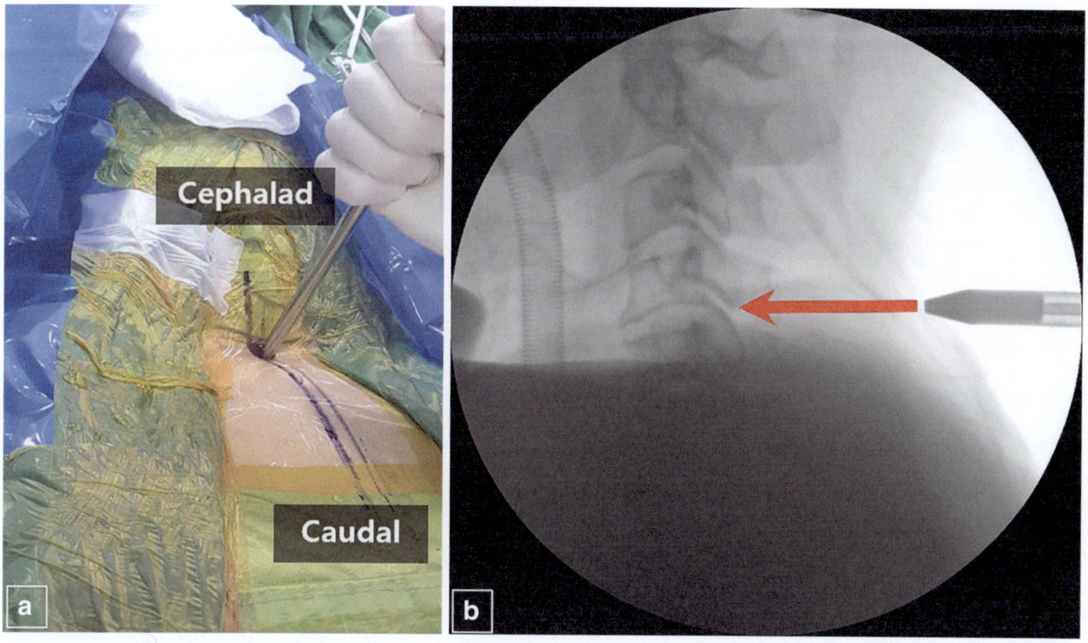


**Fig. 8** (**a**) Image of confirmation of the trajectory site. (**b**) The trajectory site is identified through the C-arm. The red arrow indicates the V-point

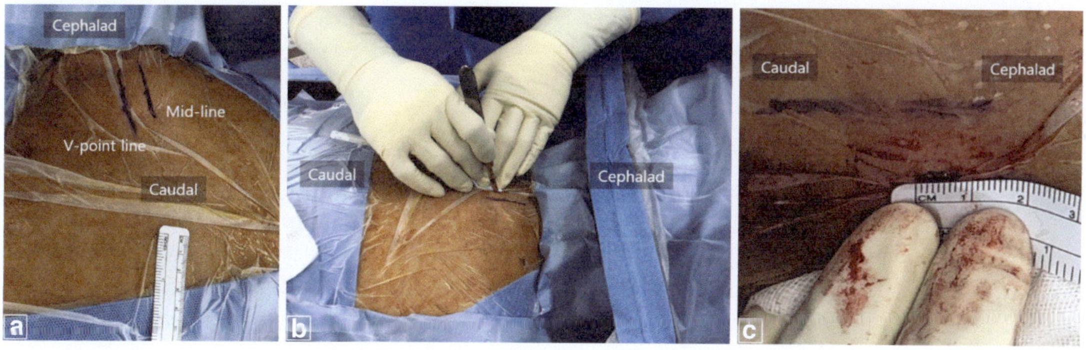


**Fig. 9** (**a, b**) Skin incision images. (**c**) A less than 1-cm skin incision is made vertically toward the V-point

3. The lateral ligamentum flavum was resected without violating the prominent venous plexus around the nerve root. Then, the lateral edge of the spinal cord and branching of the spinal nerves were identified. Bipolar radiofrequency coagulation of the venous plexus was gently performed for preparation of the desired nerve root and hernia.
4. Typically 4–6 mm in diameter of bone was removed from the lateral inferior aspect of the upper lamina followed by about 4 mm of the medial inferior portion of the inferior articular facet from the lamina–facet border (V-point) to gain access to the nerve root.
5. After foraminotomy was completed, the exiting nerve root is retracted gently with the endoscopic retractor in cephalad or caudal direction depending on its relationship with the intervertebral disc and the underlying prolapsed disc fragment is exposed. There should not be any retraction of the spinal cord to avoid significant

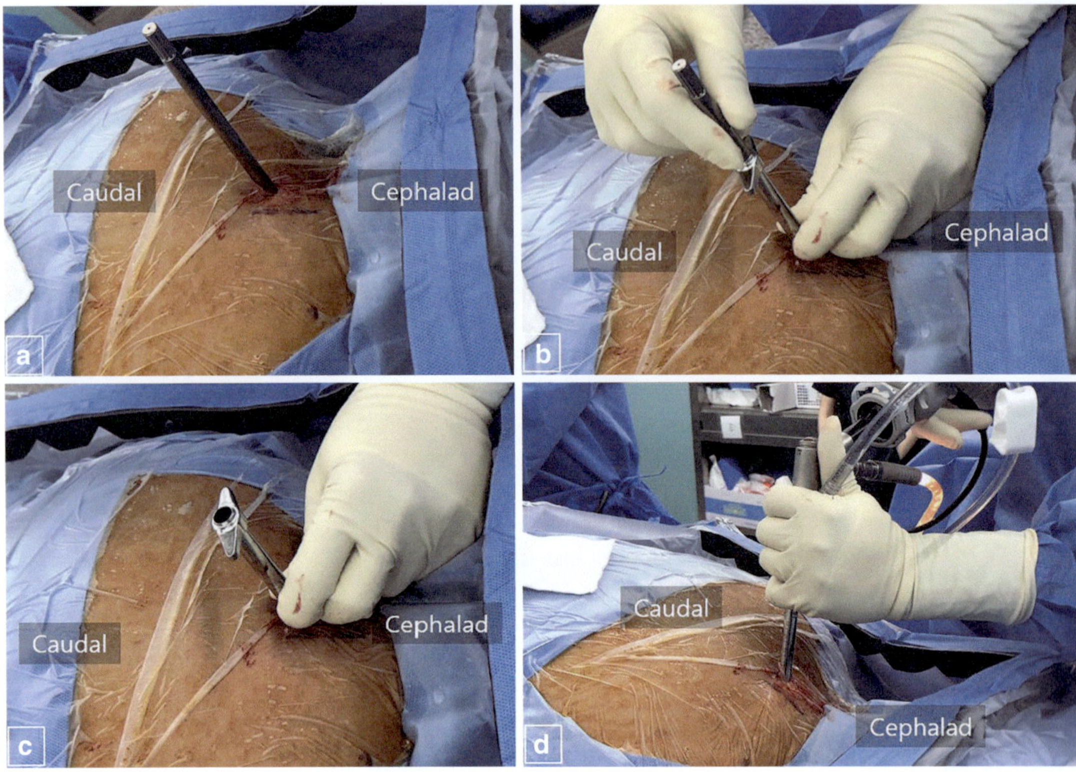


**Fig. 10** Serial images of the endoscope insertion: (**a**) obturator insertion; (**b**, **c**) working sleeve insertion; (**d**) endoscope insertion

neurological sequelae. If there is insufficient space to remove the ruptured fragments, a caudal pediculotomy can be performed to avoid damage to the nerve root or spinal cord. Additionally, if there is nerve root compression due to uncovertebral hypertrophy, decompression can be performed using a drill (Video 4).

6. The ruptured fragments were removed, and the discectomy was completed using the small-sized pituitary forceps and blunt-angled probe. The completeness of the desired nerve root decompression was identified by paying particular attention at the end of the procedure.
7. A drain was placed in the epidural space to prevent postoperative hematoma for 1 day and closed in layers with Vicryl 3–0 (Ethicon, USA) and skin staples on the skin.

- Step 4: multilevel foraminotomy and discectomy (Video 5).
  1. In case of multiple-level stenosis or disc herniation, decompression discectomy through a single-skin entry was achieved via a special technique called the sliding technique.
  2. In this technique, after completion of one level, the working sleeve was completely removed and moved cranially or caudally to the other target within the subcutaneous space under image guidance, but still within the same skin incision (Fig. 11). Skin has good elasticity and can be used to make another muscle layer tract by subfascial dissection through a single incision.
  3. Then, the same process as the foraminotomy procedure was performed in a different direction, upper or lower, for

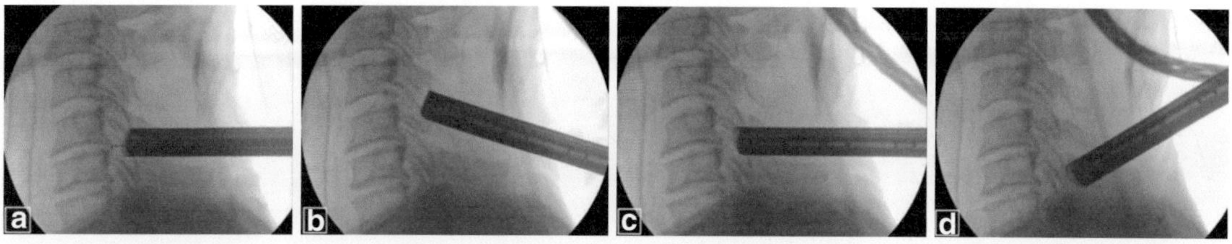

**Fig. 11** The sliding technique. After one-level decompression (**a**, **c**), the upper (**b**) or lower (**d**) interlaminar space and laminar space were confirmed under the C-arm through the same skin incision site

decompression or discectomy of the remaining cervical pathologies. When the patient's neck is extended, decompression is possible up to 4 levels.

4. After the first muscle tract, the subsequent two or three muscle tracts have an inconvenient approach angle, but do not interfere with decompression. After identification and confirmation of the V-point under the C-arm, the dilator was introduced into the created path by large forceps, and the working sleeve was inserted over the dilator. Upward and downward retraction of the skin allowed the tubular working sleeve to be placed in the V-point, where the decompression will be performed.
5. Every step of the procedure was done under image intensifier control to confirm the exact entry point. The endoscope was introduced into the lesion and subsequent procedures performed as described above.

## 6 Illustrated Cases

- Case 1: two-level foraminotomy (Fig. 12).
  - A 56-year-old male complained of right shoulder, first and second finger radiating pain refractory to conservative management. Preoperative magnetic resonance imaging (MRI) showed stenosis of C5–6 and C6–7 segment with protruded calcified disc. We performed uniportal endoscopic posterior foraminotomy. Postoperative MRI shows complete decompression.
- Case 2: three-level foraminotomy (Fig. 13).
  - A 62-year-old female presented with left shoulder and scapular radiating pain. Preoperative MRI showed severe left-side multiple stenosis (left C5–6, C6–7, and C7-T1). We performed uniportal endoscopic multiple posterior foraminotomy with one skin incision. Postoperative MR images show enough decompression without paraspinal muscle damage.
- Case 3: four-level foraminotomy (Figs. 14 and 15).
  - A 77-year-old female presented with severe neck pain, right-side shoulder-radiating pain, and gait disturbance. Preoperative MRI showed severe multiple stenosis at C3–4, C4–5, C5–6, and C6–7. We performed uniportal endoscopic multiple decompression with one skin incision by the sliding technique. Postoperative MR images show enough decompression.

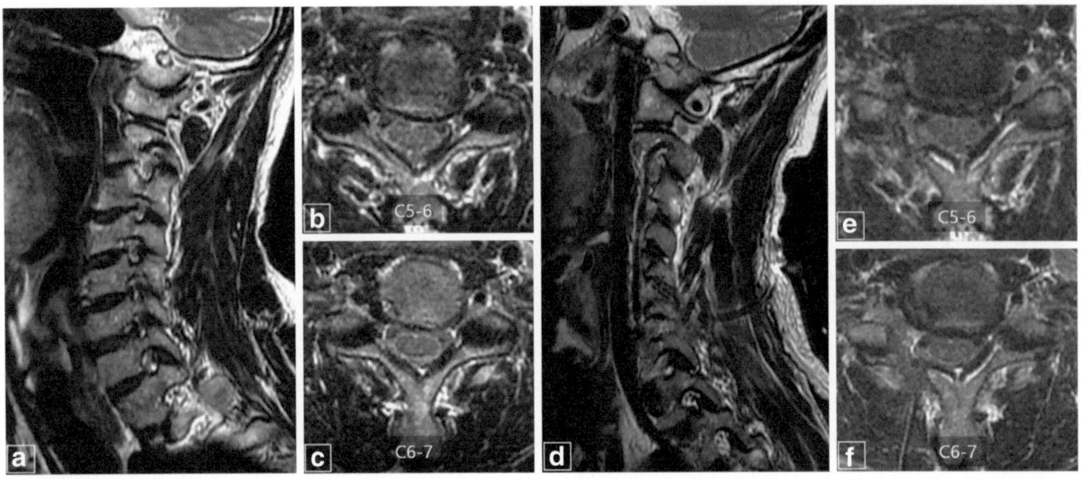


**Fig. 12** Images of case 1. (**a–c**) Preoperative MR images show cervical foraminal stenosis at the right C5–6 and C6–7. (**d–f**) Postoperative MR images show enough decompression without paraspinal muscle damage

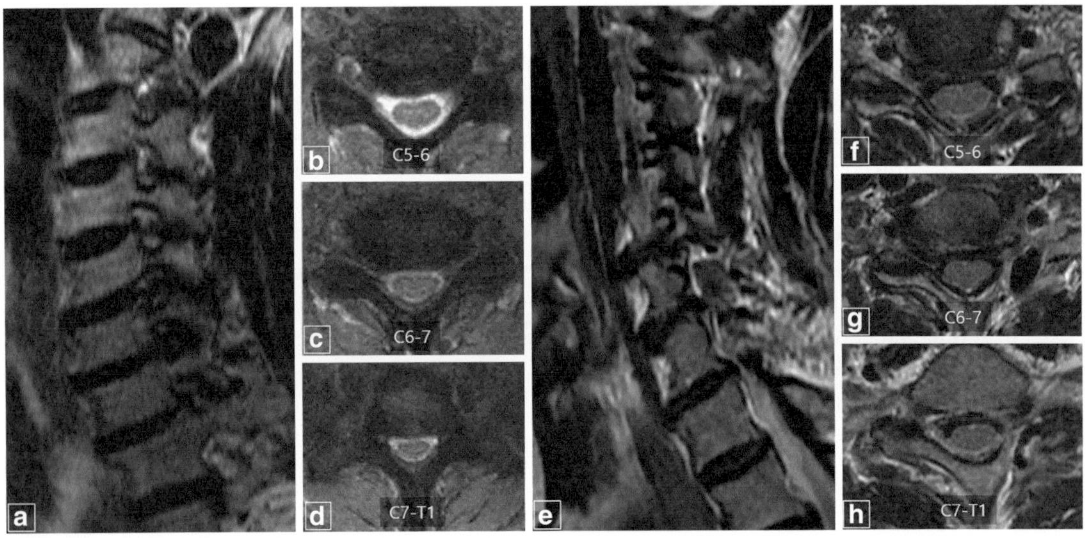


**Fig. 13** Images of case 2. (**a–d**) Preoperative MR images show cervical foraminal stenosis at the left C5–6, C6–7, and C7-T1. The sliding technique for multiple foraminal decompression with one skin incision. (**e–h**) Postoperative MRI shows enough foraminal decompression without paraspinal muscle damage

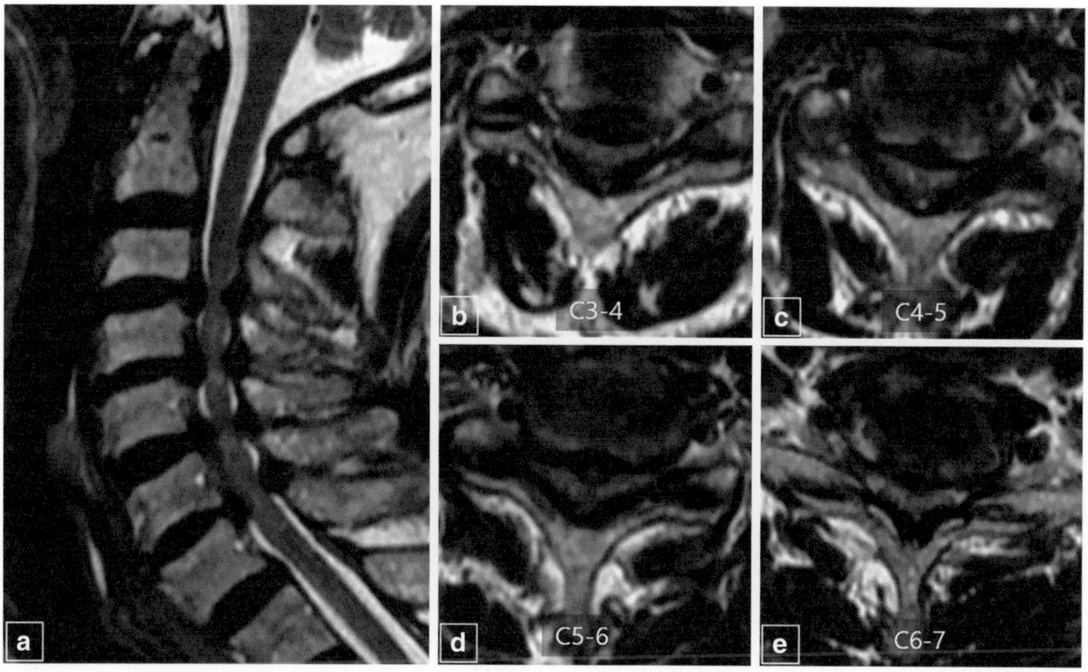


**Fig. 14** Preoperative images of case 3. Preoperative MR images show severe cervical central (**a**) and foraminal stenosis at C3–4 (**b**), C4–5 (**c**), C5–6 (**d**), and C6–7 (**e**)

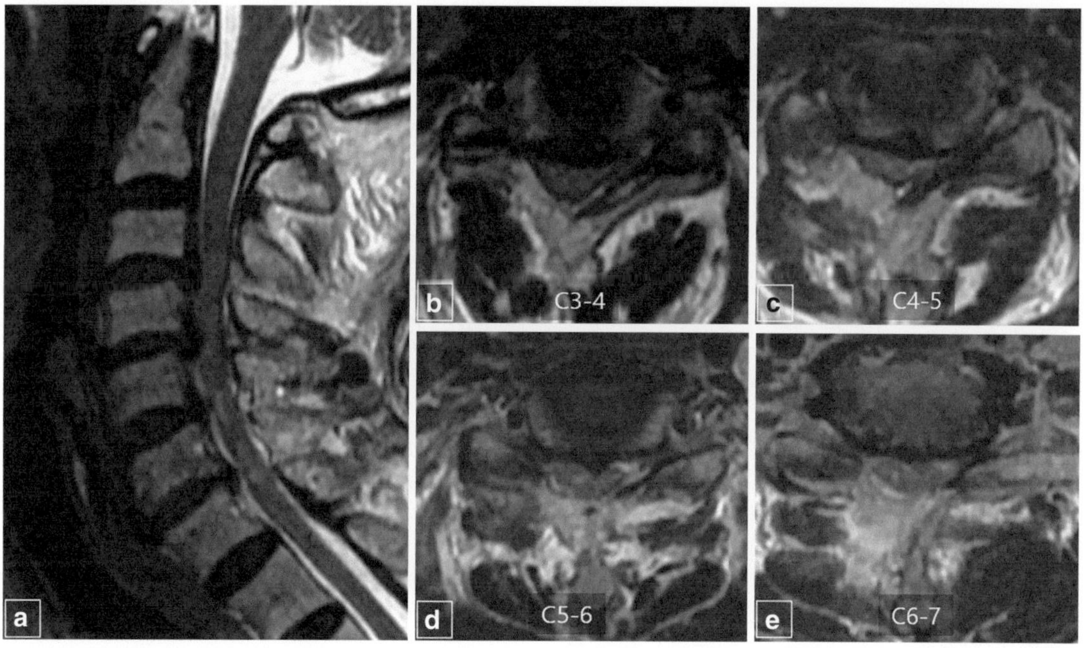


**Fig. 15** Preoperative images of case 3. Postoperative MRI shows enough multiple central canal and right-side foraminal decompression. Sagittal MRI image shows well-decompression status of central canal (**a**). Axial MRI images reveal decompression of central canal at C3–4 (**b**), C4–5 (**c**), C5–6 (**d**), and C6–7 (**e**)

## 7 Prevention and Management of Complications

One major difference and disadvantage that has to be appreciated by surgeons considering this type (the uniportal endoscopic system) of approach is that the surgical instruments are used "one-at-a-time" and long handling.

In the endoscopic surgery presented here, only one instrument is used at a time down the working channel. Continuous irrigation is helpful for both obviating the need for using suction instruments and acting as a retractor in pulsing away the dural and neural elements, but the endoscopic procedure is technically different from the microendoscopic procedure in more than just the method of visualization during the procedure. In addition, there is an endoscopic retractor that can move or protect the nerve root while using an additional instrument. When using an endoscopic retractor, root retraction should be done carefully.

Complications of PECD are affected by a steep learning curve and familiarity of the endoscopic system. Hence, we felt that a spine surgeon should perform PECD after being competent in lumbar decompression surgeries.

## 8 Discussion

The development of endoscopic techniques and, in particular, PECD technique aims to preserve posterior structures and yet achieve the similar goals of conventional posterior cervical foraminotomy. PECD is a motion-preserving procedure that focuses directly on decompression of the soft prolapsed disc and foraminal stenosis causing cervical radiculopathy [1]. With a one-step dilatation, the working channel, endoscope, and instruments were directly placed over the surface of the lamina or facet joint and placed through a less than 1 cm skin incision.

The reduction in the incision size and the direct placement of working channel without any muscle dissection can result in a reduction in blood loss, muscle disruption, bony removal, and a rapid postoperative recovery [5–7]. Furthermore, the advantages of the sliding technique for multilevel decompression might be a small incision with few skin wounds, which might be correlated with a smaller wound infection rate.

Patients with symptomatic cervical radiculopathy due to foraminal stenosis or disc herniations can be effectively managed with either a traditional open or a minimally invasive foraminotomy, and here we describe an endoscopic technique for performing a multilevel posterior cervical foraminotomy that highlights the nuances of a procedure that offers both advantages and challenges to the spine surgeon who is trying to take advantage of the newest advances in the growing technology available in minimally invasive spine surgery.

## References

1. Wu PH, Kim HS, Lee YJ, Kim DH, Lee JH, Yang KH, et al. Posterior endoscopic cervical foramiotomy and discectomy: clinical and radiological computer tomography evaluation on the bony effect of decompression with 2 years follow-up. Eur Spine J. 2021;30(2):534–46.
2. Zhang C, Wu J, Xu C, Zheng W, Pan Y, Li C, et al. Minimally invasive full-endoscopic posterior cervical Foraminotomy assisted by O-arm-based navigation. Pain Physician. 2018;21(3):E215–E23.
3. Kim M, Kim HS, Oh SW, Adsul NM, Singh R, Kashlan ON, et al. Evolution of spinal endoscopic surgery. Neurospine. 2019;16(1):6–14.
4. Ruetten S, Komp M, Merk H, Godolias G. Use of newly developed instruments and endoscopes: full-endoscopic resection of lumbar disc herniations via the interlaminar and lateral transforaminal approach. J Neurosurg Spine. 2007;6(6):521–30.
5. Lim KT, Nam HGW, Kim SB, Kim HS, Park JS, Park CK. Therapeutic feasibility of full endoscopic decompression in one- to three-level Lumbar Canal stenosis via a single skin port using a new endoscopic system, percutaneous Stenoscopic lumbar decompression. Asian Spine J. 2019;13(2):272–82.
6. Nam HGW, Kim HS, Lee DK, Park CK, Lim KT. Percutaneous Stenoscopic lumbar decompression with Paramedian approach for Foraminal/Extraforaminal lesions. Asian Spine J. 2019;13(4):672–81.
7. Zhang C, Wu J, Zheng W, Li C, Zhou Y. Posterior endoscopic cervical decompression: review and technical note. Neurospine. 2020;17(Suppl 1):S74–80.

# Posterior Full Endoscopic Cervical Foraminotomy and Discectomy Using the Partial Pediculotomy and Partial Vertebrectomy

Chang-Il Ju, Pang Hung Wu, Hyeun Sung Kim, and Il-Tae Jang

**Abstract**

Cervical radiculopathy is a common cervical spine condition leading to significant disability from nerve root dysfunction. Conservative therapy is recommended for at least 6 weeks in the treatment of cervical radiculopathy without myelopathy.

For patients with unilateral cervical radiculopathy refractory to conservative management from lateral disc herniation or degenerative spondylotic foraminal stenosis, a posterior endoscopic cervical foraminotomy should be considered.

Percutaneous endoscopic cervical discectomy (PECD) for decompression of cervical nerve roots is a well-established, minimally invasive surgery for cervical radiculopathy.

This endoscopic cervical posterior technique is further advanced, and if partial pediculotomy and vertebrectomy are additionally performed, decompression of foraminal stenosis, which has been difficult in the past, becomes possible. The surgical outcomes with this technique are equivalent to any other technique, approach-related tissue damage is minimized, and tissue preservation is maximized. The uniportal full endoscopic PPPV approach for posterior endoscopic cervical foraminotomy and discectomy improved radiological and clinical outcomes, providing a safe, alternative technique in posterior cervical decompression with a low rate of complications.

However, there may be a long learning curve for proficiency in endoscopic techniques.

In this chapter, the authors have tried to introduce the surgical technique of this full endoscopic cervical foraminotomy and discectomy using the partial pediculotomy and vertebrectomy in cervical foraminal pathology and briefly review surgical indications, outcomes, and other relevant issues.

**Keywords**

Foraminotomy · Pediculotomy
Vertebrotomy · Cervical · Endoscopy

**Supplementary Information** The online version contains supplementary material available at https://doi.org/10.1007/978-981-99-1133-2_5.

C.-I. Ju
Department of Neurosurgery, Chosun University Hospital, Gwangju, South Korea

P. H. Wu
National University Health System, JurongHealth Campus, Orthopaedic Surgery, Singapore, Singapore

H. S. Kim (✉) · I.-T. Jang
Department of Neurosurgery, Spine Center, Gangnam Nanoori Hospital, Seoul, South Korea



H. S. Kim et al. (eds.), *Advanced Technique of Endoscopic Cervical and Thoracic Spine Surgery*,
https://doi.org/10.1007/978-981-99-1133-2_5

# 1 Advantages of This Approach

Cervical radiculopathy is usually caused by compression of the nerve root due to lateral disc herniation or degenerative stenosis of the cervical intervertebral foramen. Surgical decompression is an effective treatment method when conservative methods fail to relieve pain or when significant weakness occurs in the upper extremity muscles supplied by the compressed nerve root [1–3]. Anterior cervical discectomy and fusion (ACDF) and cervical artificial disc replacement (TDR) were the standard of care of reference [4]. Morbidity due to anterior cervical spine surgery ranged from 13.2% to 19.3%, and pseudoarthrosis and adjacent segment disease were the most common postoperative complications [5].

Posterior cervical foraminotomy has become increasingly popular as an alternative to ACDF, reducing problems associated with fusion, and has the added benefit of preserving motion with equally good clinical outcomes [6–8].

Posterior cervical foraminotomy is a motion-preserving technique first described by Spurling and Scovillein 1944 [9]. Today, however, it can be done using advanced minimally invasive techniques that minimize incisions, result in less bleeding, and provide an effect equivalent to open surgery, significantly reducing the length of hospital stay and return to daily activities after surgery. In addition, the treatment cost is also reduced [10–12].

In this chapter, the authors tried to do their best for readers to understand how to handle this endoscopic system in cervical foraminal stenosis by demonstrating the figures of each surgical step and decompression of the main pathology followed, as well as presenting the overview of this surgical technique by briefly reviewing surgical indication, outcome, and other relevant issues.

## 1.1 Advantages

- A cervical posterior approach rather than an anterior approach reduces the risk of esophageal or airway damage and allows cervical nerve decompression to be performed posteriorly.
- It minimizes the damage to the ipsilateral paraspinal muscles and soft tissues at the cervical surgical site and completely preserves the contralateral cervical anatomical structures.
- It preserves the posterior tension band by preventing damage to the posterior ligament complex (superior supraspinatus, interspinous ligament, and facet joint capsule) to maintain the normal integrity of the cervical spine.
- Because only the cervical exiting nerve can be decompressed without performing anterior fusion, it is possible to preserve the normal range of motion of neck after surgery.
- The postoperative recovery is quick regardless of age, and the rehabilitation period can be shortened.

# 2 Indications and Contraindications

## 2.1 Clinical Indications

1. Cervical radiculopathy with defined neurological disturbance (sensory disorder, reflex abnormality, motor weakness).
2. Cervicogenic headache or discogenic axial pain from soft cervical disc herniation.
3. Persistent cervical radiculopathy after nerve root block.
4. Unsuccessful conservative therapy for at least 6 weeks.

## 2.2 Radiological Indications

1. Cervical disc herniation around the foraminal area demonstrated on computed tomography (CT) and/or magnetic resonance imaging (MRI).
2. No definite segmental instability on dynamic radiography (flexion-extension view).
3. Foraminal stenosis with disc space narrowing.

### 2.3 Contraindications

1. Ossification of the posterior longitudinal ligament or cervical stenosis.
2. Myelopathy or severe neurological deficit.
3. Cervical spondylolisthesis or segmental instability.
4. Other pathological conditions, such as fracture, tumor, or active infection.

### 2.4 Relative Contraindications

1. Severe foraminal stenosis above the C4–5 level.
2. Multilevel cervical spondylosis with myelopathic change.

## 3 Anesthesia and Position

The procedure is performed under general anesthesia for ease of patient positioning and immobilization. The patient is placed in prone position on a radiolucent table with Wilson's frame.

In posterior cervical spine surgery, the Mayfield head clamp is commonly used to provide a rigid, stable position of the head throughout the procedure. The use of the Mayfield head clamp has been associated with skull fractures, lacerations, air embolisms, and epidural hematoma.

However, the posterior cervical endoscopic surgery can be performed without Mayfield head clamp; this method has several advantages such as reducing the head fixation equipment and the additional risk of complications resulting from skeletal traction during surgery.

This posterior cervical endoscopic spine surgery can be performed safely and effectively with three-point plaster traction technique without the risks associated with skeletal traction.

Patients received general anesthesia and were positioned prone on a Wilson frame with the shoulder strapped and neck flexed in a slight reverse Trendelenburg position using the three-point plaster traction technique on head, shoulder, and back without the use of a Mayfield clamp to increase interlaminar space of the cervical spine (Table 1). The patient's face was positioned in a commercial anesthesia pillow foam supporting bony prominence, with space created for the eyes, nose, and mouth. The head attachment was tilted down slightly, allowing cervical spine flexion, and secured with plaster. The patient's arms were padded and tucked longitudinally next to them. The anterior superior iliac spine and knees were padded, and hips and knees were flexed slightly. Both the shoulders were strapped to pull down the shoulder slightly without pressure on the brachial plexus and finally strapped on the back to reduce skin fold (Fig. 1).

**Table 1** Comparison of anesthesia methods and advantages and disadvantages during full endoscopic spinal surgery

| Anesthesia | Local | Epidural | General |
|---|---|---|---|
| Comfortable | – | + | +++ |
| Intraoperative relax | – | + | +++ |
| Motor block | – | + | +++ |
| Sensory block | – | + | +++ |
| Neural irritation | ++ | + | – |
| Wake-up | ++ | + | – |

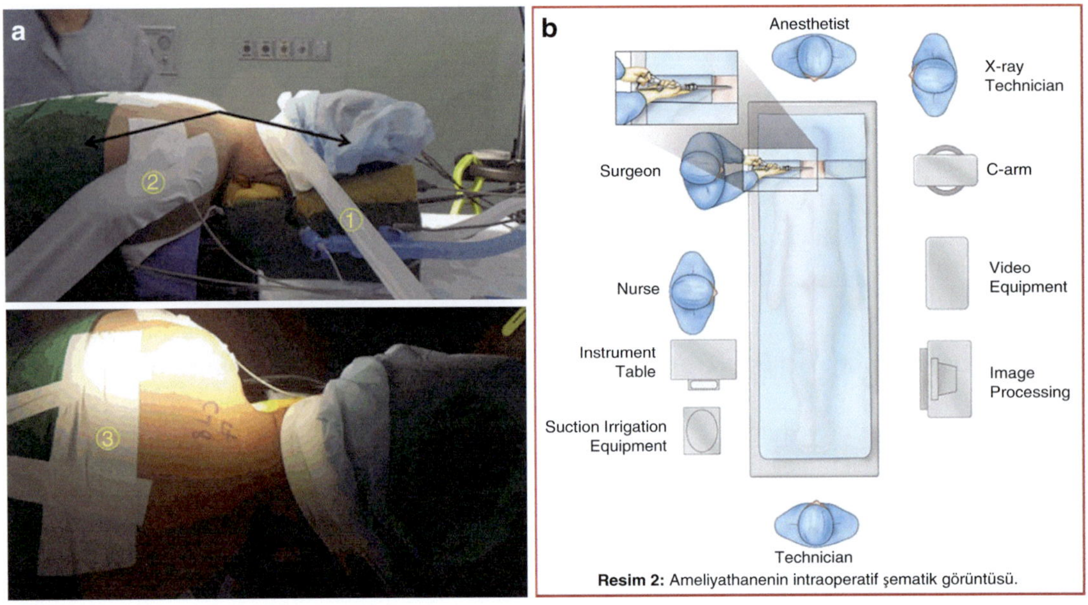


**Fig. 1** Patients are positioned prone with their heads secured without a radiolucent Mayfield head holder. The patient's face was positioned in a commercial anesthesia pillow foam supporting bony prominence, with space created for the eyes, nose, and mouth (**a**). Standard operation room setup (**b**)

## 4 Special Instruments (Fig. 2)

1. Guidewire.
2. Obturator, serial dilators, and working cannula 7.3 mm with a bevel tip.
3. Endoscope with 30° viewing angle, outer diameter 6.5 mm, working channel diameter 3.7 mm, and working length 208 mm (used in traditional Lumbar transforaminal approach).
4. High-speed endoscopic drill with 3.5 mm diamond tip.
5. Radiofrequency ablator with probe.
6. Endoscopic Kerrison's rongeurs.
7. Endoscopic disc forceps.
8. Endoscopic bone cutter.
9. Endoscopic blunt bent tip probe.

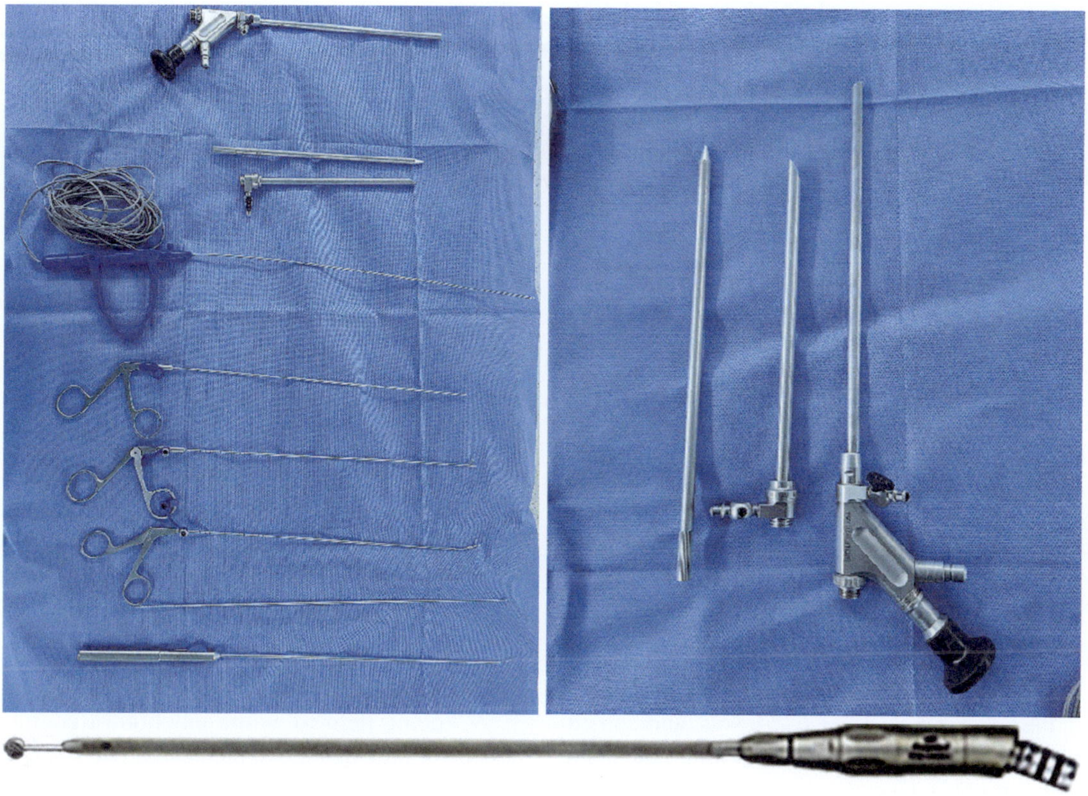

**Fig. 2** Endoscopic instrument and diamond endoscopic drill

## 5 Procedures

### 5.1 Anatomical Consideration

The cervical intervertebral foramen extends from the inferior aspect of the pedicle to the superior aspect of the pedicle of the inferior vertebrae. The anterior wall of the foramen is formed by the uncinate process, the posterolateral aspect of the intervertebral disc, and the adjoining vertebral body. The facet joint, along with the superior articular process of the lower vertebra, forms the posterior wall of the foramen. The nerve root enters the foramen medially at the medial border of the rostral and caudal pedicle and exits the foramen laterally as it passes the lateral margin of the rostral and caudal pedicles. In the sagittal oblique plane, the nerve roots are seen to lie below a line drawn from the tip of the uncinate process to the tip of the superior articular process.

The V-point (including the inferior margin of the cephalic lamina, the medial junction of the inferior and superior facet joints, and the superior margin of the caudal lamina) is the anatomical landmark for the beginning of bone drilling [13, 14]. In the middle-aged group, the dura width and the interlaminar width decreased in the same direction so that we can predict the relative position between the lateral dura edge and the V-point with less remarkable errors. In the old-aged group (the 70 s), significant changes in two parameters were found, the dura width increased in the C4–5, C5–6, and C6–7 levels, but interlaminar width decreased according to aging. These results mean that the lateral dura edge

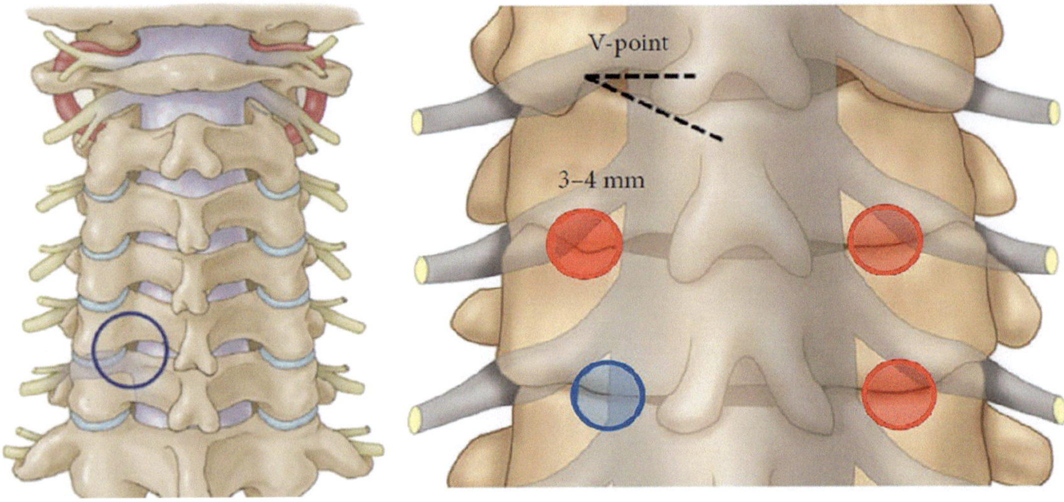


**Fig. 3** The circled area indicates the degree of bone removal. After bone removal, we can usually first identify the exiting nerve root, the free axillary epidural space, and the dura lateral margin (red circle). On the other hand, when the dura margin is extended to the lateral region, it is difficult to secure free epidural space because the dura lateral margin occupies most of the surgical space after bone removal (blue circle) [15]

would be more laterally located than the V-point in the C4–5, C5–6, and C6–7 levels, and considerable attention is required not to injure the nerve structures [15]. (Fig. 3) Another essential considering point is the surgical position of the cervical spine curvature. Insufficient neck flexion induces the V-point to move more medially, and insufficient bony removal would be done more than the predicted extent [15].

## 5.2 Step 1. Entry Point Marking

- The skin marking of the entry point was performed at a site about 3–4 cm lateral to the midline under fluoroscopy of the guide AP and lateral view.
- Targeting point is the V-point of the intersection of intervertebral disc space and medial border of facet joint junction in the AP view, and the facet joint is on the correct level in the lateral view (Fig. 4).
- This is an anatomical landmark called the "V"-point, defined as the junction of confluence of the cranial and the caudal laminofacet in a V-shape.

## 5.3 Step 2. Approach and Docking

- After making a vertical or transverse 8-mm skin incision at the ipsilateral side in "V"-point, an obturator that served as a guide for the 4.7-mm outer diameter working sleeve was advanced into the V-point and docked (Fig. 5a, b).
- The tip position was confirmed with fluoroscopy.
- A 30° viewing angle, 7.3-mm outer diameter, and 4.7-mm working channel (Joimax GmbH, Karlsruhe, Germany) were used for the procedure under continuous normal saline irrigation of 25 mmHg pressure (Fig. 5c, d).
- Hemostasis and soft-tissue dissection were done with a radiofrequency probe (Ellman's

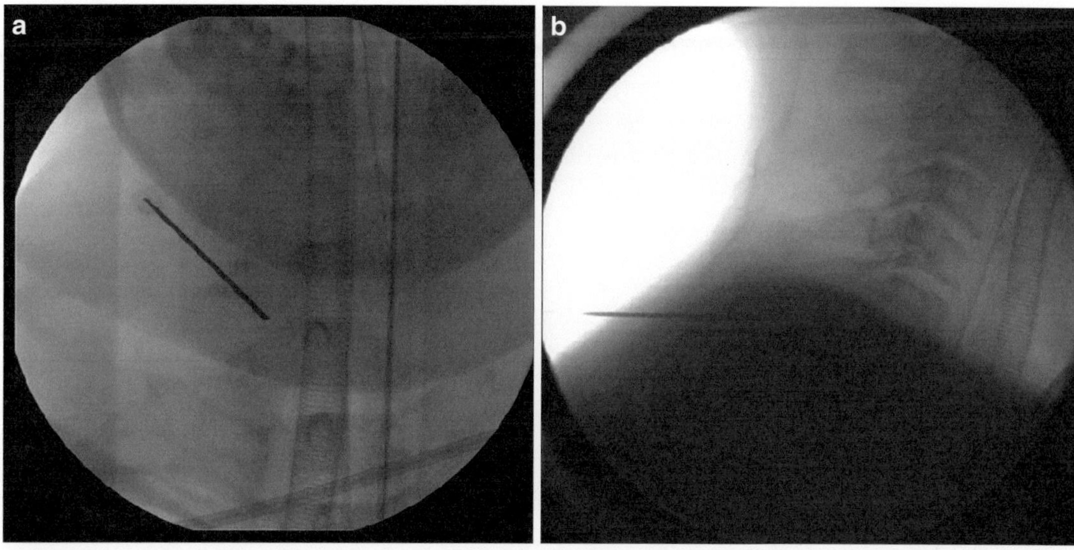


**Fig. 4** The skin marking of the entry point was performed at a site about 3–4 cm lateral to the midline under fluoroscopy of the guide AP and lateral view. Targeting point is the V-point in the AP view (**a**), and the facet joint on the correct level in the lateral view (**b**)

bipolar radiofrequency electrocoagulator; elliquence, Baldwin, New York, USA) and endoscopic forceps.

## 5.4 Step 3. Bony Decompression with Foraminotomy (Video 1)

- If the docking of the endoscope to the V-point is confirmed on the fluoroscopic view, check the V-point that the upper and lower lamina meets in the endoscopic view.
- The anatomical structure to start is the medial aspect of the lateral mass and facet joint, start working from the cephalad laminofacet site first. Drilling with a long, straight 3.5-mm diameter, coarse diamond high-speed drill (Primado High-Speed Drill System; NSK, Nakanishi, Japan) is used to create a working window depending on the size of herniated material and degree of foraminal stenosis (Fig. 6).
- Typically, 3–5-mm diameter of bone was removed in a circular fashion from the lateral inferior aspect of the upper lamina followed by approximately 3 mm of the medial inferior portion of the upper facet from the laminofacet border ("V"-point).
- Then, drilling on the about 3–5-mm diameter of the superomedial corner of the medial aspect of superior articular facet of lower vertebra lying close to the dorsal aspect of the nerve root, which leads to the proximal portion of the nerve root (Fig. 7).
- Before doing this procedure, tilting the patient toward the operator makes it easier for the surgeon to work with the medial aspect of the facet from the medial side of the cervical lamina to the facet joint.
- A 3.5-mm diamond drill was used for all bone removal and forceps, and punches were used for loose bone fragments.

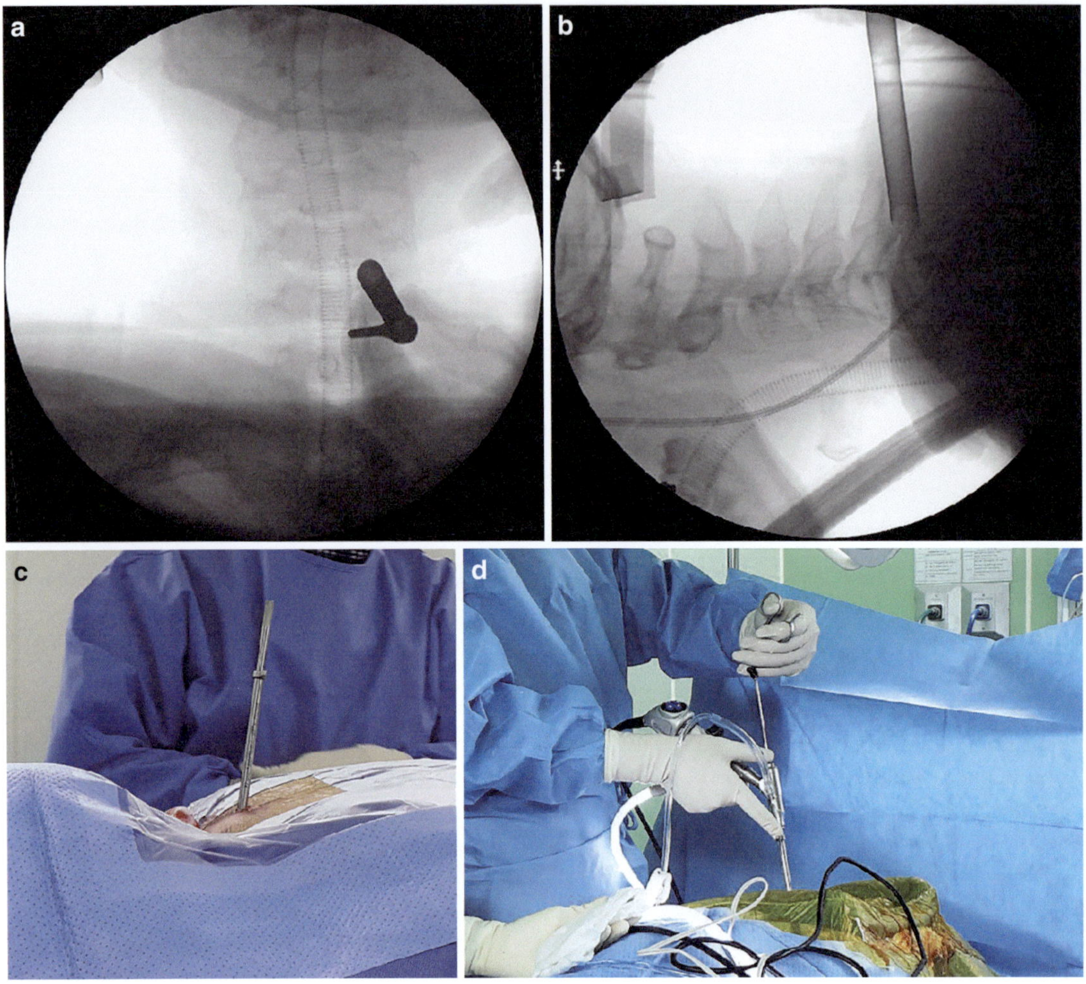


**Fig. 5** After making a vertical or transverse 8-mm skin incision at the ipsilateral side in "V"-point, an obturator that served as a guide for the 4.7-mm outer diameter working sleeve was advanced into the V-point and docked (**a**, **b**). 30° viewing angle, 7.3 mm outer diameter, and 4.7 mm working channel (Joimax GmbH, Karlsruhe, Germany) were used for the procedure under continuous normal saline irrigation of 25 mmHg pressure (**c**, **d**)

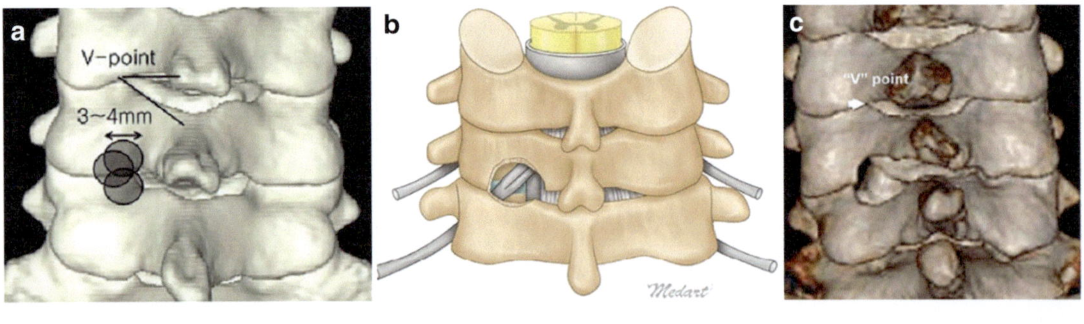


**Fig. 6** A 3–5-mm diameter of bone was removed in a circular fashion from the lateral inferior aspect of the upper lamina followed by approximately 3 mm of the medial inferior portion of the upper facet from the laminofacet border ("V"-point). Then, drilling on the about 3–5-mm diameter of the superomedial corner of the medial aspect of the superior articular facet of the lower vertebra lying close to the dorsal aspect of the nerve root, which leads to the proximal portion of the nerve root. (**a**, **b**) Postoperative cervical CT shows the bone drilling area in the laminofacet area (**c**)

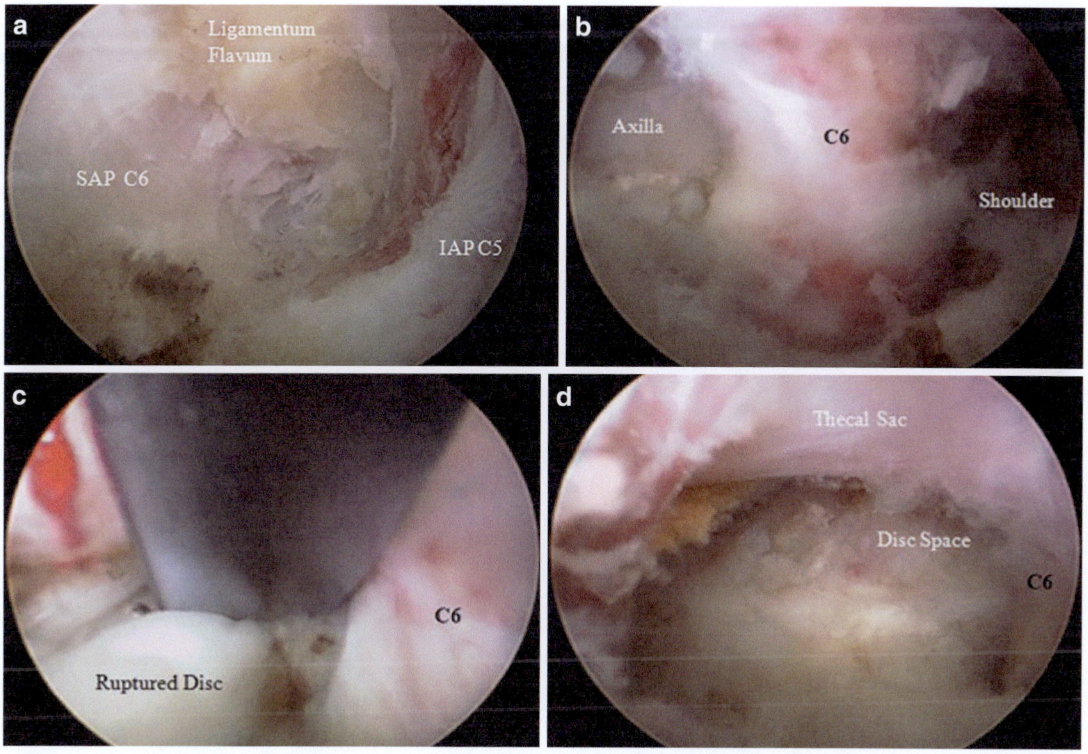


**Fig. 7** In the endoscopic view, after bone drilling, C5 inferior articular process and C6 superior articular process were partially removed, and the ligamentum flavum was observed as the medial part of the widened V-point (**a**). The C6 exiting nerve root is observed, and it can be confirmed that the compressed nerve protrudes from the prolapse of the intervertebral disc (**b**). The C6 nerve root is carefully retracted, the ruptured disc comes out from the bottom, and it can be easily removed. (**c**) After the prolapsed disc is removed, the compressed C6 exiting nerve root is decompressed and epidural space and disc space can be confirmed (**d**)

## 5.5 Step 4. Complete Exiting Nerve Root Decompression with Vertebrectomy (Video 1)

- After posterior foraminotomy and exposure of the exiting nerve root and spinal cord, the working cannula is shifted to the center of the upper medial side of the pedicle, and drilling on the pedicle 3–5-mm deeper than the nerve site to create a working space below the exiting nerve root to access the herniated disc area (Fig. 8).
- Surgical procedure in this way allows cervical discectomy with a minimal nerve traction.
- In the case of central disc herniation in the preoperative MRI, more nerve retractions are required. However, excessive retractions can cause nerve damage.
- More nerve retraction is required if the disc is located in the center of the preoperative MRI. However, in this case, excessive retraction can cause nerve damage.
- Therefore, an advanced technique to access the central disc with minimal nerve retractions

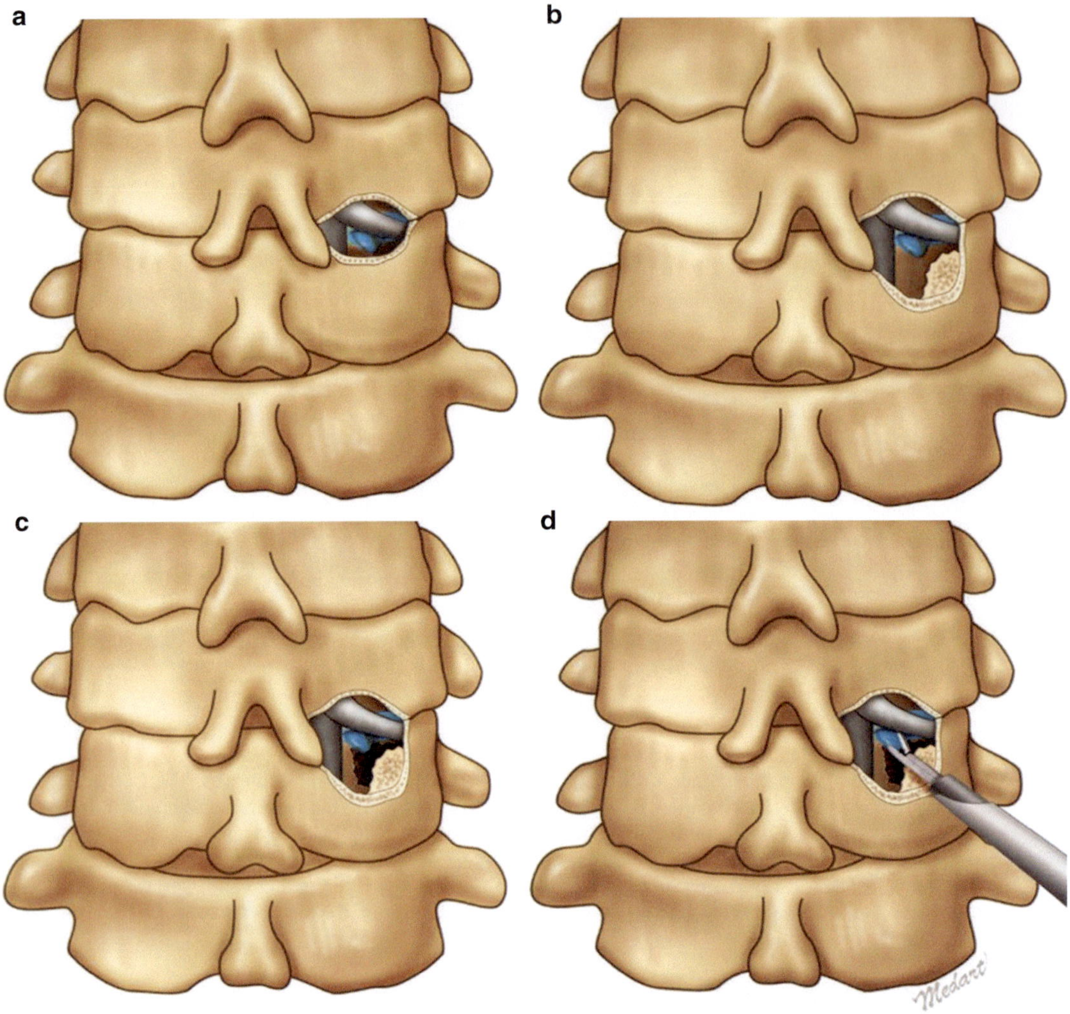


**Fig. 8** Schematic diagram of surgery step-by-step process of complete exiting nerve root decompression with vertebrectomy. Bony decompression and foraminotomy (**a**), drilling on the pedicle 3–5 mm deeper than the nerve site to create a working space below the exiting nerve root to access the herniated disc area (**b**), partial pediculotomy and vertebrectomy (**c**), the disc space can be created by a natural retraction of the exiting nerve root, and the prolapsed disc can be removed easily with endoscopic forceps and a Kerrison rongeur (**d**)

as possible is required, and the partial pediculotomy and vertebrectomy are the most effective and useful methods for this procedure (Fig. 9).

- Also, in addition, using this method, it is possible to completely and effectively decompress the nerve roots in the intervertebral foramen.
- After drilling on the pedicle underneath the neural elements to secure a working space in a central location, the lateral part of the corpus of the caudal cervical vertebra was drilled to provide access to the central disc without a significant neural retraction (Fig. 10).

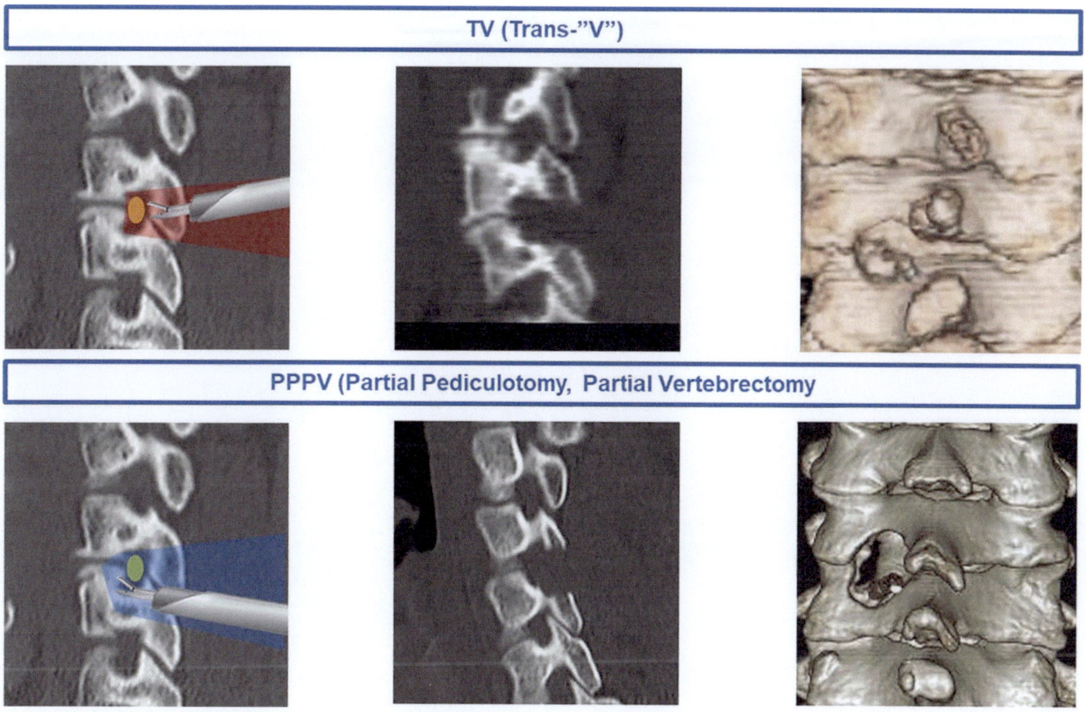


**Fig. 9** Diagrams showing the concept of partial pediculotomy and partial vertebrectomy for posterior endoscopic cervical foraminotomy with subneural epidural space creation. Drilling and decompression were performed in the cone shape (blue). Drilling the medial superior part of the pedicle and lateral superior part of the corpus of the caudal vertebra created a subneural epidural space sufficient for the working instruments to access the lateral one-third of the intervertebral disc space without a significant, if any, neural retraction

- After working on the bone with a drill, a forceps or cutter is carefully inserted into the subneural space created on the ventral side of the neural elements, and the disc material and osteophytes are carefully accessed and removed with forceps.
- After the axilla of the spinal cord and exiting nerve root are identified in endoscopic view, the working cannula was carefully rotated with the open bevel facing away from the axilla of the spinal cord (Fig. 11).
- In this way, the disc space can be created by a natural retraction of the exiting nerve root, and the prolapsed disc can be removed easily with endoscopic forceps and a Kerrison rongeur.
- Radiofrequency electrocautery was often used to obtain the operative endoscopic view with hemostasis and help in gently releasing the adhesion of the neural elements from the disc. Uncovertebral hypertrophy was removed by grinding with a drill or cutting with a cutter.
- After all procedures are finalized, in the endoscopic view, nerve elements pulsate freely under full decompression.
- Finally, the skin is sutured and the decision to insert a drainage tube is made according to the bleeding during surgery.

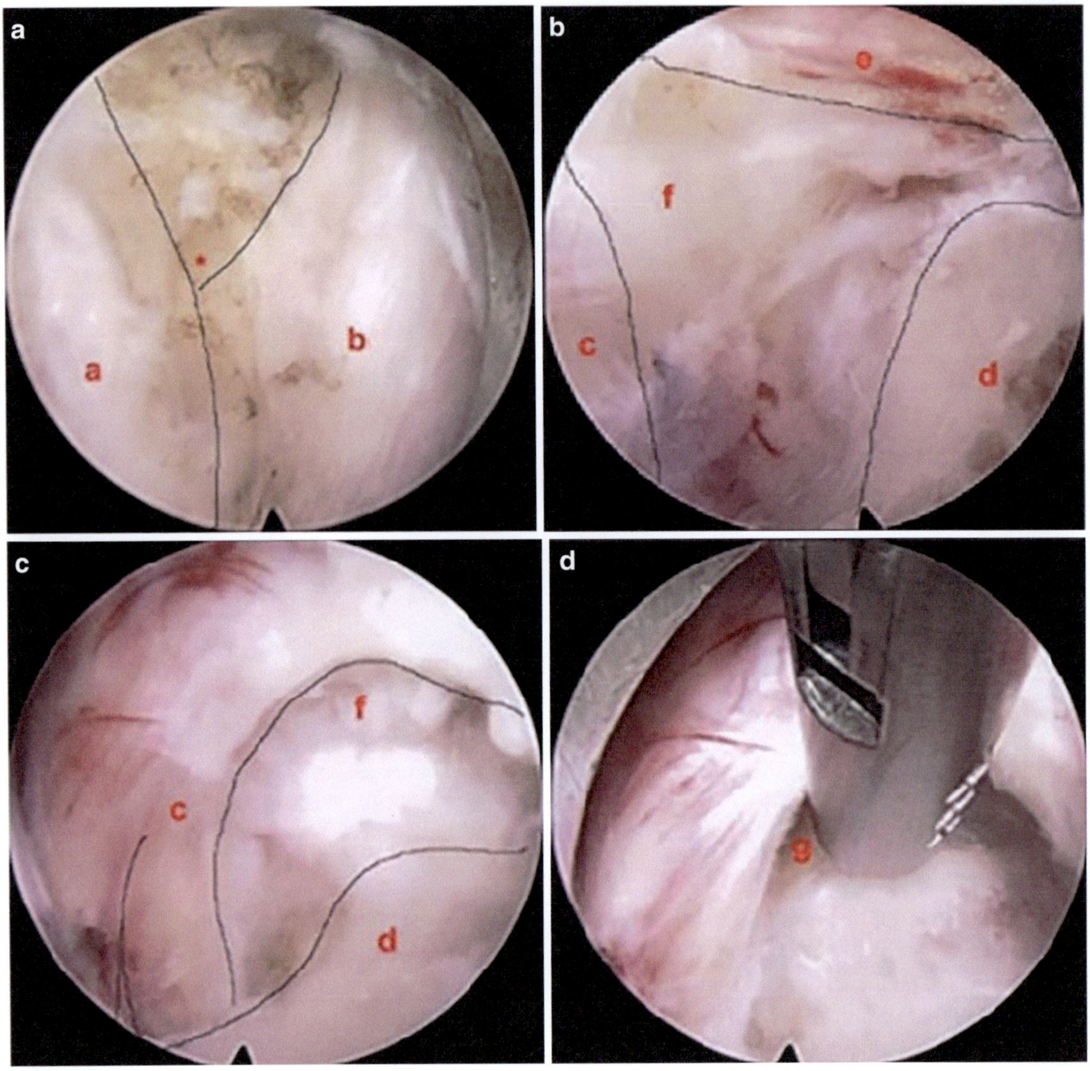


**Fig. 10** Endoscopic surgical view images of four steps of the partial pediculotomy and partial vertebrectomy approach for posterior endoscopic cervical foraminotomy. Docking and soft-tissue dissection exposing the V-point of the laminofacet junction, which was the landmark for drilling for the partial pediculotomy and partial vertebrectomy approach for posterior endoscopic cervical foraminotomy (**a**). After endoscopic drilling to complete cervical foraminotomy, the inferior and medial aspects of the left C5 nerve root (axilla) were exposed, and the pedicle was located intimately with the axilla of the C5 exit nerve root (**b**). Endoscopically, the medial superior part of the pedicle (medial pediculotomy) and the lateral superior part of the corpus of caudal vertebra helped create a subneural epidural working space to expose the C4–C5 intervertebral disc space, then, the prolapsed intervertebral disc at C4–C5 disc space under the axilla of the C5 exit nerve root was exposed (**c**). After removal of the prolapsed disc, the pulsating exit nerve root and dura of spinal cord under irrigation fluid were observed (**d**)

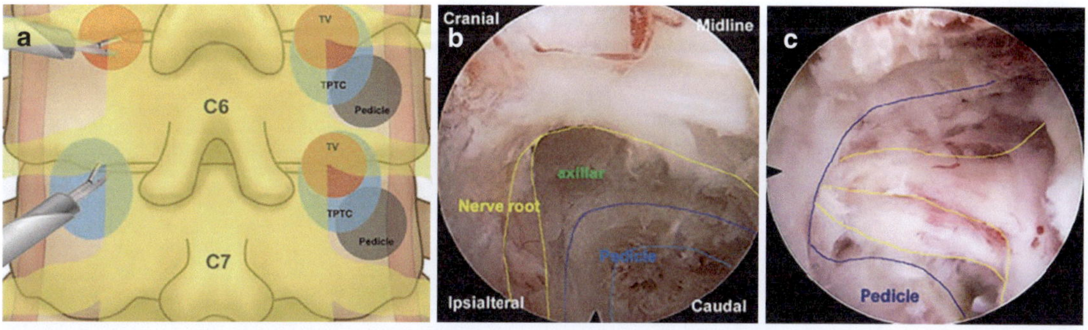


**Fig. 11** Schematic diagram of anatomy of partial pediculotomy and partial vertebrectomy (**a**). In the posterior foraminotomy (small orange circle), it is difficult to remove the intervertebral disc in the intervertebral foramen due to the difficulty in retraction of the exiting nerve root, and complete decompression of the exiting nerve is difficult in foraminal stenosis (**b**). However, when partial pediculotomy and partial vertebrectomy are performed (blue circle), complete decompression of the exiting nerve root is possible in the intervertebral foramen, and the remaining disc material without nerve root retraction can be completely removed by securing space below the nerve root (**c**)

# 6 Illustrated Cases

## 6.1 Case 1 (Fig. 12)

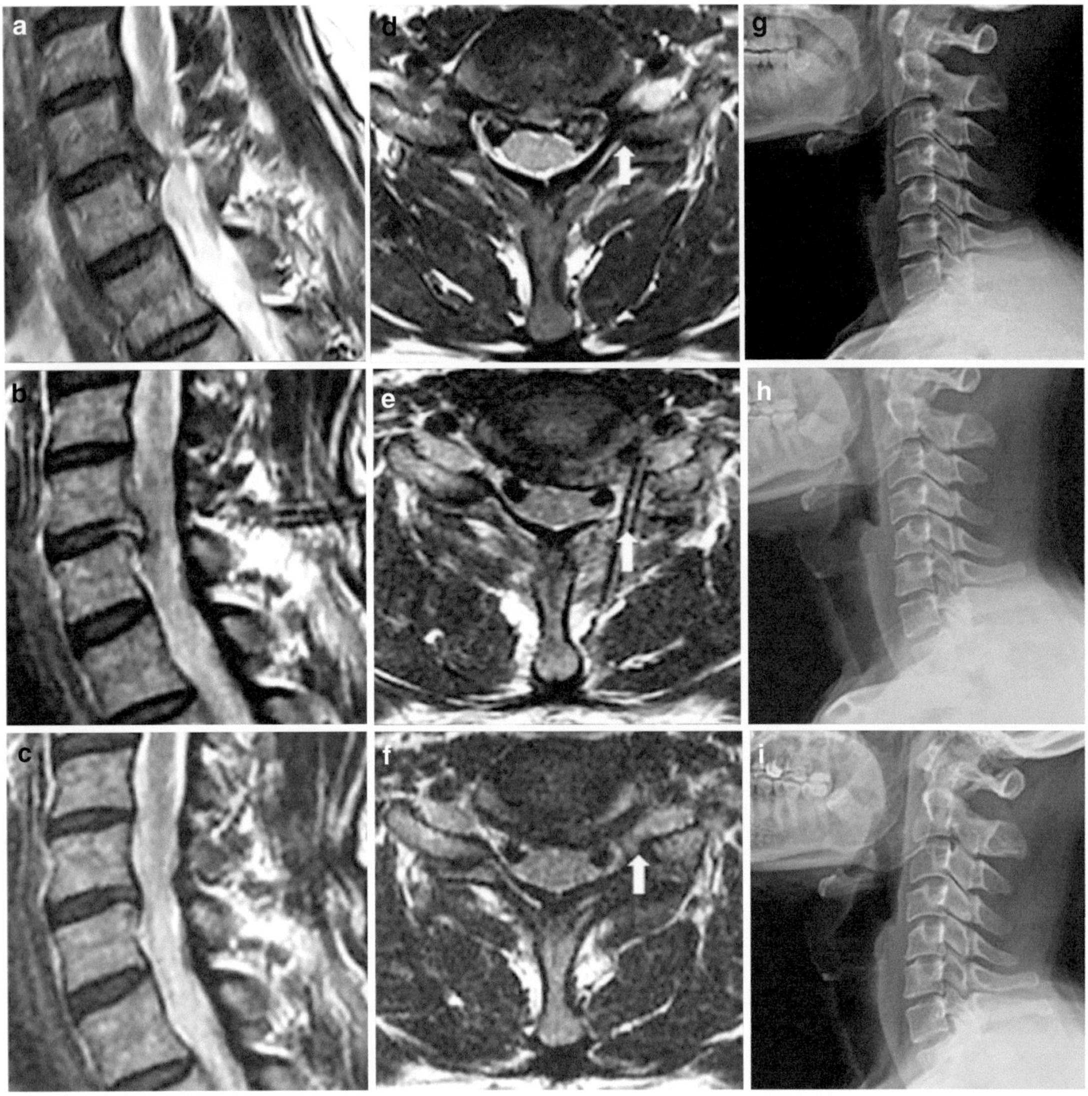


**Fig. 12** Images of a 43-year-old man with subacute onset of a left shoulder weakness with deltoid and biceps flexion strength of grade 2. He had recovered completely 2 months after left C4–C5 partial pediculotomy and partial vertebrectomy for posterior endoscopic cervical foraminotomy. Preoperative magnetic resonance imaging (MRI) studies showing a large prolapsed intervertebral disc in left C4–C5 abutting the exit nerve root of left C5 (**a**, **d**). Early postoperative MRI studies showing decompression of the left C4–C5 foramen with removal of the prolapsed left C4–C5 disc space (**b**, **e**). MRI studies at 6 months of follow-up showing some reconstitution of the medial laminofacet joint with no recurrence of the left C4–C5 intervertebral disc space (**c**, **f**). Lateral view of C-spine shows no changes in alignment of preoperative, postoperative, and final follow-up for 6 months (**g**–**i**)

## 6.2 Case 2 (Fig. 13)

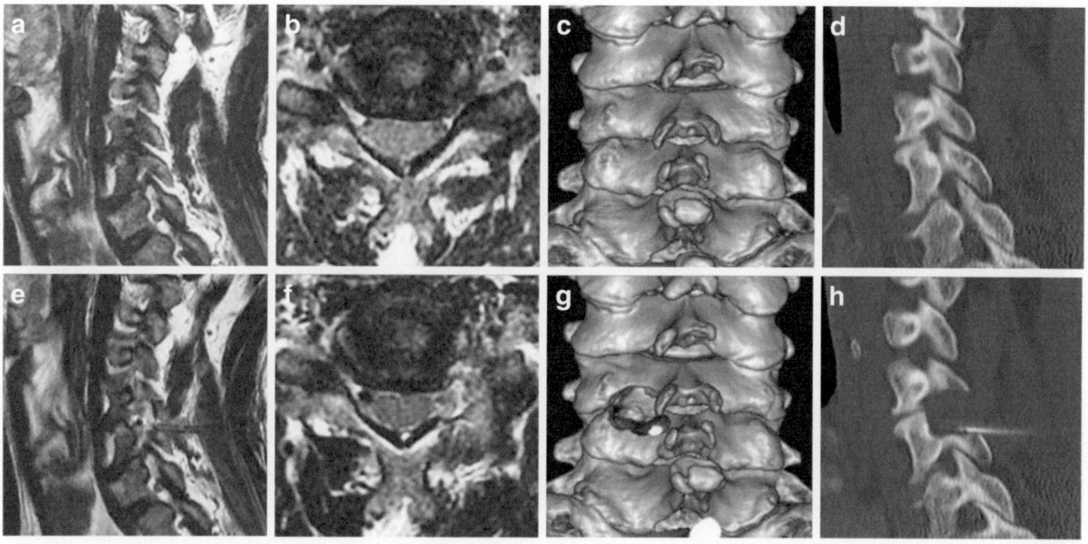


**Fig. 13** A 66-year-old man with subacute onset of left arm radiating pain with tingling sensation weakness of wrist drop is presented. He recovered completely 2 months after left C5–6 partial pediculotomy and partial vertebrectomy approach for posterior endoscopic cervical foraminotomy and discectomy (PPPV PECF). Preoperative magnetic resonance imaging (MRI) scan showed a foraminal intervertebral disc in left C5–6 abutting the exit nerve root of left C6. (**a**, **b**) Preoperative computed tomography (CT) scan showed mild uncovertebral joint hypertrophy with narrowing of the left C5–6 foramen. (**c**, **d**) Early postoperative MRI showed decompression of left C5–6 foramen with removal of prolapsed left C5–6 disc space (**e**, **f**). Postoperative CT showed wide posterior cervical foraminotomy with decompression of left C5–6, and upper half of the left C6 pedicle was drilled to expose the disc space of left C5–6 (**g**, **h**)

# 7 Prevention and Management of Complications

## 7.1 Instability (Fig. 14)

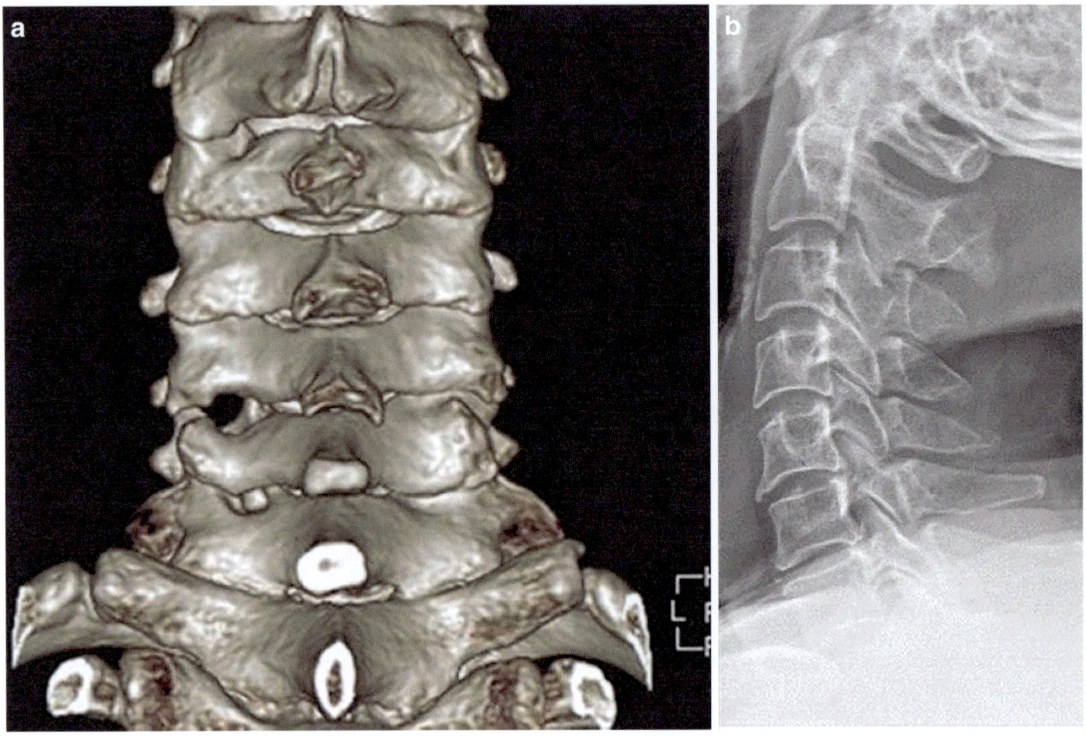


**Fig. 14** (**a**) Excessive laminofacet removal can cause facet joint injury, which can lead to instability. (**b**) Preserving the lateral third of the possible laminofacet area during surgery can prevent instability

## 7.2 C5 Nerve Palsy (Fig. 15)

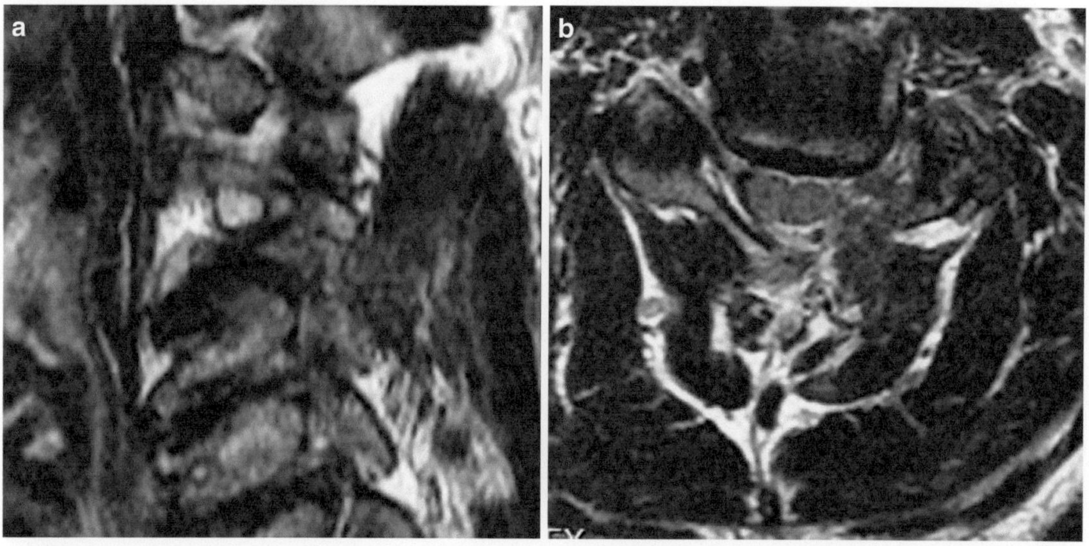

**Fig. 15** Although relatively few in the lower cervical area, C5 nerve palsy often occurs in the mid-cervical area (C3–4-5). (**a**) As with posterior cervical decompression, postoperative posterior cord shift with nerve tethering at the superior facet or uncovertebral joint, cord ischemia second blood flow reduced due to radicular artery traction, and surgical trauma can occur as causes (**b**)

## 7.3 Spinal Cord Injury (Fig. 16)

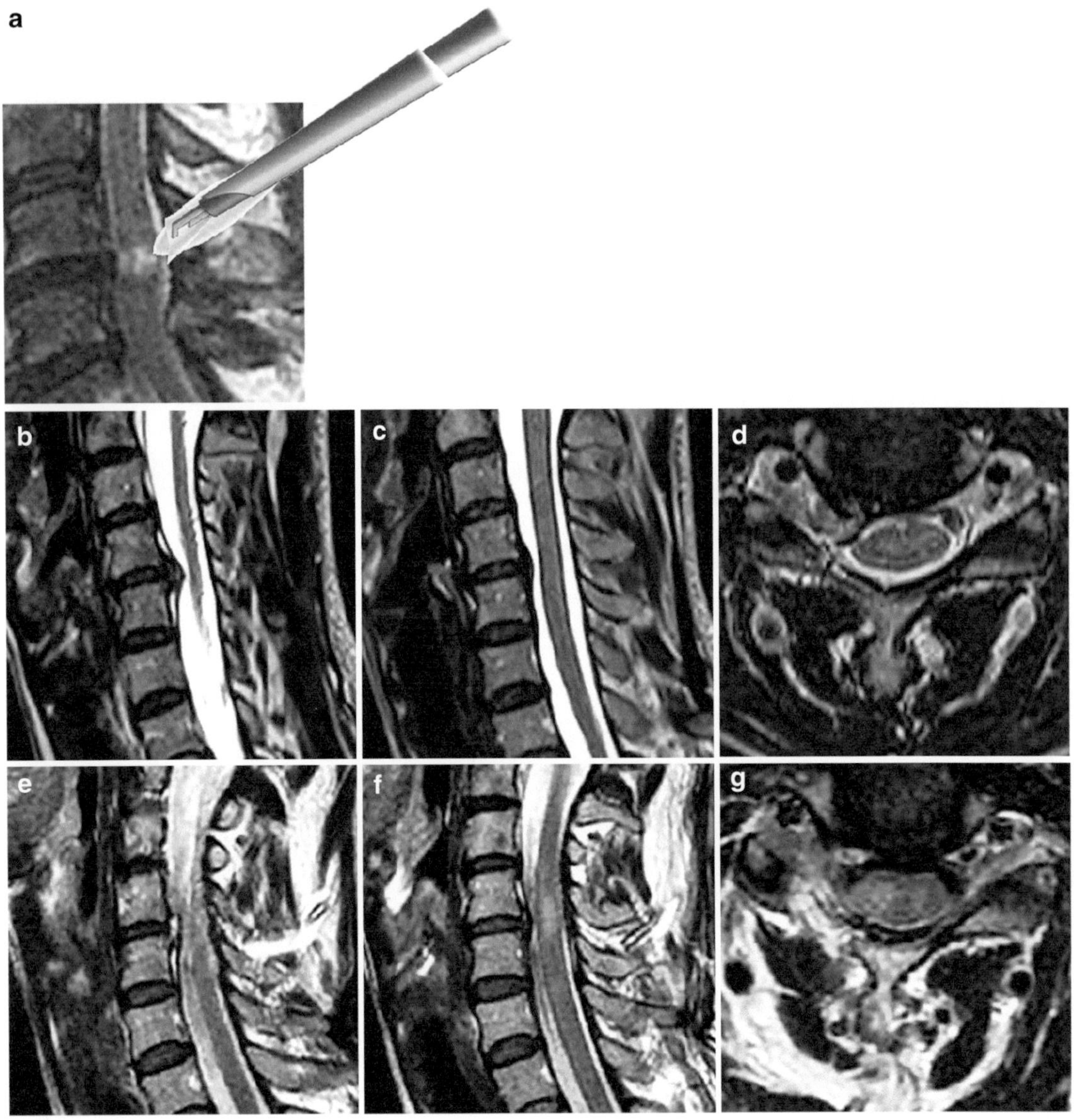

**Fig. 16** During full endoscopic cervical surgery, various surgical procedures must be performed by inserting various surgical instruments in the narrow surgical field near the spinal cord in a narrow endoscopic view, so be very careful not to injure the spinal cord. (**a**) Both punching and drilling can cause spinal cord injury, (**b–d**) and irrigation to secure the surgical field of view can also cause spinal cord injury if high pressure is applied to the spinal cord for a long time (**e–g**)

## 8 Discussion (Surgical Tips and Pitfall)

Cervical radiculopathy is a common cervical spine condition leading to significant disability from nerve root dysfunction. Conservative therapy is recommended for 6 weeks for cervical radiculopathy without myelopathy.

Full endoscopic cervical posterior decompression is becoming popular as a soft-tissue-conserving minimally invasive technique for cervical foraminal decompression and discectomy for a prolapsed intervertebral disc and foraminal stenosis. However, full endoscopic posterior cervical foraminotomy and discectomy may cause the neurological complications associated with the spinal cord and exiting nerve root retraction, and in most cases, it causes transient neurological symptoms, but in severe neural damage, severe uncontrollable radiculopathic pain, as well as paralysis with muscle atrophy, can occur. Also, incomplete decompression is a main cause of residual radicular pain; on the other hand, aggressive excess bone removal of cervical laminofacet area leads to instability due to failure of the facet joint.

Therefore, it is of utmost importance to safely decompress the nerve root during full endoscopic posterior cervical foraminotomy and discectomy. Endoscopic surgical technique of drilling 3–5 mm on the medial one-third of the pedicle and corpus ventral to the spinal cord and exiting nerve root could create space for efficient discectomy and uncus decompression without nerve root retraction and preserve the stability of the spinal segment.

The partial pediculotomy and partial vertebrectomy approach (PPPV) for posterior cervical foraminotomy and discectomy (PECF) is a useful technique for creating a space ventral to the neural elements and helping prevent the complications resulting from neural retraction using the endoscopic working channel.

## References


1. Henderson Charles M, Hennessy Robert G, ShueyHenry M, et al. Posterior-lateral foraminotomy as anexclusive operative technique for cervical radiculopathy: a review of 846 consecutively operated cases. Neurosurgery. 1983;13(5):504–12.
2. Krupp W, Schattke H, Mu¨ke R. Clinical results of the foraminotomy as described by Frykholm for thetreatment of lateral cervical disc herniation. Acta Neurochir. 1990;107(1–2):22–9.
3. Aldrich F. Posterolateral microdiscectomy for cervical monoradiculopathy caused by posterolateralsoft cervical disc sequestration. J Neurosurg. 1990;72(3):370–7.
4. Grieve JP, Kitchen ND, Moore AJ, et al. Results ofposterior cervical foraminotomy for treatment of cervical spondylitic radiculopathy. Br J Neurosurg. 2009;14(1):40–3.
5. Epstein NE. A review of complication rates foranterior cervical diskectomy and fusion (ACDF). Surg Neurol Int. 2019;10:100.
6. Selvanathan SK, Beagrie C, Thomson S, et al. Anterior cervical discectomy and fusion versusposterior cervical foraminotomy in the treatmentof brachialgia: the Leeds spinal unit experience(2008-2013). Acta Neurochir. 2015;157:1595–600.
7. Lee DG, Park CK, Lee DC. Clinical and radiological results of posterior cervical foraminotomy attwo or three levels: a 3-year follow-up. Acta Neurochir. 2017;159:2369–77.
8. Papavero L, Kothe R. Minimally invasive posterior-cervical foraminotomy for treatment of radiculopathy: an effective, time-tested, and costefficient motion-preservation technique. Oper Orthop Traumatol. 2018;30:36–45.
9. Spurling RG, Scoville WB. Lateral rupture of the cervical intervertebral disc: a common cause of shoulder and arm pain. Surg Gynecol Obstet. 1944;78:350–8.
10. Gala VC, O'Toole JE, Voyadzis JM, et al. Posterior minimally invasive approaches for the cervical spine. Orthop Clin North Am. 2007;38:339–49. [5] Fessler RG, Khoo LT. Minimally invasive cervical microendoscopicforaminotomy: an initial clinical experience. Neurosurgery2002;51(5 Suppl):S37–45
11. Siddiqui A, Yonemura KS. Posterior cervical microendoscopic diskectomy and laminoforaminotomy. In: Kim DH, Fessler RG, Regan JJ, editors. Endoscopic spine surgery and instrumentation: percutaneous procedures. New York, NY: Thieme; 2005. p. 66–73.
12. Adamson TE. Microendoscopic posterior cervical laminoforaminotomy for unilateral radiculopathy: results of a new technique in 100cases. J Neurosurg. 2001;95(1 Suppl):51–7.

13. Del Curto D, Kim JS, Lee SH. Minimally invasive posterior cervical microforaminotomy in the lower cervical spine and C-T junction assisted by O-arm-based navigation. Comput Aided Surg. 2013;18:76–83.
14. Kim JS, Eun SS, Prada N, et al. Modified transcorporeal anterior cervical microforaminotomy assisted by O-arm-based navigation: a technical case report. Eur Spine J. 2011;20(Suppl 2):S147–52.
15. Kim JY, Kim DH, Lee YJ, Jeon JB, Choi SY, Kim HS, Jang IT. Anatomical importance between neural structure and bony landmark: clinical importance for posterior endoscopic cervical Foraminotomy. Neurospine. 2021;18(1):139–46. https://doi.org/10.14245/ns.2040440.220.

# Uniportal Full Endoscopic Posterior Cervical Decompressive Laminectomy

Ji Yeon Kim, Dong Chan Lee, and Hyeun Sung Kim

**Abstract**

Endoscopic posterior cervical decompression obviates the need for extensor muscle dissection and disruption of the posterior spinous process–ligament–muscle complex and can prevent post-laminectomy kyphosis. With the development of the fine endoscopic diamond drill, safe bone drilling can be performed over the dura until the free end of the ligamentum flavum is exposed and the detached ligamentum flavum is removed without manipulation. Multiple pathologies in adjacent cervical levels can be treated with a single incision on the skin. Therefore, the uniportal endoscopic posterior cervical approach may have the advantage of minimal invasiveness compared to biportal endoscopic surgery or open minimally invasive surgery.

**Supplementary Information** The online version contains supplementary material available at https://doi.org/10.1007/978-981-99-1133-2_6.

J. Y. Kim · D. C. Lee (✉)
Department of Neurosurgery, Spine Center, Wiltse Memorial Hospital, Anyang, South Korea

H. S. Kim
Department of Neurosurgery, Spine Center, Nanoori Gangnam Hospital, Seoul, South Korea

**Keywords**

Endoscopy · Uniportal · Stenosis Laminectomy · Cervical

## 1 Advantages of the Uniportal Endoscopic Approach for Posterior Cervical Decompressive Laminectomy

Various minimally invasive surgical methods, such as selective laminectomy and microendoscopic laminoplasty, have been developed to preserve the cervical extensor muscles [1–3]. Endoscopic posterior cervical decompression obviates the need for extensor muscle dissection and disruption of the posterior spinous process–ligament–muscle complex and can prevent post-laminectomy kyphosis [4]. It does not require the sacrifice of a cervical motion segment, thereby reducing the need for additional fusion. Jian et al. [5] reported favorable clinical and radiological outcomes following full-endoscopic posterior cervical unilateral laminotomy for bilateral decompression (ULBD) to treat cervical canal stenosis.

Recently, Kim et al. [6] described the novel technique of biportal endoscopic ULBD with "circumferential drilling and en bloc removal" using optimized instruments to treat cervical spondylotic myelopathy.



H. S. Kim et al. (eds.), *Advanced Technique of Endoscopic Cervical and Thoracic Spine Surgery*,
https://doi.org/10.1007/978-981-99-1133-2_6

Uniportal endoscopic spine surgery has limitations in using various instruments compared to biportal endoscopic surgery. However, with the development of the fine endoscopic diamond drill, we can perform delicate bone drilling over the dura without additional pressure to the spinal cord and remove the ligamentum flavum as the final surgical step to avoid spinal cord injury due to early dural exposure. Furthermore, with canal decompression, symptomatic foraminal stenosis can be decompressed simultaneously [7], and multiple pathologies at adjacent levels can be treated by creating only a single incision on the skin In this context, the uniportal endoscopic posterior cervical approach may have the advantage of minimal invasiveness compared to biportal endoscopic surgery or open minimally invasive surgery.

## 2 Indications and Contraindications

Uniportal endoscopic ULBD can be considered for selective patients with one or two levels of cervical stenosis.

- Indications
  1. Cervical canal stenosis due to hypertrophied ligamentum flavum with or without myelopathy.
  2. Cervical canal stenosis with concomitant foraminal stenosis or foraminal disc herniation.
  3. Cervical canal stenosis with ossification of the posterior longitudinal ligament (OPLL) in less than 50% of the spinal canal.
- Relative contraindications
  1. Multiple-level cervical canal stenosis involving more than three levels.
  2. Cervical canal stenosis with central disc herniation.
  3. Higher cervical level above the C3–4.
- Contraindications
  1. Cervical canal stenosis with segmental instability.
  2. Cervical canal stenosis with OPLL involving more than 50% of the spinal canal.
  3. Cervical canal stenosis with prominent central disc herniation.
  4. Cervical canal stenosis with prominent ossification of the ligamentum flavum (OLF).
  5. Severe cervical canal stenosis that has higher chance of cervical cord injury.

In cases of contraindication, conventional anterior cervical discectomy and fusion (ACDF) or posterior cervical surgery, such as laminoplasty or laminectomy, can be considered instead of the posterior endoscopic approach. ACDF can be proposed when a herniated disc causes persistent pain or symptomatic segmental instability following posterior endoscopic decompression.

## 3 Anesthesia and Position

The patient underwent surgery under general anesthesia in the prone position on a radiolucent Wilson frame for posterior surgery equipped with a chest bar. A compression-free sponge device was placed under the patient's face, and the neck was slightly flexed. A slightly flexed neck position was maintained using a skin tape and without skull fixation. This is also the surgical position recommended for posterior endoscopic cervical foraminotomy and discectomy.

## 4 Special Instruments

Endoscopic decompression surgery utilizes an endoscopic system with the 30° viewing angle, 7.3-mm outer diameter, 251-mm-length endoscope or an interlaminar endoscopic system with the 12° viewing angle, an 8.4 mm outer diameter, 120-mm-long endoscope (Fig. 1a, b).

A compressed spinal cord is vulnerable and may be injured upon slight pressure by the instruments. The 3.5-mm and 3.0-mm endoscopic diamond drills are essential for safe laminar drilling to expose the free end of the ligament flavum (Fig. 1c, d).

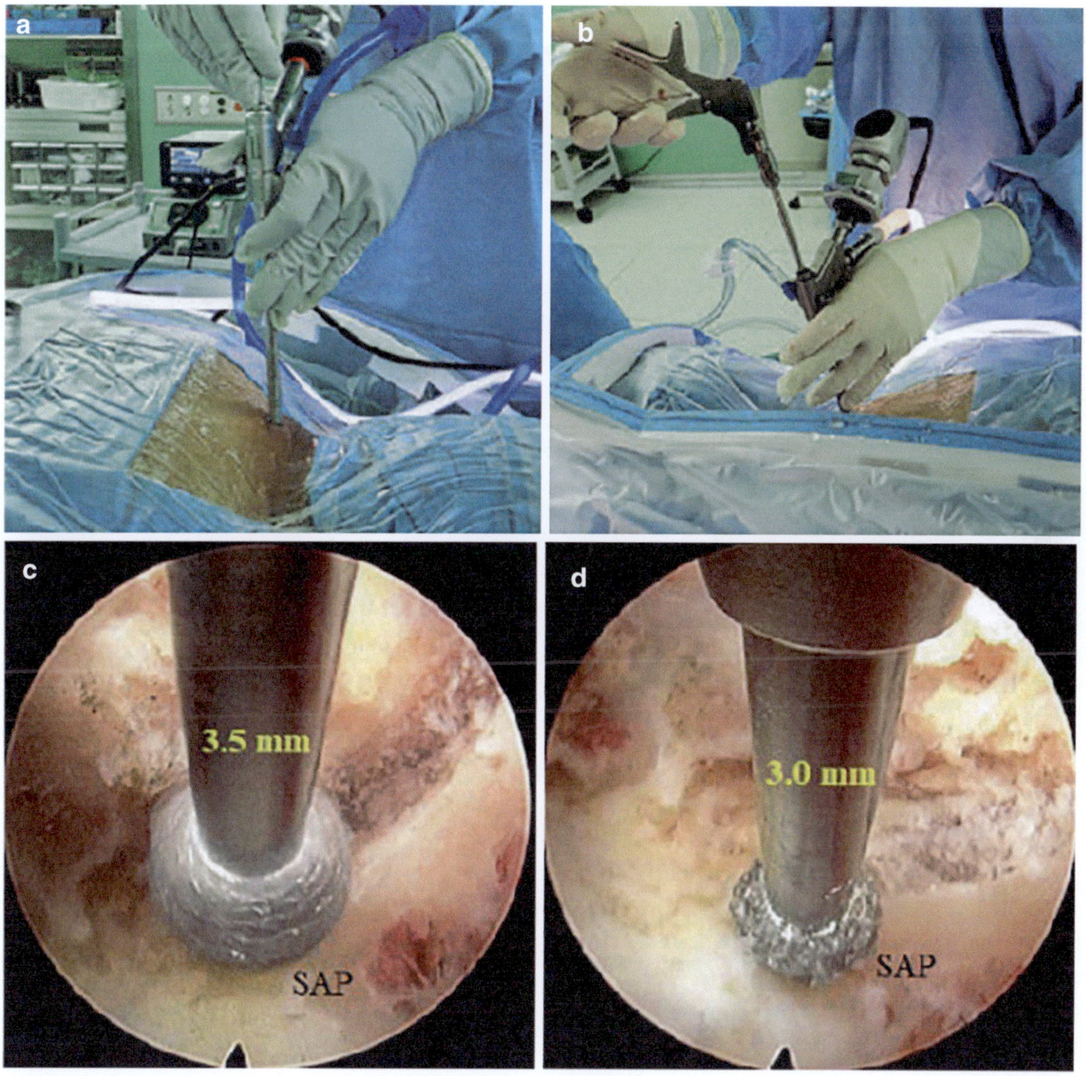


**Fig. 1** Surgical equipment. (**a**) A small diameter endoscopic system with 30° viewing angle, 7.3-mm outer diameter, and 251-mm-length. (**b**) An interlaminar endoscopic system with the 12° viewing angle, an 8.4-mm outer diameter, and 120-mm-long. Endoscopic diamond drills. (**c**) 3.5-mm diameter. (**d**) 3.0-mm diameter. A 3.0-mm diamond drill offers more delicate bone drilling overlying the dura and ligamentum flavum, especially at the tip of the superior articular process (SAP). IAP: inferior articular process

## 5 Surgical Steps of the Uniportal Endoscopic Posterior Cervical Approach for Bilateral Canal Stenosis

The surgical procedure is elaborated with an illustrated case of a left-sided approach for C5–6 ULBD (Fig. 2).

### 5.1 Making the Skin Entry and Inserting the Working Cannula

Under image intensification, fluoroscopic confirmation of the level was performed with the insertion of spinal needles in the target area. We usually make skin incision on the uncovertebral

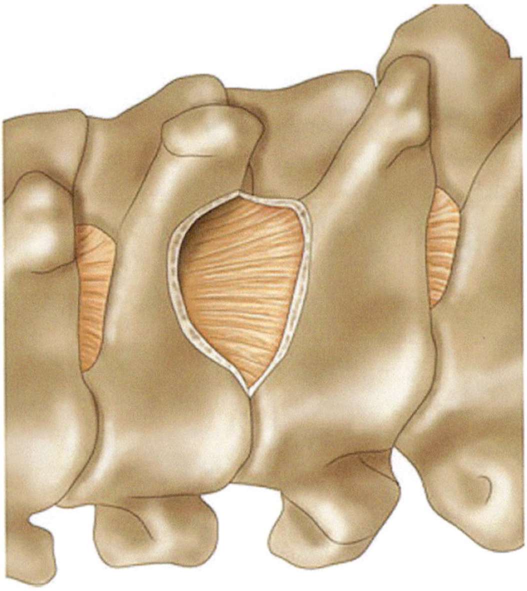

**Fig. 2** Illustration of uniportal endoscopic unilateral laminotomy for bilateral decompression at the C5–6 level through the left-sided approach to treat cervical canal stenosis

joint line for posterior endoscopic cervical foraminotomy (Fig. 3a). However, skin incision should be created on the medial pedicle line to perform bilateral decompression more safely while avoiding spinal cord injury by accessing the instruments on the contralateral side with a shallow angle (Fig. 3b). Medially moved skin entry points offer the inclinatory surgical route by undercutting the facet joint during foraminotomy in the case of combined foraminal stenosis (Fig. 3b). As shown on the lateral X-ray images, skin incision was made on the plane of the involved intervertebral disc for single-level decompression (Fig. 3c) and created on the pedicle line between the two adjacent targeted lesions (Fig. 3d). A longitudinal linear skin incision of approximately 1 cm, parallel to the muscle fiber, is critical for free movement of the endoscopic system. Serial dilators were inserted through the skin incision site, and a working cannula was inserted along the serial dilator.

## 5.2 Soft Tissue Dissection to Expose the Targeted Lamina and Interlaminar Window (Video 1)

Incidental instrument insertion into the interlaminar area before clear identification can cause penetration of the ligamentum flavum and spinal cord injury. Therefore, the working cannula should be docked on bony structures, such as the facet joint or adjacent lamina, instead of the interlaminar window. The position of the needle, serial dilators, and working cannula should be confirmed using intraoperative radiography. We exposed the whole part of the targeted laminas and interlaminar window before bone drilling using a radiofrequency (RF) probe (Fig. 4a).

## 5.3 Partial Laminotomy Along the Caudal Border of the Upper-Level Lamina (Video 2)

A partial laminotomy was performed along the inferior border of the upper-level (C5) lamina using a fine endoscopic drill until the proximal free margin of the ligamentum flavum was exposed (Fig. 4b–e). Drilling of the midline part of the lamina (C5) facilitated easy access to the contralateral side of the interlaminar area (Fig. 4d, e). Subsequently, the laminotomy was extended to the medial border of the contralateral facet joint (Fig. 4f).

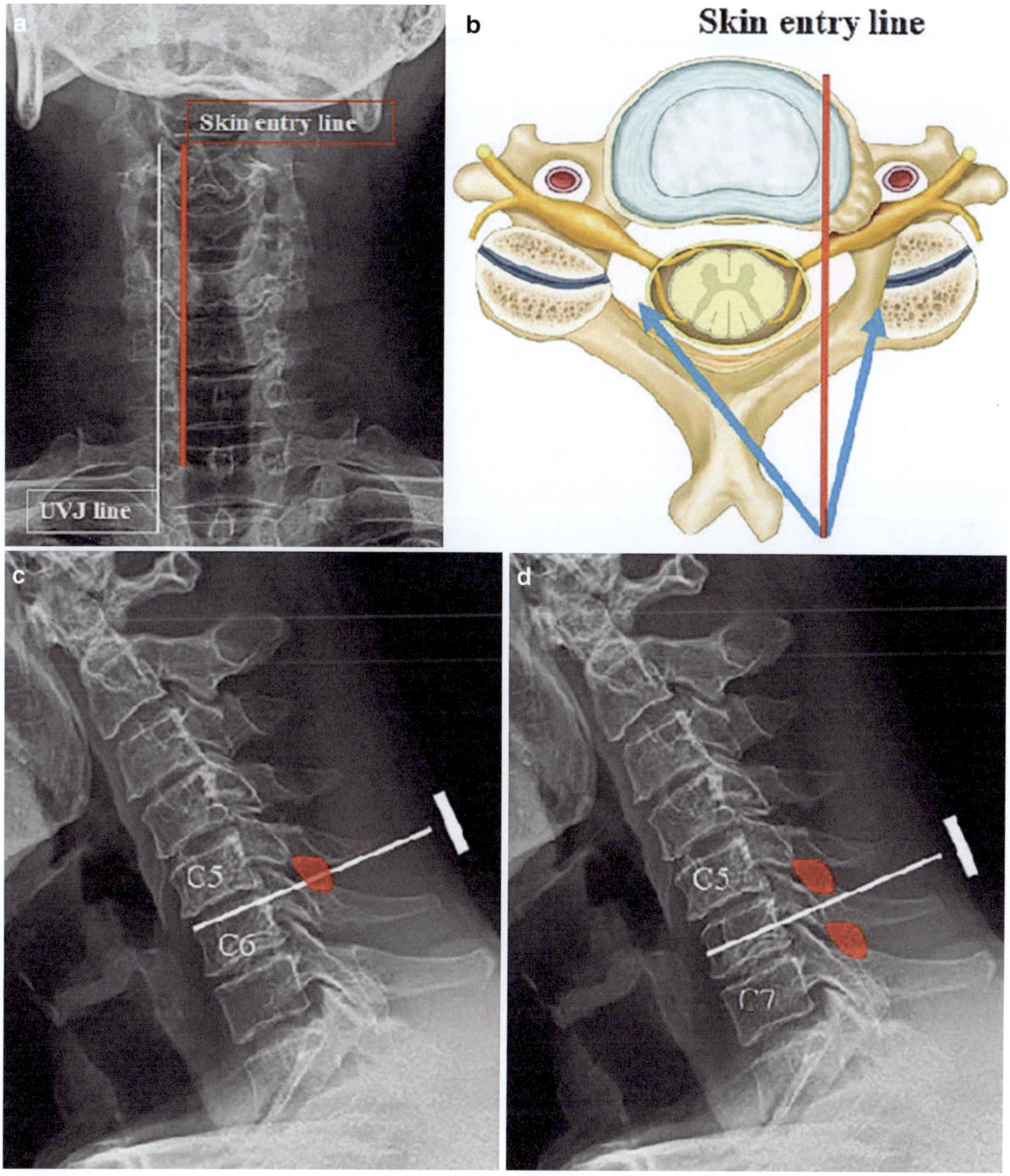


**Fig. 3** Skin entry points of uniportal endoscopic posterior cervical approach for canal decompression and foraminotomy. (**a**, **b**) Skin entry should be made on the medial pedicular line (bold red line) instead of the uncovertebral joint (UVJ) line (white line). Skin entry points for single-level decompression (**c**) and adjacent levels operation (**d**) are displayed on the lateral X-ray images (red circular areas: target lesions for decompression)

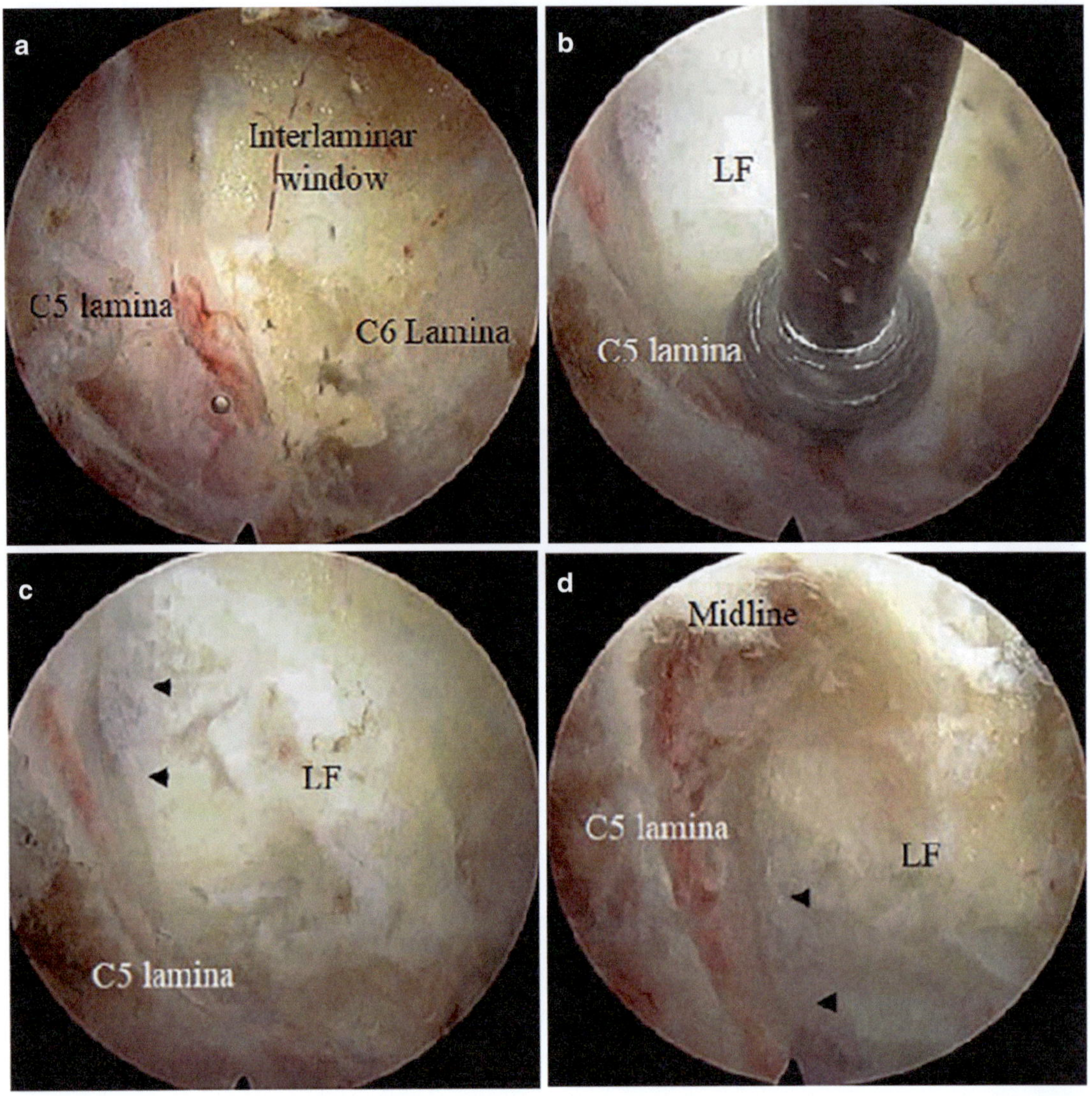


**Fig. 4** Intraoperative endoscopic view of the posterior cervical unilateral laminotomy for bilateral decompression at the C5–6 level of the left-sided approach. (**a**) Adjacent lamia and interlaminar window were exposed after soft tissue dissection. (**b–d**) Ipsilateral laminotomy of the upper-level lamina (black arrowheads: proximal end of the ligamentum flavum (LF). (**d**) Midline lamina blocked the endoscopic view, so the contralateral side cannot be seen. (**e**, **f**) Contralateral sublaminar space was exposed after drilling the midline lamina. (**g**) Ipsilateral laminotomy of the lower-level lamina. (**h**) The contralateral medial border of the superior articular process (SAP) should be drilled for successful neural decompression (white dotted line: contour of the SAP). (**i–l**) The boundary of the circumferential laminotomy was confirmed (white flower marks: contralateral facet joint space). (**m**) The ligamentum flavum was detached from the bony margin. (**n**) Careful epidural dissection was performed. (**o**, **p**) Additional removing of the ligamentum flavum at the contralateral corner of the interlaminar window. (**q**) A completely decompressed dural sac was confirmed after removing the hypertrophied ligamentum flavum. *LF* ligamentum flavum, *SAP* superior articular process, *IAP* inferior articular process

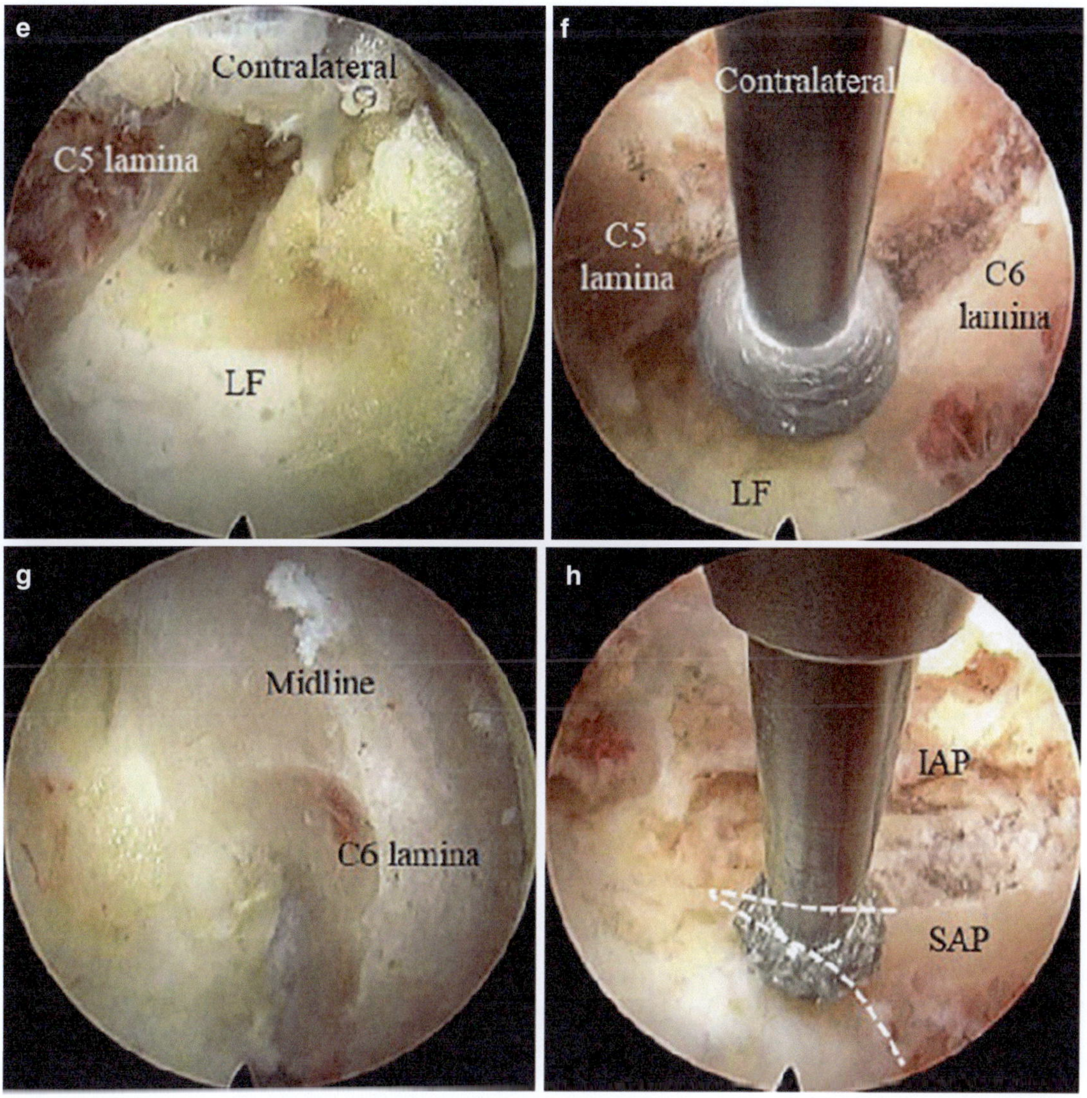


**Fig. 4** (continued)

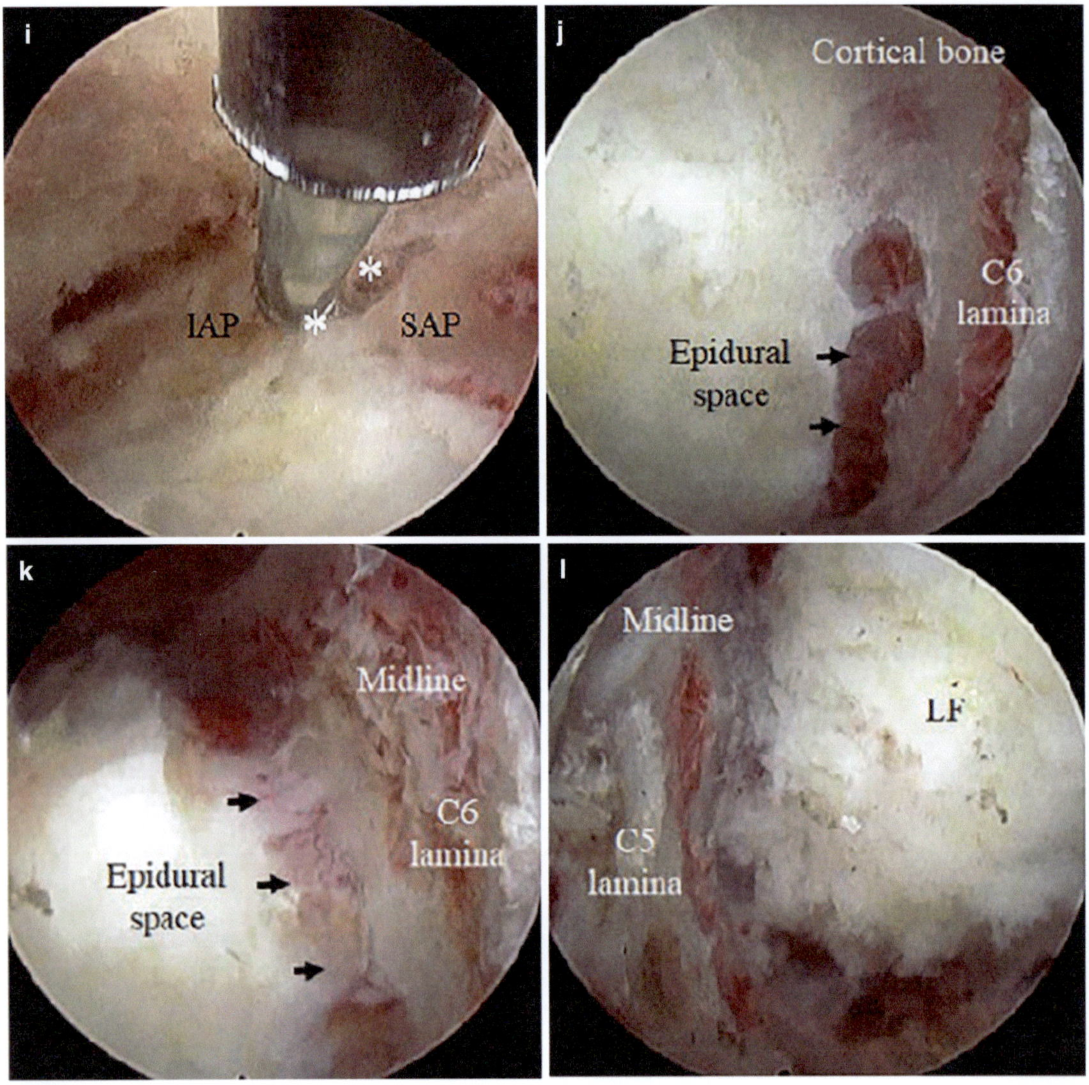


**Fig. 4** (continued)

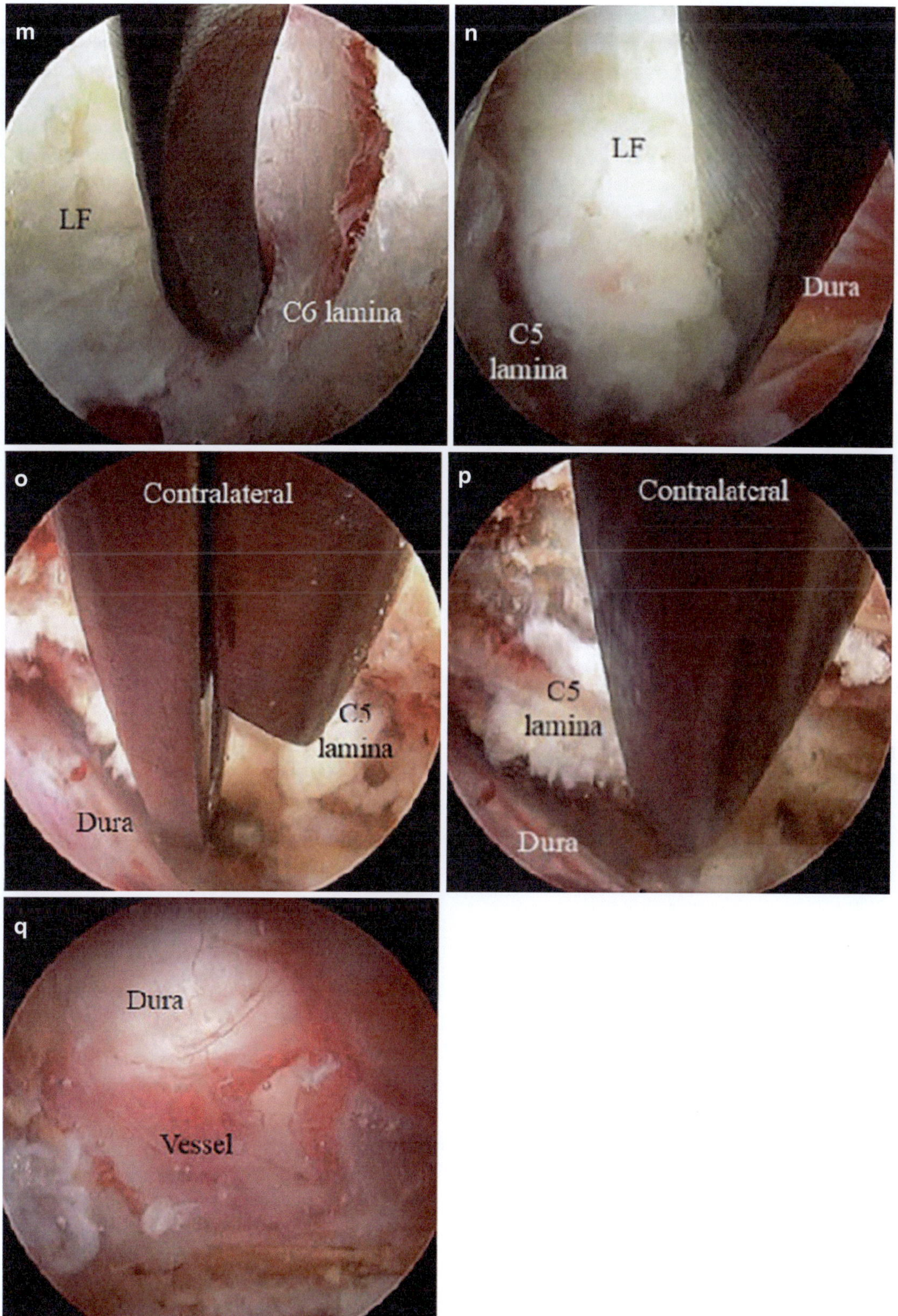


**Fig. 4** (continued)

### 5.4 Partial Laminotomy Along the Cranial Border of the Lower-Level Lamina (Video 3)

A partial laminotomy was performed along the superior border of the lower-level (C6) lamina using an endoscopic diamond drill until the bilateral distal free margin of the ligamentum flavum was confirmed (Fig. 4g, h). A 3.0-mm endoscopic drill enhanced delicate bony drilling in the contralateral corner (Fig. 4h). The contralateral end point of the drilling was the medial tip of the superior articular process (SAP) (Fig. 4i).

### 5.5 Detachment and Removing of Hypertrophied Ligamentum Flavum (Video 4)

After confirming the laminotomy area, the remaining inner cortical bone was further drilled, until it resembled thin paper, and proximal and distal free margins of the ligamentum flavum were separated from the bony margin (Figs. 4j–l). Subsequently, the ligamentum flavum was detached from the laminotomy sites, and epidural dissection was performed simultaneously using a fine dissector (Fig. 4m, n). The secured ligamentum flavum was removed using endoscopic forceps, and the remaining part at the contralateral corner was removed using a 1.0-mm endoscopic punch without manipulating the dura (Fig. 4o, p). The dura was sufficiently expanded, and free dural pulsation was confirmed (Fig. 4q). Diffuse epidural bleeding was controlled using a hemostatic agent rather than a radiofrequency (RF) probe. A drainage catheter was inserted to prevent postoperative epidural hematoma.

### 5.6 Essential Surgical Steps to Access the Contralateral Area

The midline part of the lamina blocked the endoscopic view, so we were not able to visualize the contralateral sublaminar space (Fig. 5a, c). Therefore, sufficient bony drilling is essential to access the contralateral sublaminar area (Fig. 5b, d, e).

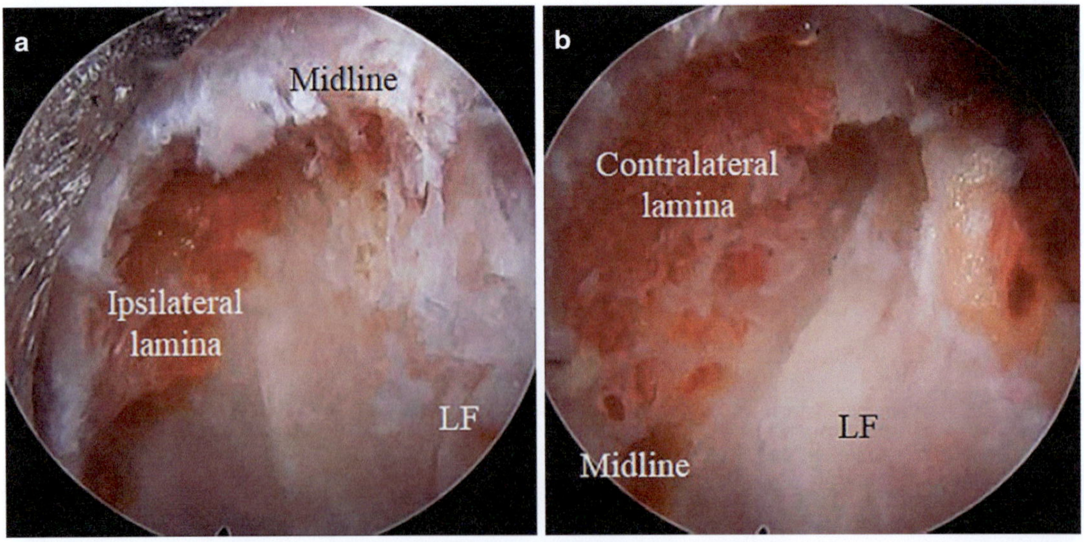


**Fig. 5** Critical steps of midline laminar drilling to access the contralateral area. (**a**) Midline part of the upper-level lamina blocked the endoscopic view. (**b**) The contralateral sublaminar area was exposed after midline drilling. (**c**) The midline part of the lower-level lamina cut off the vision to the contralateral area. (**d**) The contralateral area, including the medial facet joint border, was confirmed after midline drilling. (**e**) The extent of midline laminar drilling to complete the contralateral canal decompression. *LF* ligamentum flavum

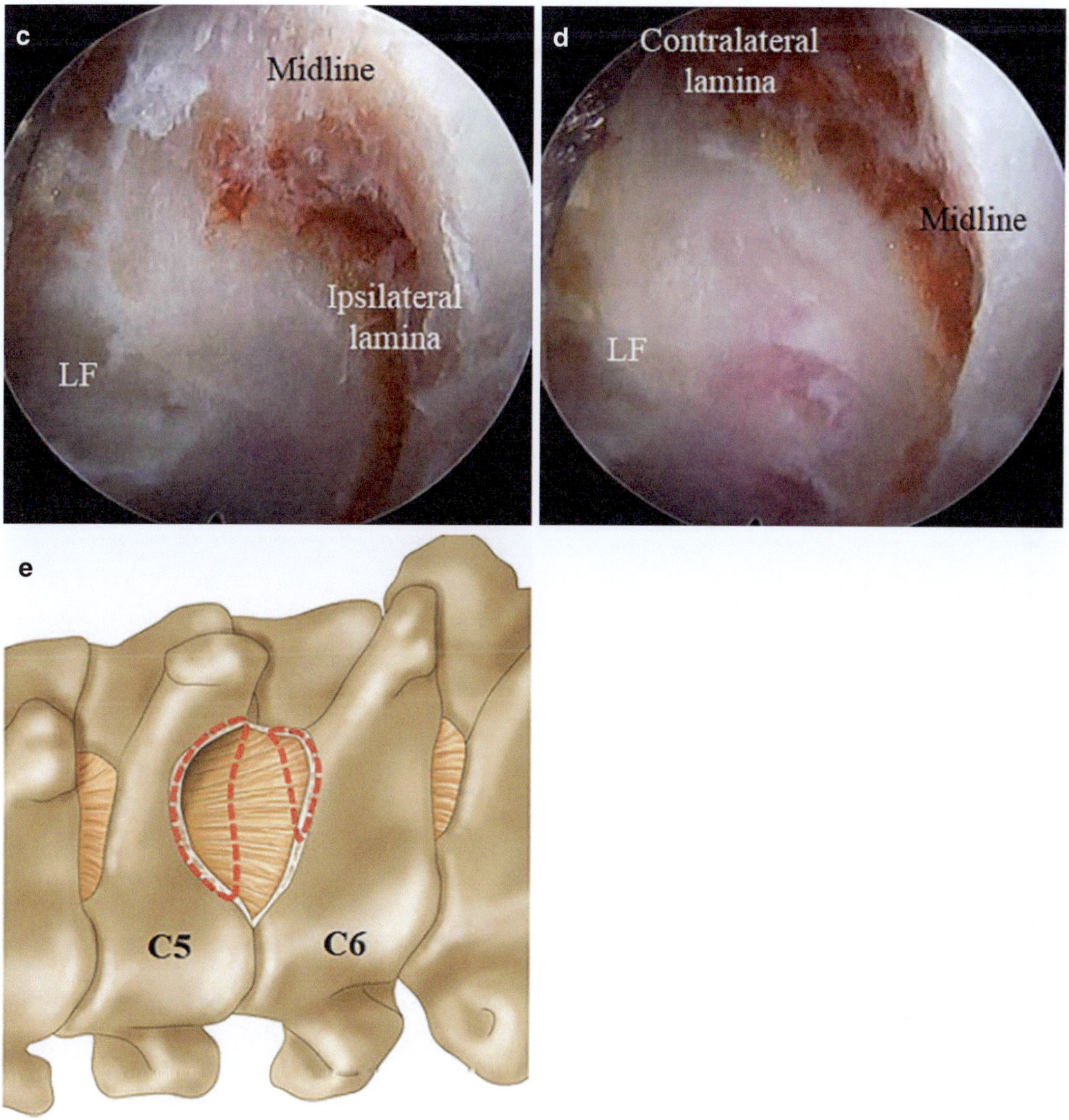


**Fig. 5** (continued)

## 6 Surgical Steps for Combined Pathologies of the Cervical Canal and Foraminal Stenosis (Videos 5 and 6)

In the illustrated case, the patient had bilateral canal stenosis at the C5–6 level and unilateral canal stenosis with foraminal stenosis on the left side of the C6–7 level (Fig. 6). We performed uniportal endoscopic ULBD at the C5–6 level and unilateral decompression with foraminotomy at the C6–7 level. One skin entry was created on the C6 pedicle line for two-level decompression surgery (Fig. 3d).

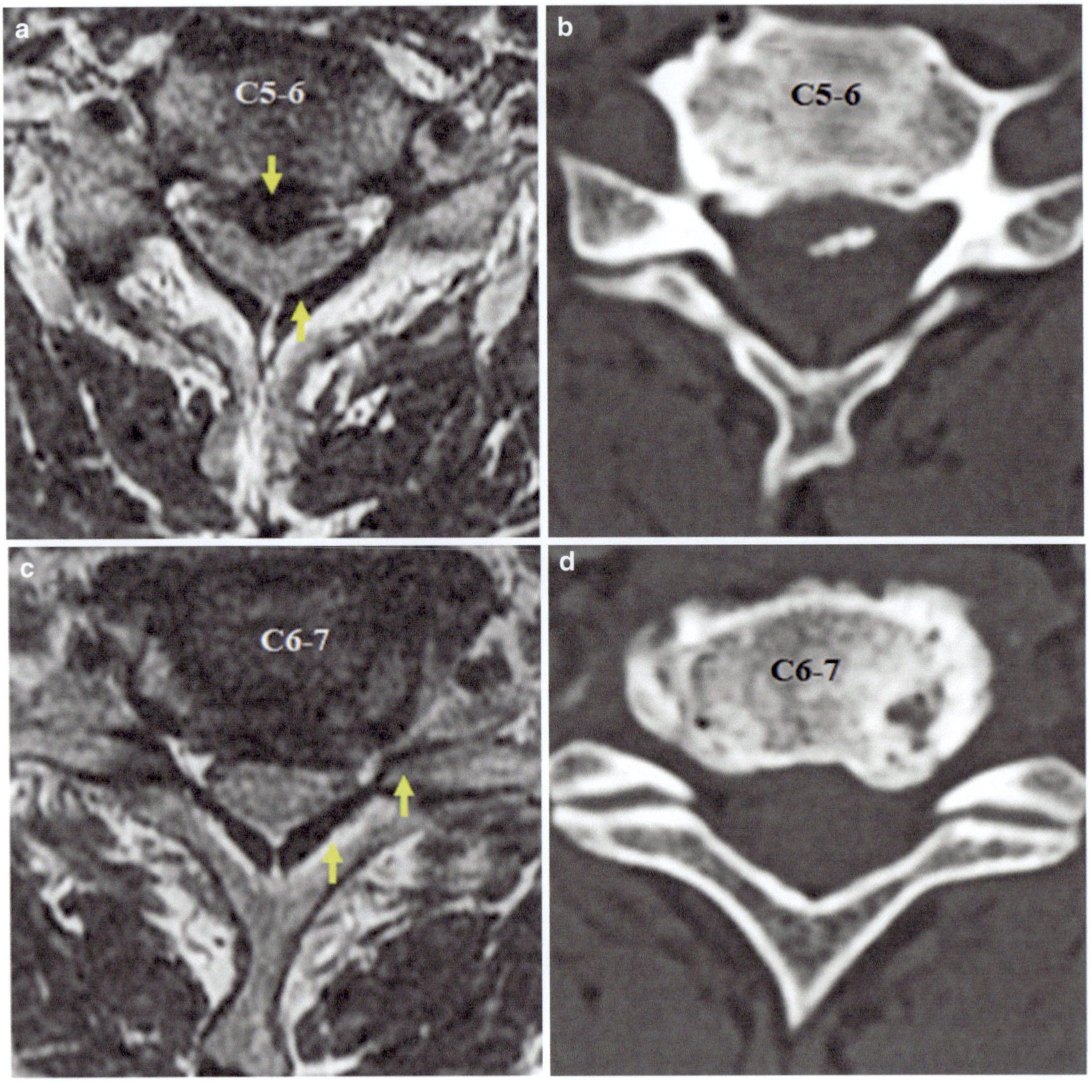


**Fig. 6** A case of symptomatic cervical canal stenosis with foraminal stenosis in the two adjacent cervical levels. (**a**, **b**) Bilateral canal stenosis with calcified central herniated disc at the C5–6 level. (**c**, **d**) Left unilateral canal stenosis with foraminal stenosis at the C6–7 level. (**e**) Prominent calcified disc and hypertrophied ligamentum flavum compressing the spinal cord at the C5–6 level. Yellow arrows indicate the lesions

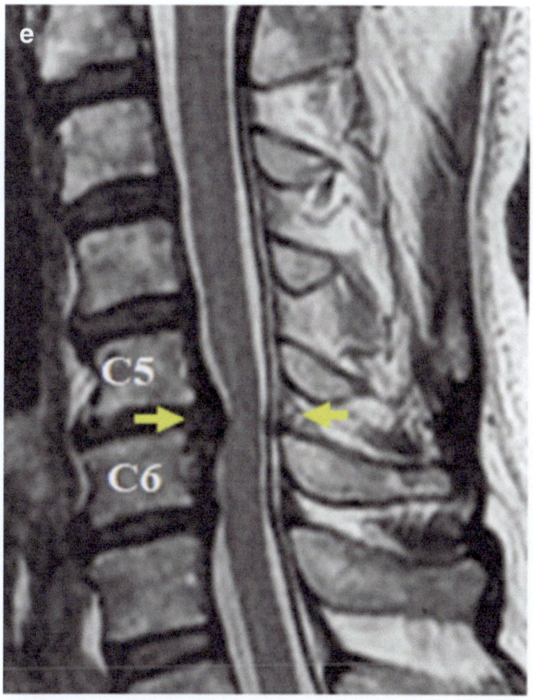


**Fig. 6** (continued)

## 7 Left Uniportal Endoscopic Posterior Cervical Approach for ULBD at the C5–6 Level (Video 5)

The same procedures were performed as elaborated above (Fig. 7).

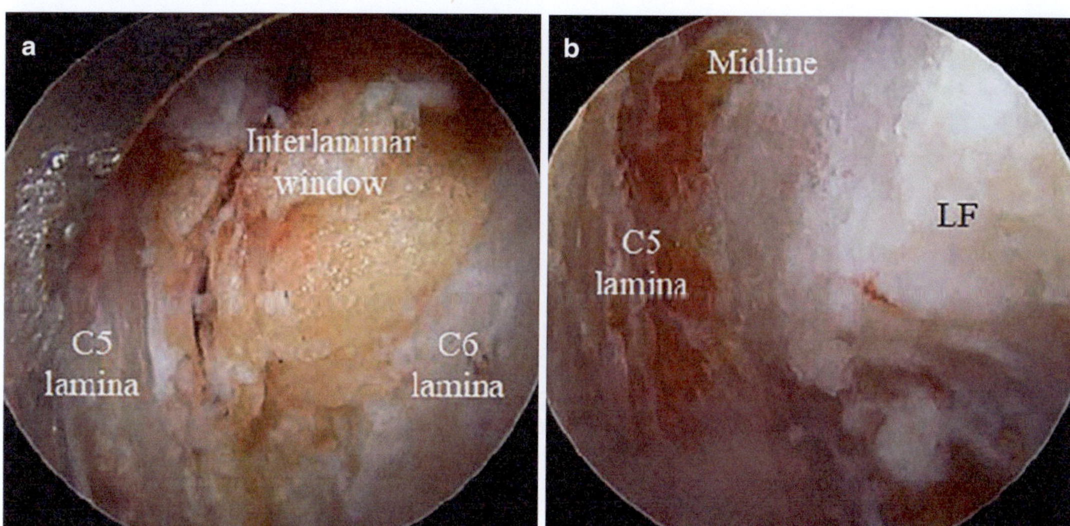


**Fig. 7** Surgical steps and postoperative images of the endoscopic posterior cervical unilateral laminotomy for bilateral decompression at the C5–6 level of the left-sided approach. (**a**–**c**) Partial laminotomy along the inferior border of the upper-level lamina. (**d**–**f**) Partial laminotomy along the superior border of the lower-level lamina (white flower mark: the tip of SAP). (**g**, **h**) Detachment of the ligamentum flavum. (**i**, **j**) Removing the ligamentum flavum using forceps. (**k**) Complete neural decompression is confirmed. (**l**, **n**) Bilateral canal stenosis was successfully resolved (red arrow). (**m**) Contralateral sublaminar drilling was extended to the contralateral superior articular process (*) while preserving the spinous process and contralateral lamina (yellow dotted line: the surgical route of sublaminar drilling)

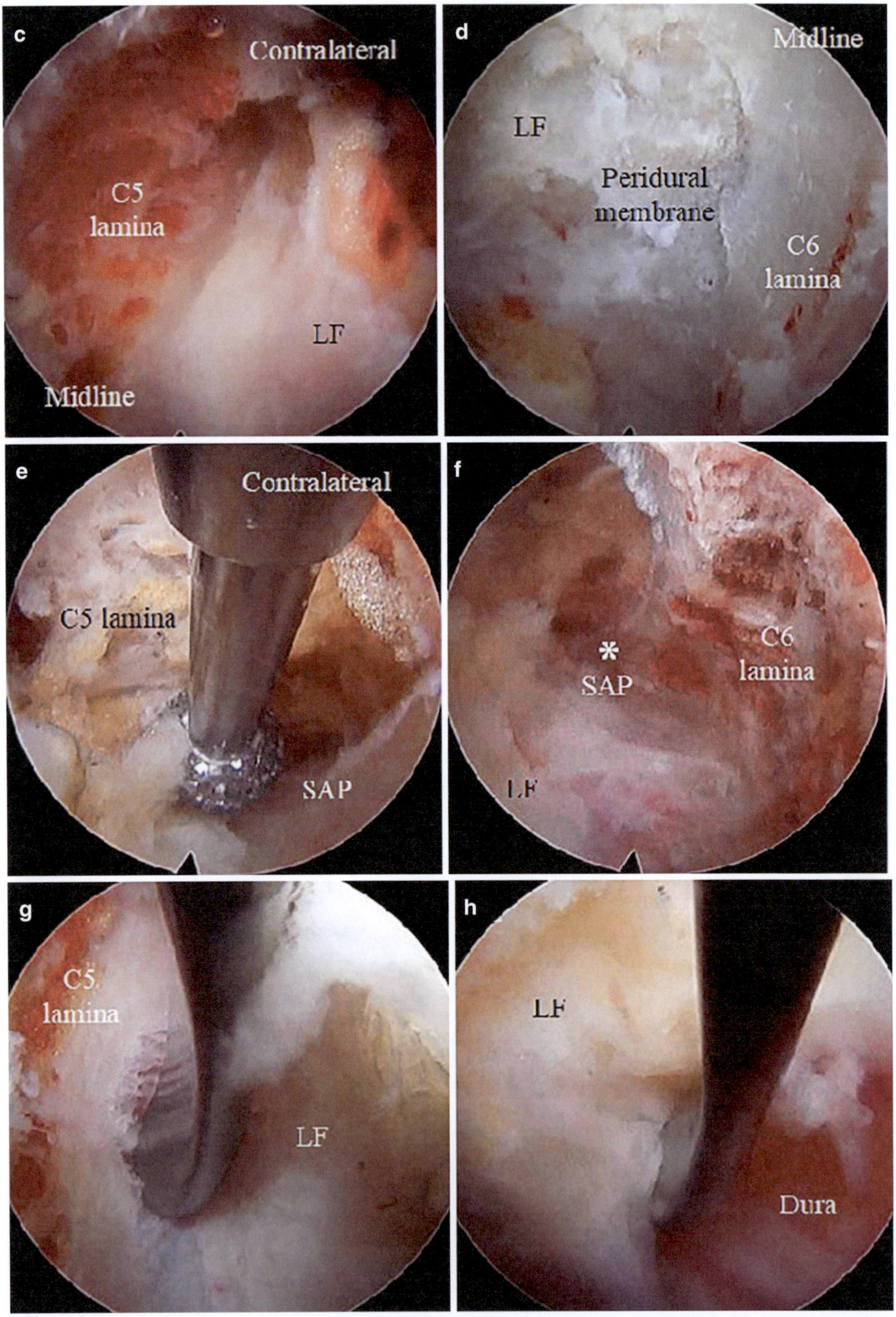


**Fig. 7** (continued)

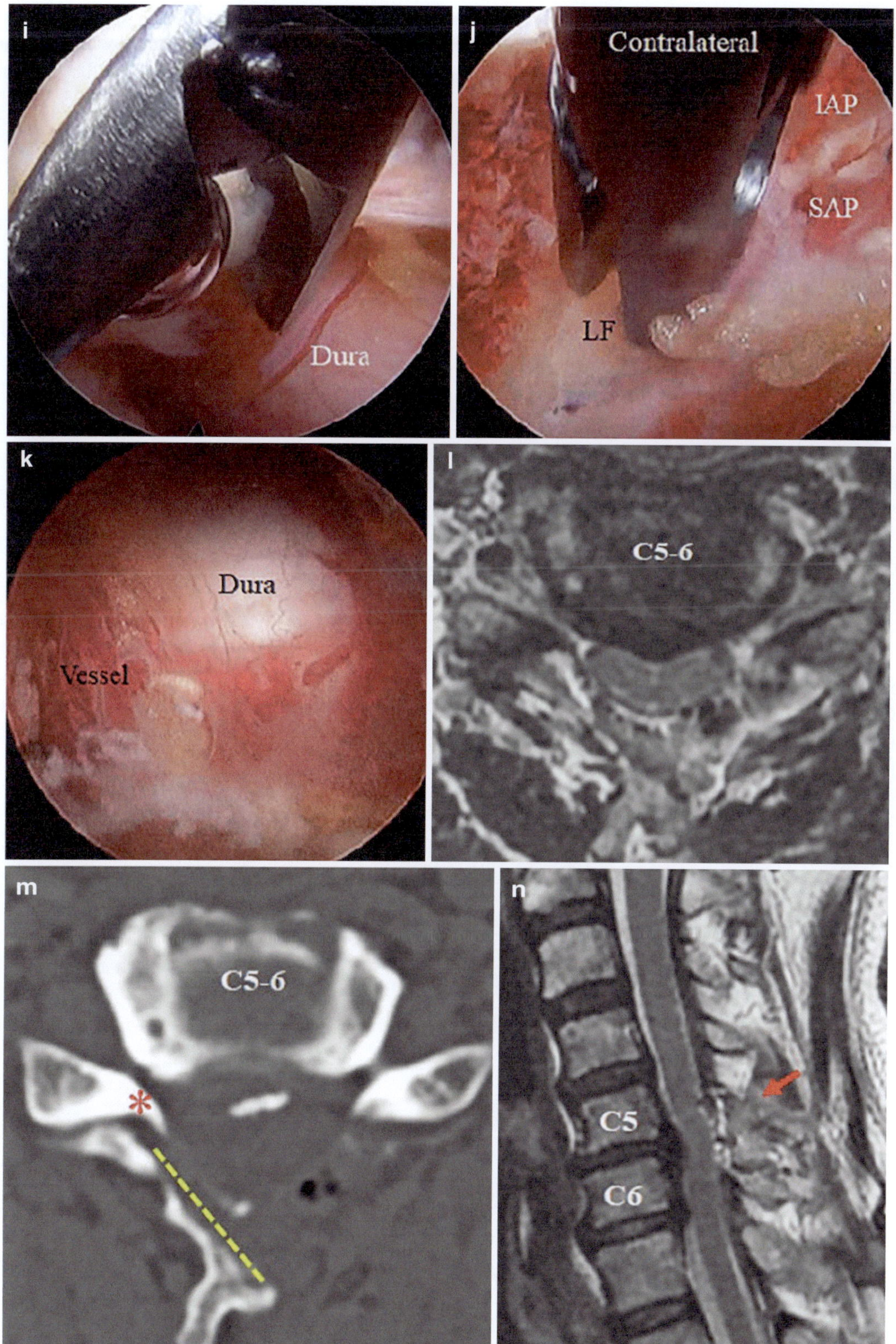


**Fig. 7** (continued)

## 8 Left Uniportal Endoscopic Posterior Cervical Approach for Unilateral Canal Decompression and Foraminotomy at the C6–7 Level

### 8.1 Ipsilateral Laminotomy to Free the Hypertrophied Ligamentum Flavum (Video 6)

Ipsilateral laminotomy was performed along the inferior border of the upper-level (C6) lamina (Fig. 8a, b) and the superior border of the lower-level (C7) lamina (Fig. 8c, d) using a fine endoscopic drill until the proximal and distal free margin of the ligamentum flavum was exposed.

### 8.2 Foraminotomy to Remove the Bony Spur and Herniated Disc (Video 6)

Hypertrophied SAP was thinned using an endoscopic drill and removed with a 1.0-mm endoscopic punch (Fig. 8e, f). After detaching the ligamentum flavum from the medial border of the facet joint (Fig. 8g), foraminal discectomy and bony spur drilling were performed while protecting the nerve root using a bevel of the working cannula (Fig. 8h, i).

### 8.3 Removal of the Hypertrophied Ligamentum Flavum (Video 6)

Subsequently, the detached ligamentum flavum was removed using fine forceps and punches (Fig. 8j). The adjacent laminotomy area in the C5–6 level was found, and the remaining ligamentum flavum was removed (Fig. 8k). Finally, sufficiently expanded dura and decompressed nerve roots were confirmed (Fig. 8l, m, n).

### 8.4 Extent of Bony Removal

We described the boundary of bony removal using the 3D spine model (Fig. 9a). Furthermore, we confirmed the extent of the laminotomy and foraminotomy area of adjacent operating levels during the follow-up period using postoperative 3D spine computed tomography (CT) (Fig. 9b).

**Fig. 8** Surgical steps and postoperative images of the endoscopic posterior cervical unilateral laminotomy and foraminotomy at the C6–7 level. (**a–d**) Ipsilateral circumferential laminotomy was performed using the endoscopic drill. (**e–i**) Foraminotomy and foraminal discectomy were successfully undergone. (**j–l**) Detached LF was removed, and sufficient neural decompression was confirmed (*: upper-level laminotomy area, *: bony spur removed space). (**m, n**) Postoperative images show a well-decompressed spinal canal and foraminal area

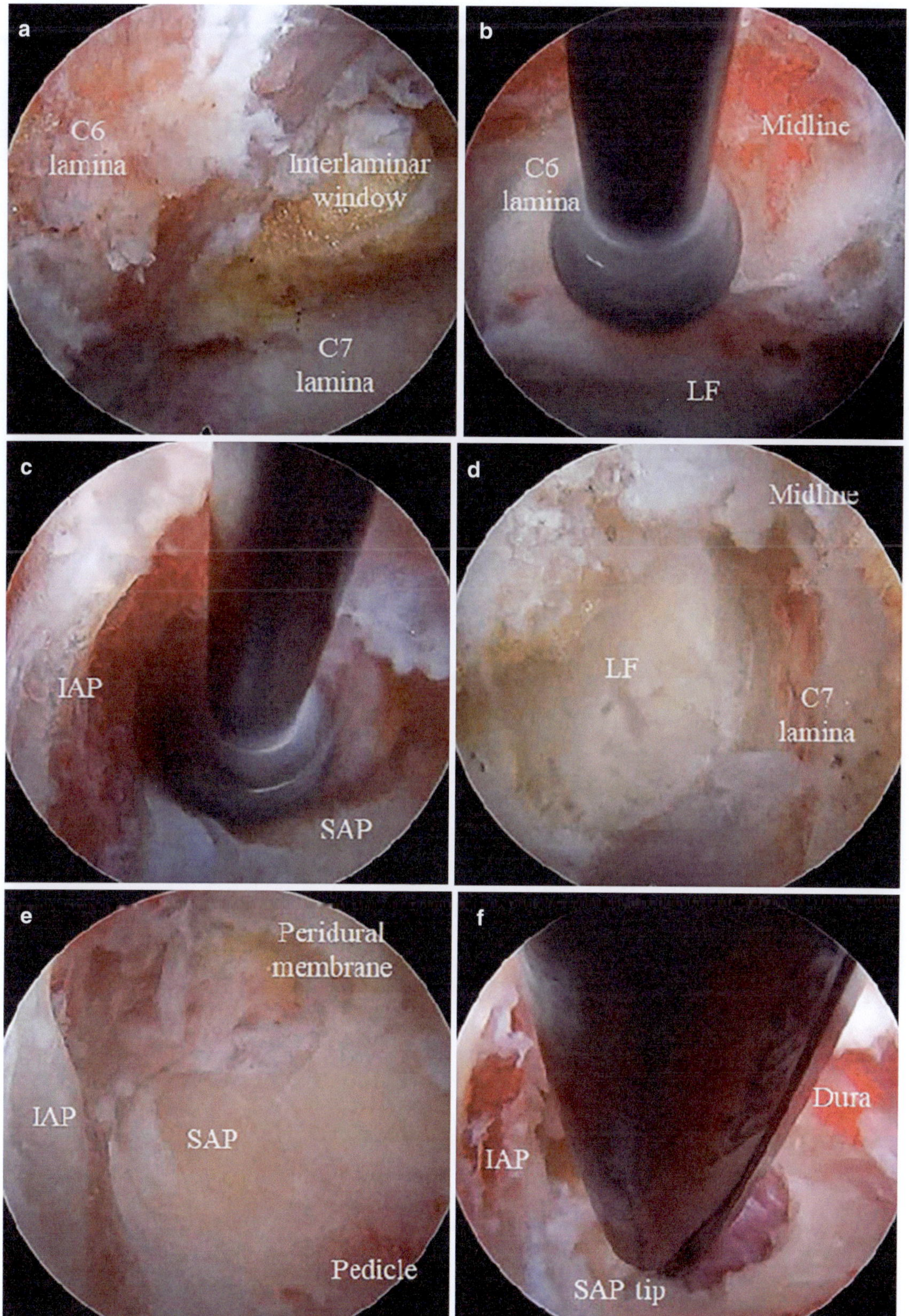
a
C6
lamina
Interlaminar
window
C7
lamina
b
C6
lamina
Midline
LF
c
IAP
SAP
d
Midline
LF
C7
lamina
e
Peridural
membrane
IAP
SAP
Pedicle
f
Dura
IAP
SAP tip

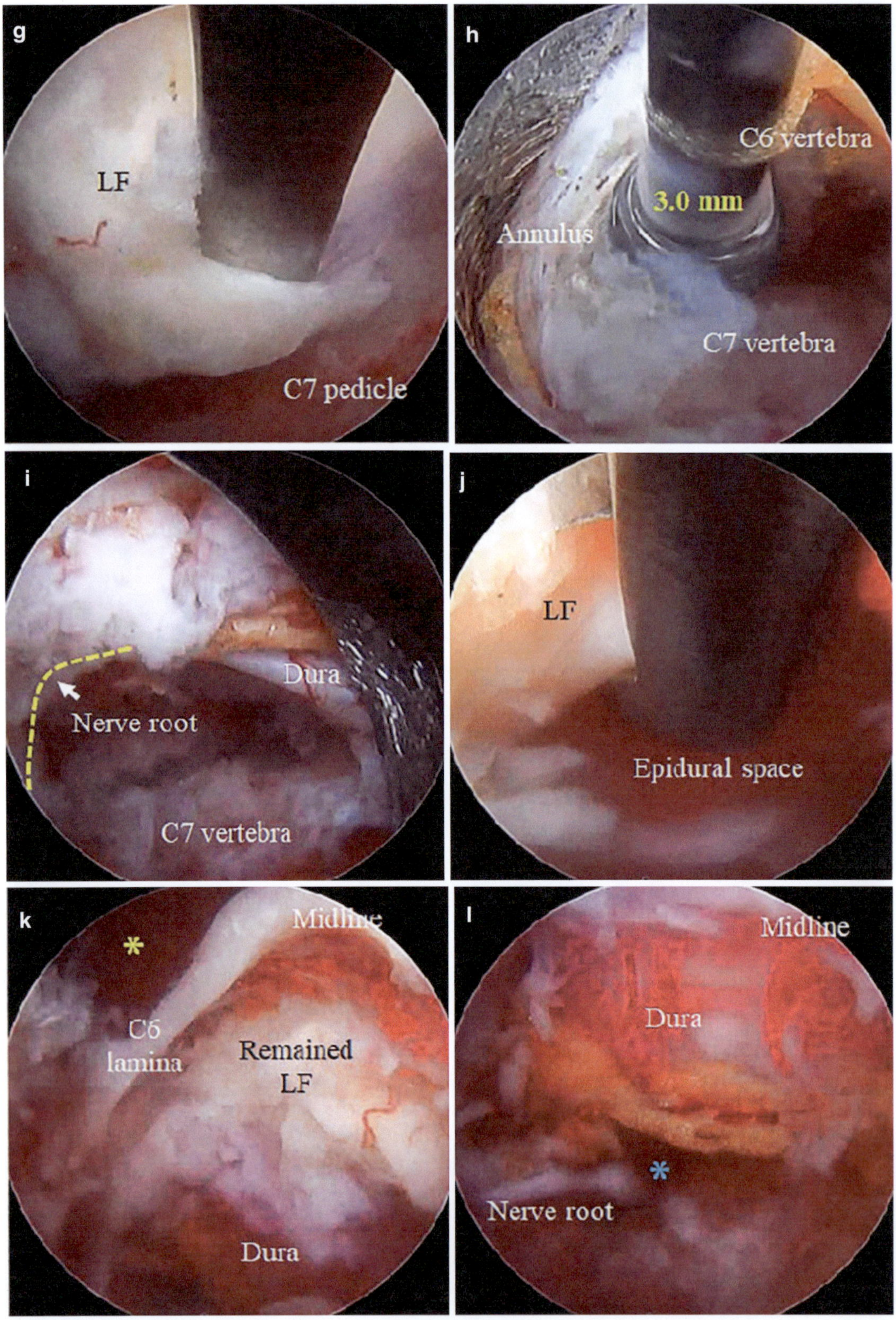


**Fig. 8** (continued)

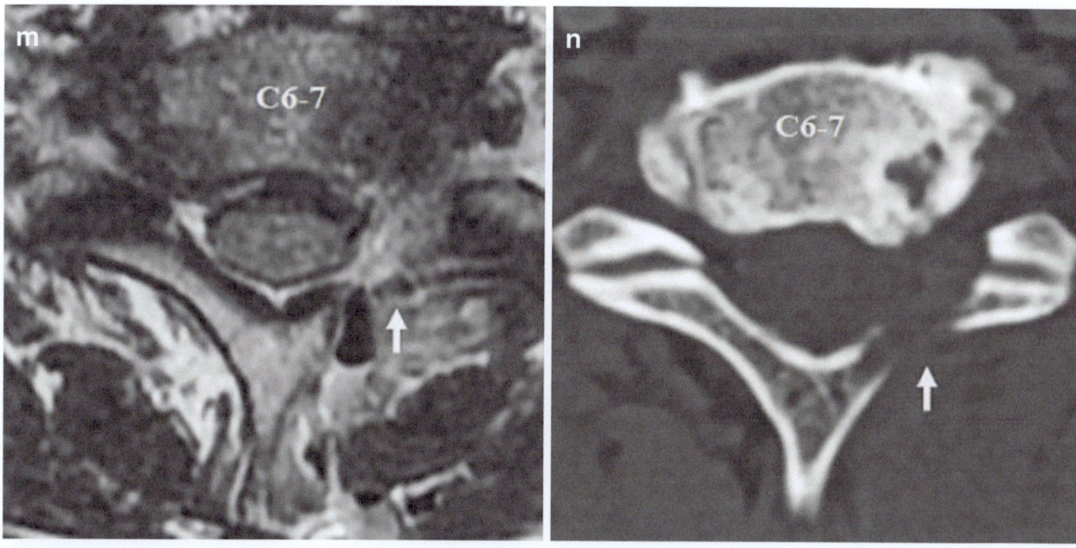


**Fig. 8** (continued)

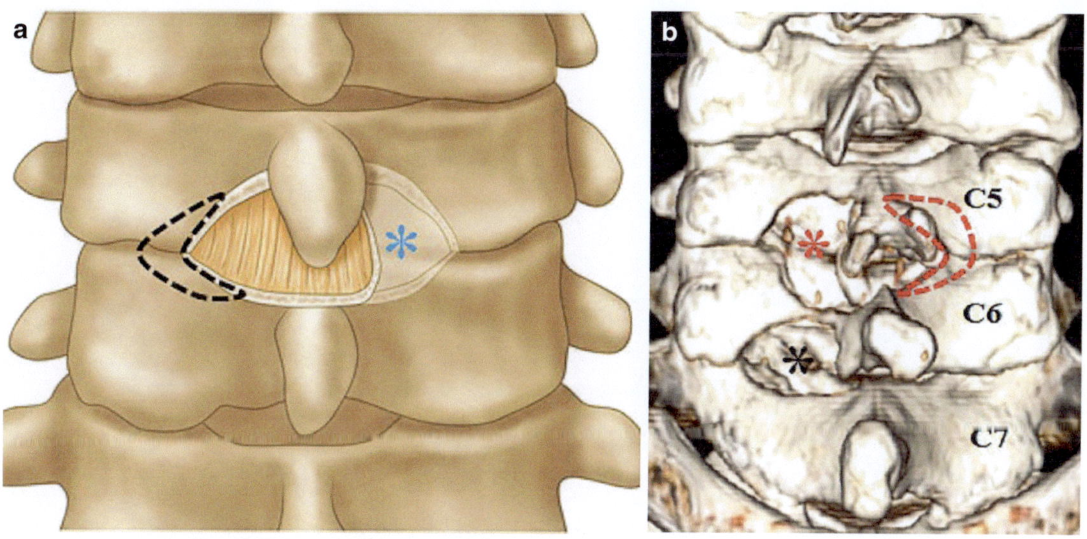


**Fig. 9** The extent of the laminotomy and foraminotomy. (**a**) Illustration shows the boundary of the laminotomy after endoscopic posterior unilateral laminotomy for bilateral decompression (ULBD). The contralateral sublaminar bone was drilled while preserving the outer cortical bone (*). Additional foraminotomy can be performed simultaneously (black dotted area). (**b**) Postoperative 3D spine CT image reveals the boundary of the laminotomy after ULBD at the C5–6 level (*) and unilateral decompression with foraminotomy at the C6–7 level (*). The contralateral sublaminar bony drilling area is shown by a red dotted line at the C5–6 level

## 9 Illustrated Cases

**Case 1** A 60-year-old man presented with insidious-onset motor weakness, which gradually progressed in the lower extremities. He complained of radicular pain in the left upper arm. He underwent artificial disc replacement surgery at the C4–5 level seven years ago. Preoperative magnetic resonance (MR) and CT images reveal central cervical stenosis at the C4–5 levels, which compressed the spinal cord secondary to ligamentum flavum hypertrophy (Fig. 10a–c). We performed the left-sided approach of uniportal endoscopic ULBD and ipsilateral foraminotomy

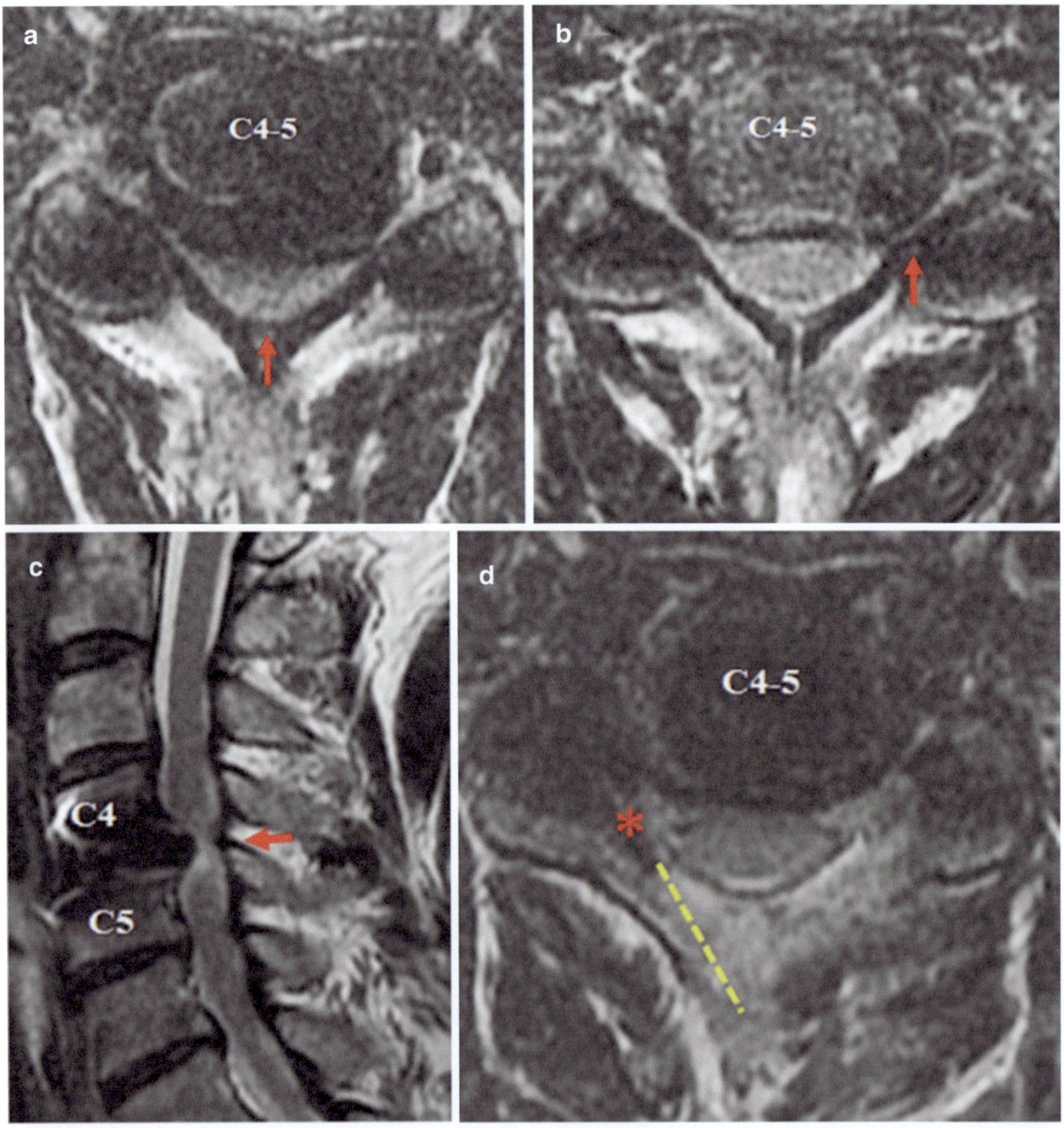


**Fig. 10** Left uniportal endoscopic approach to treat the combined pathologies of bilateral cervical canal stenosis and ipsilateral symptomatic foraminal stenosis at the C4–5 level. (**a**–**c**) Preoperative T2-weighted MR images show cervical canal stenosis and left foraminal stenosis (red arrows) at the C4–5 level. (**d**, **e**) Postoperative MR images reveal sufficiently decompressed bilateral spinal canal and left foraminal area (*: Contralateral superior articular process, yellow dotted line: a trajectory of the sublaminar bony drilling). (**f**) There is no definite segmental instability shown on the preoperative X-ray images. (**g**) Postoperative X-ray image reveals the contour of the laminotomy (yellow arrow). (**h**) A fully decompressed dural sac was found after ligamentum flavum removal

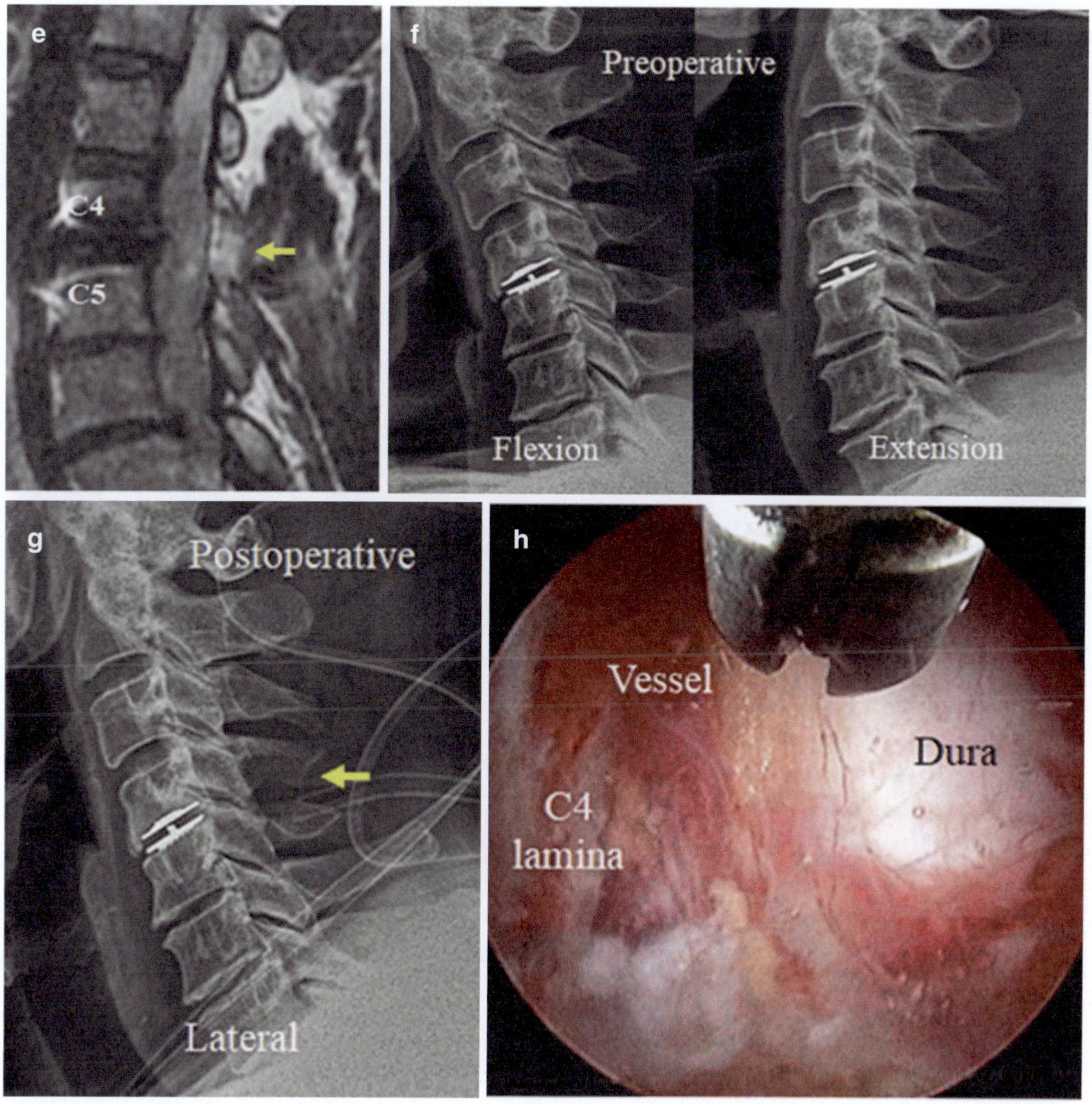


**Fig. 10** (continued)

at the C4–5 level. Postoperative MR images show sufficient decompression of the dural sac with well-preserved bilateral facet joints and contralateral lamina (Fig. 10d, e). No definite segmental instability was visible on pre-and postoperative X-ray images (Fig. 10f, g). Intraoperative images reveal a fully decompressed dural sac (Fig. 10h). Myelopathic symptoms and radiating arm pain gradually improved after surgery.

**Case 2** A 52-year-old man presented with gradual progression of motor weakness in the lower and upper extremities. The patient complained of posterior neck and shoulder pain, which was intractable to conservative treatments. Preoperative MR and CT images reveal a calcified central herniated disc and hypertrophied ligamentum flavum, which compressed the spinal cord and induced a signal change at the C3–4 level (Fig. 11a–d). We performed the right-sided approach of uniportal endoscopic ULBD and ipsilateral foraminotomy at the C3–4 level. Postoperative MR and X-ray images show sufficient decompression of the dural sac with well-preserved bilateral facet joints and contralateral lamina (Fig. 11e–h). Postoperatively, the symptoms of neurologic deficits and neck pain improved.

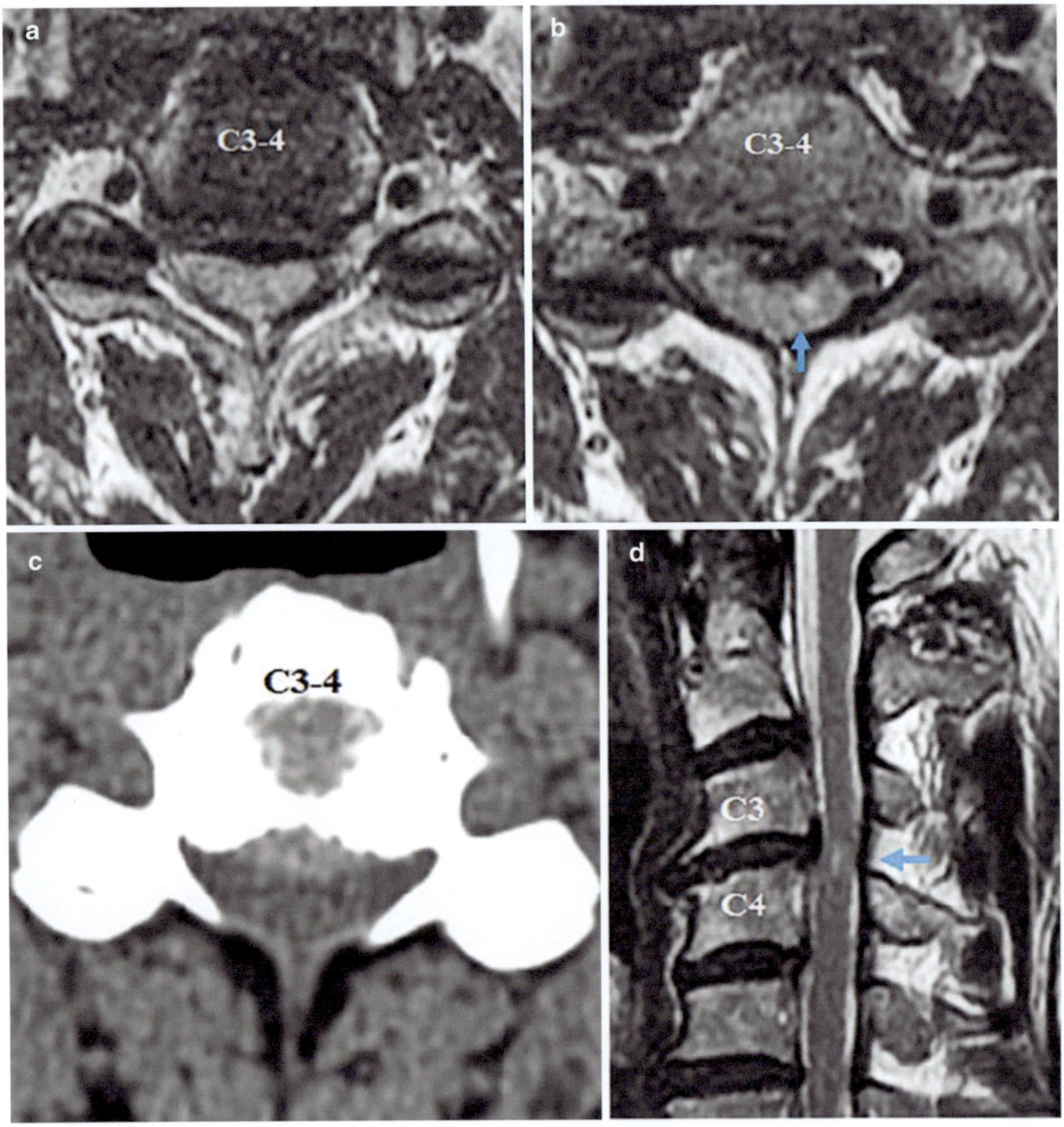


**Fig. 11** Right uniportal endoscopic approach to treat the combined pathologies of bilateral spinal canal stenosis and ipsilateral foraminal stenosis at the C4–5 level. (**a**–**d**) Preoperative T2-weighted MR and CT images show cervical canal stenosis with the spinal cord signal change (blue arrow) at the C4–5 level. (**e**–**g**) Postoperative MR images reveal sufficiently decompressed bilateral spinal canal and right foraminal area (red arrows) (*: contralateral superior articular process, red dotted line: a trajectory of the sublaminar bony drilling). (**h**) Postoperative X-ray image reveals the contour of the laminotomy (red arrow)

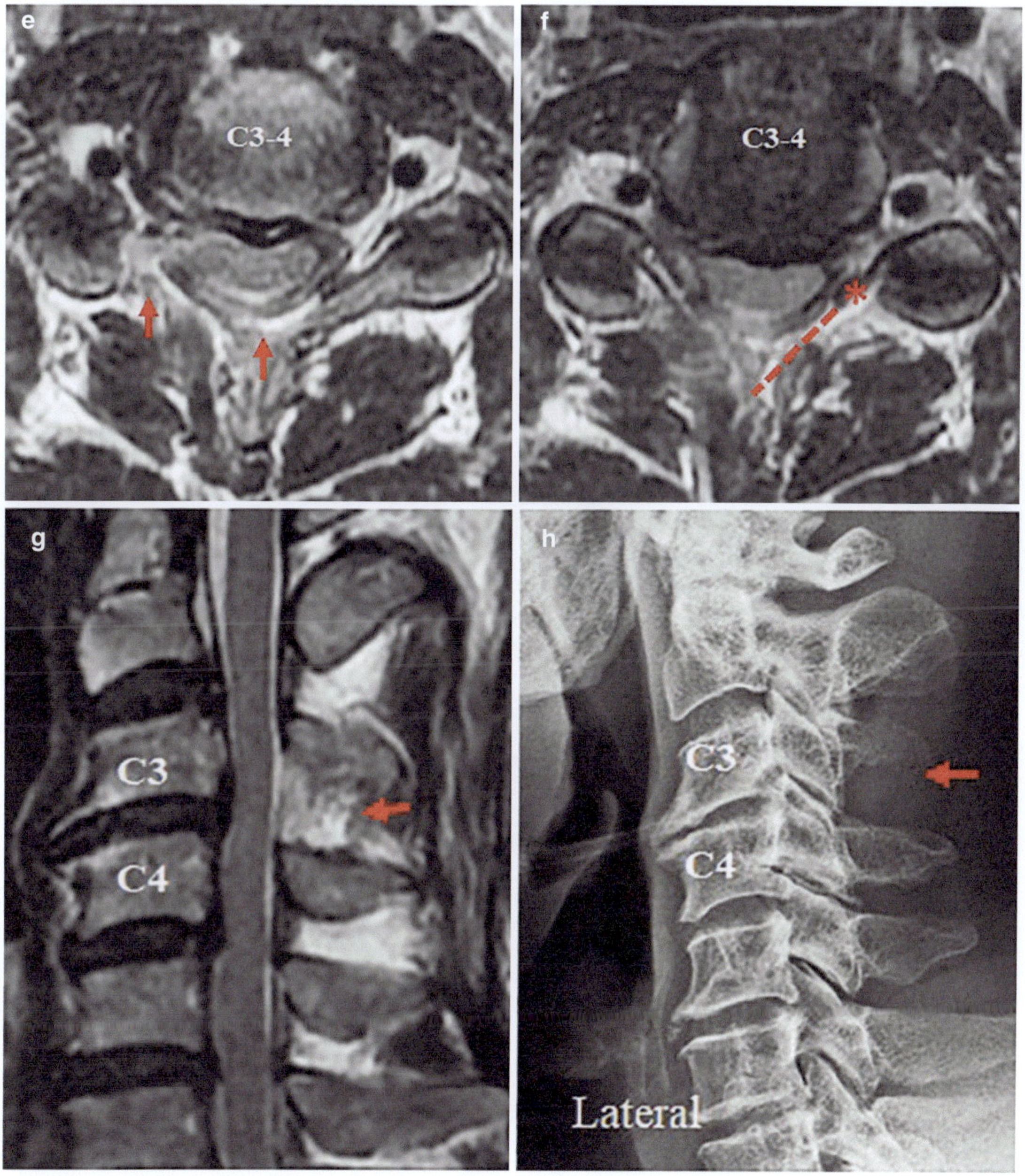


**Fig. 11** (continued)

**Case 3** A 43-year-old man presented with gradual progression of motor weakness in the lower extremities and upper back and left arm pain despite two years of conservative treatment. Preoperative MR and CT images show left unilateral cervical canal stenosis with foraminal stenosis at the C5–6 level and bilateral canal stenosis at the C7-T1 level (Fig. 12a–f). We performed the left-sided approach of uniportal endoscopic ipsilateral decompression with foraminotomy at the C5–6 level and ULBD with ipsilateral foraminotomy at the C7-T1 level. Postoperative MR and CT images show sufficient decompression of the dural sac and exiting

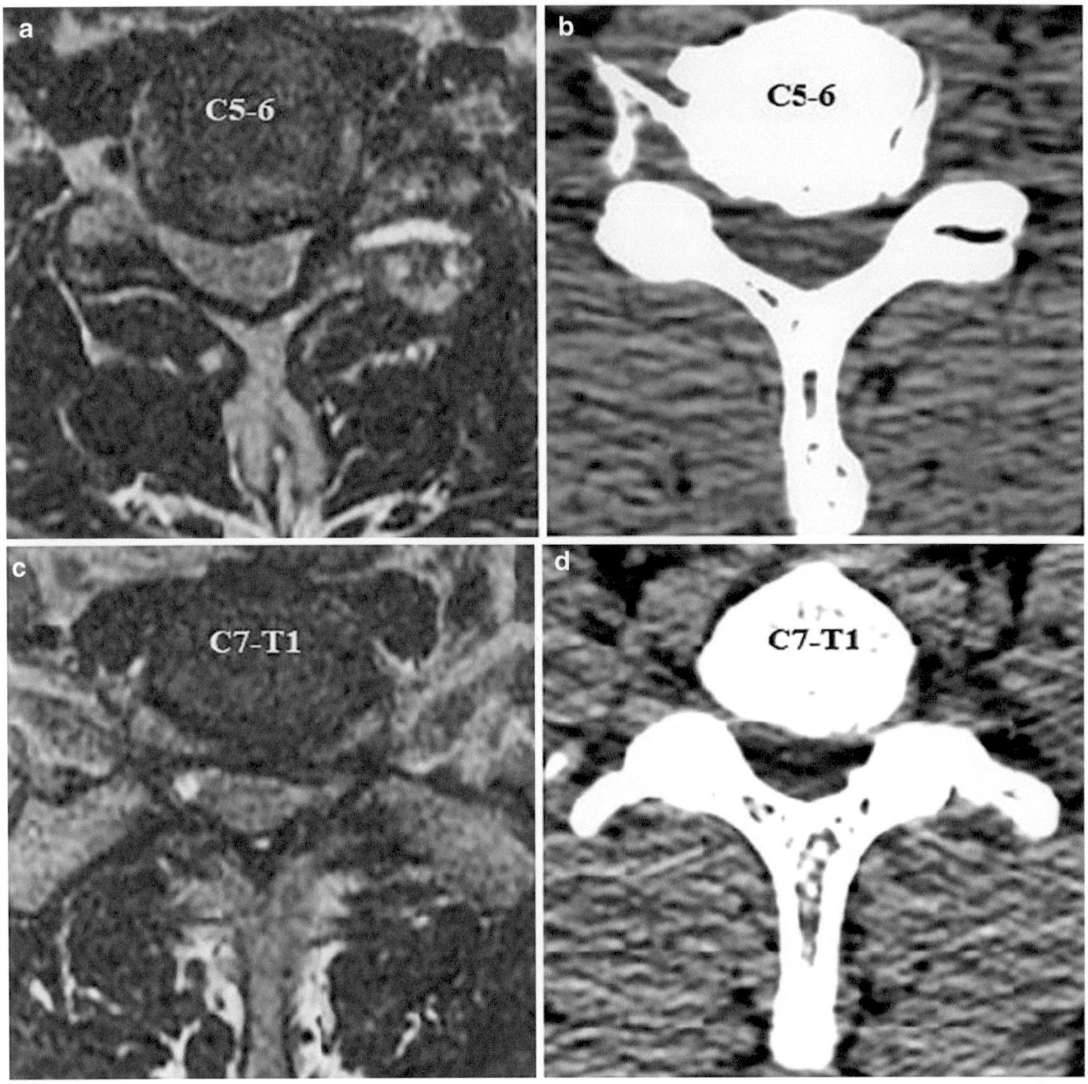


**Fig. 12** An uniportal endoscopic posterior cervical approach for combined pathologies of cervical canal stenosis and foraminal stenosis in two jumping levels. (**a–f**) Preoperative T2-weighted MR and CT images show spinal canal stenosis combined with foraminal stenosis at the C5–6 and C7-T1 levels (yellow arrows). (**g–l**) Postoperative MR and CT images reveal adequately decompressed spinal canal at both cervical levels (*: contralateral superior articular process, red dotted line: a trajectory of the sublaminar bony drilling). (**m**) Narrowed foramina in both levels are sufficiently expanded on the postoperative CT image. (**n**) Postoperative 3D spine CT image shows the extent of the laminotomy (red dotted area: boundary of the contralateral sublaminar drilling). (**o**) Postoperative X-ray images do not indicate segmental instability

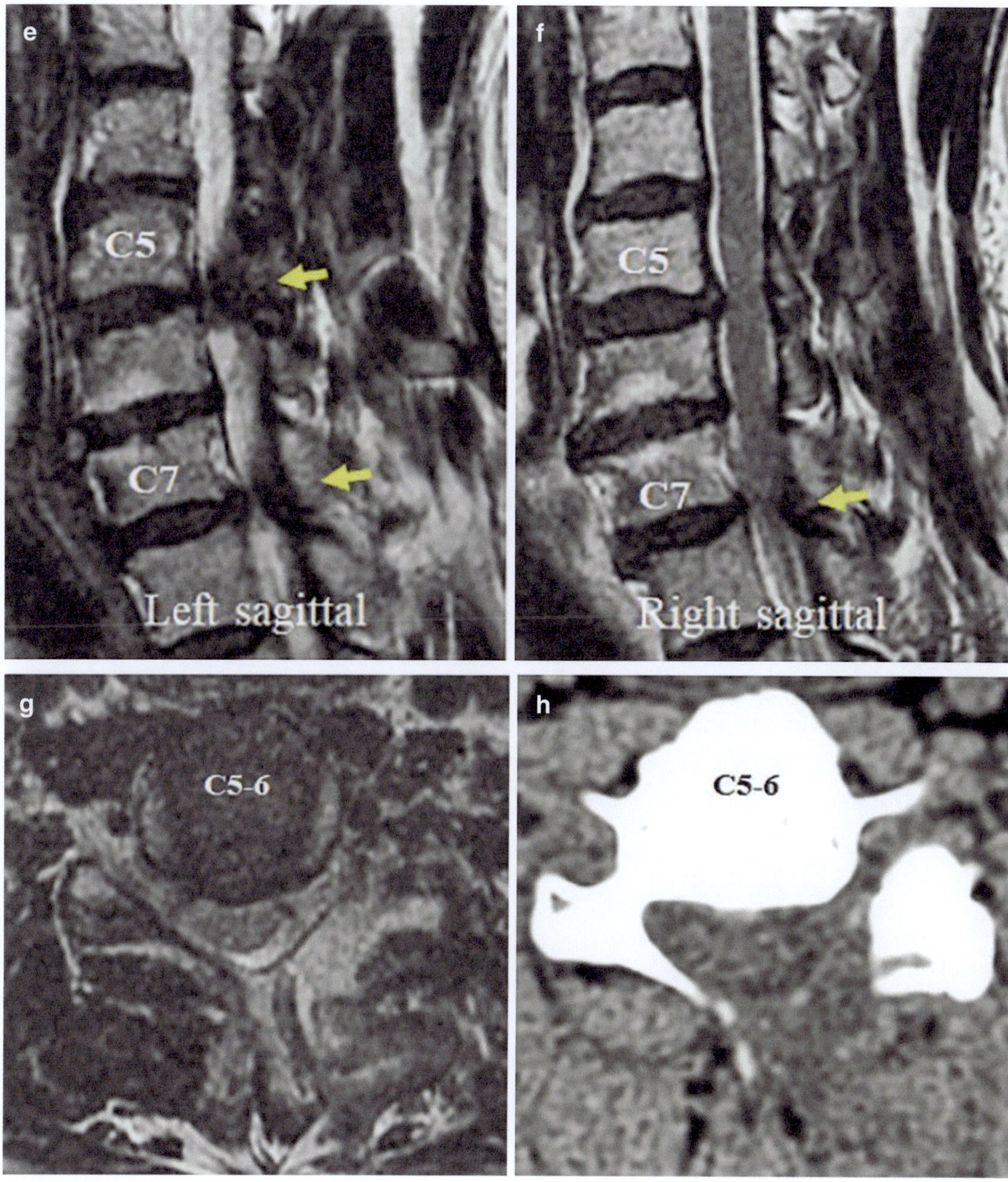


**Fig. 12** (continued)

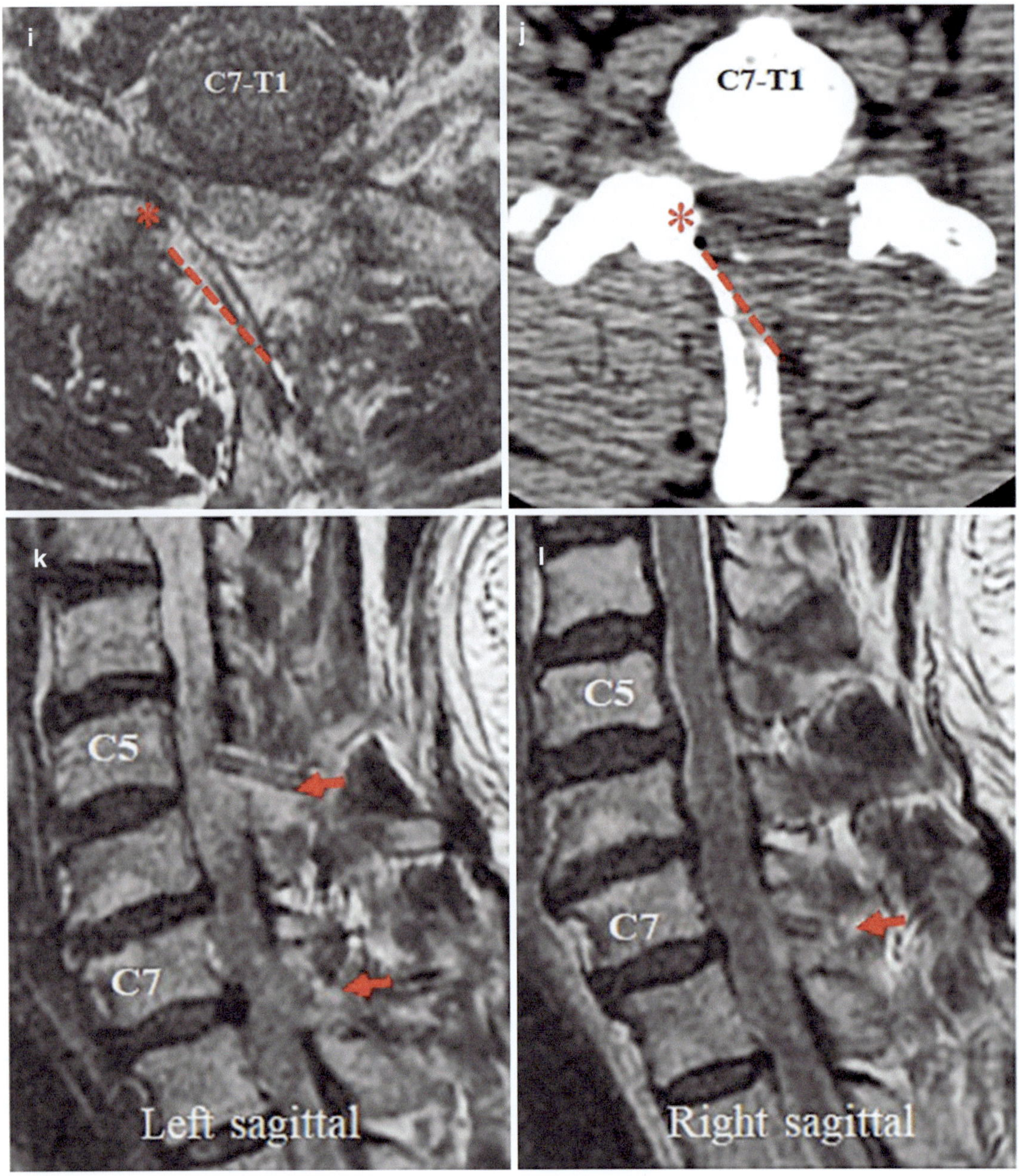


**Fig. 12** (continued)

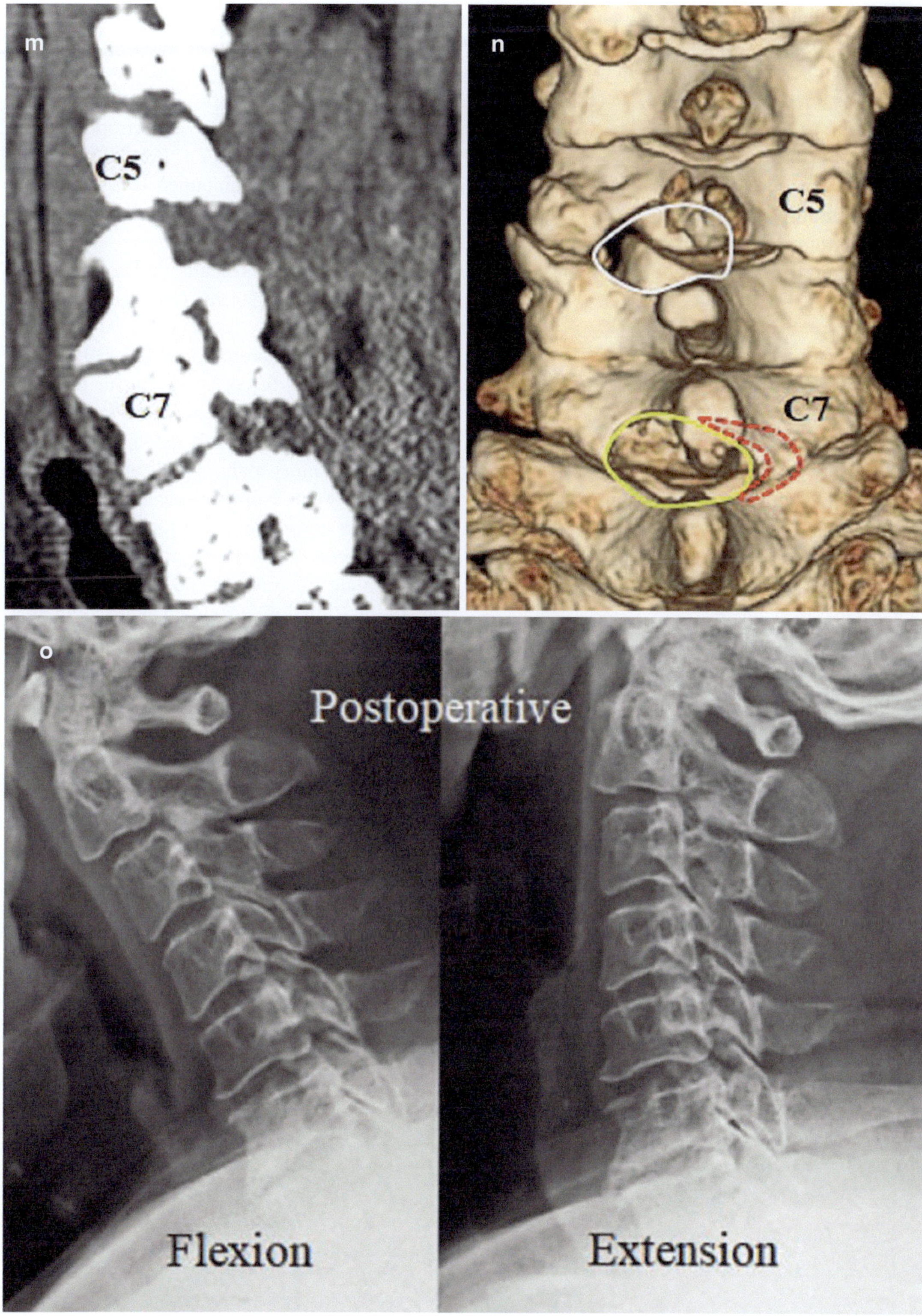


**Fig. 12** (continued)

nerve root while preserving the facet joints and contralateral lamina (Fig. 12g–m). We successfully decompressed the contralateral corner by confirming the contralateral SAP (Fig. 12i, j). The extent of the laminotomy was confirmed using a postoperative 3D spine CT image (Fig. 12n). Postoperatively, there was no postoperative instability on dynamic X-ray (Fig. 12o), and the symptoms of neurological deficits and arm pain improved significantly.

## 10 Prevention and Management of Complications (Videos 7 and 8)

The best way to avoid serious complications is to maintain the surgical steps and appropriate indications. Uniportal endoscopic ULBD could be considered for selected patients with one or two levels of cervical stenosis that satisfied the indications described above.

Coagulation of the exposed epidural vessel using the RF probe can decrease massive epidural bleeding during detachment of the ligamentum flavum from the dura (Fig. 13a). However, the massive use of RF in epidural vessels may induce spinal cord injury, and we recommend a foamy hemostatic agent for diffuse and multifocal epidural bleeding. A drainage catheter was inserted to prevent postoperative epidural hematoma, and the drainage bag was kept under negative pressure for approximately 2 days after surgery.

Wide laminotomy, including the midline part of the upper- and lower-level lamina, is essential to obtain the space for advancing the working cannula to the contralateral sublaminar space. Narrow midline bony drilling induces additional spinal cord compression by the advancing, working cannula's bevel, while the spinal cord is severely compressed by the hypertrophied ligamentum flavum (Video 7). Furthermore, the bevel tip should be maintained away from the spinal cord to avoid additional neural compression (Fig. 13b).

Pressing the drill vertically on the rigid inner cortical bone with a strong force can cause the drill to bounce and cause severe spinal cord injury (Video 8). Therefore, careful drilling with adequate pressing force, according to the bone density, is critical for preventing the bouncing of the drill. Continuous high-speed drilling can cause thermal injury to the spinal cord. Therefore, short-intermittent drilling is essential for the thinning of inner cortical to avoid thermal injury.

It is difficult to access the endoscope close to the contralateral corner of the interlaminar window. In this situation, a zoomed endoscopic view can help identify the structures, especially in the drilling of the contralateral SAP (Fig. 13c, d).

Continuous saline infusion pressure in the spinal cord may increase epidural pressure and induce spinal cord injury [8]. We should carefully monitor the good patency of the saline outflow and recommend saline infusion pressures below 30 mmHg.

If incidental durotomy occurs during endoscopic surgery, the hole should be repaired using a fibrin sealant patch. However, if endoscopic repair fails, open microscopic surgery should be performed for complete dural repair.

Intraoperative electrophysiological monitoring may prevent iatrogenic spinal cord injury.

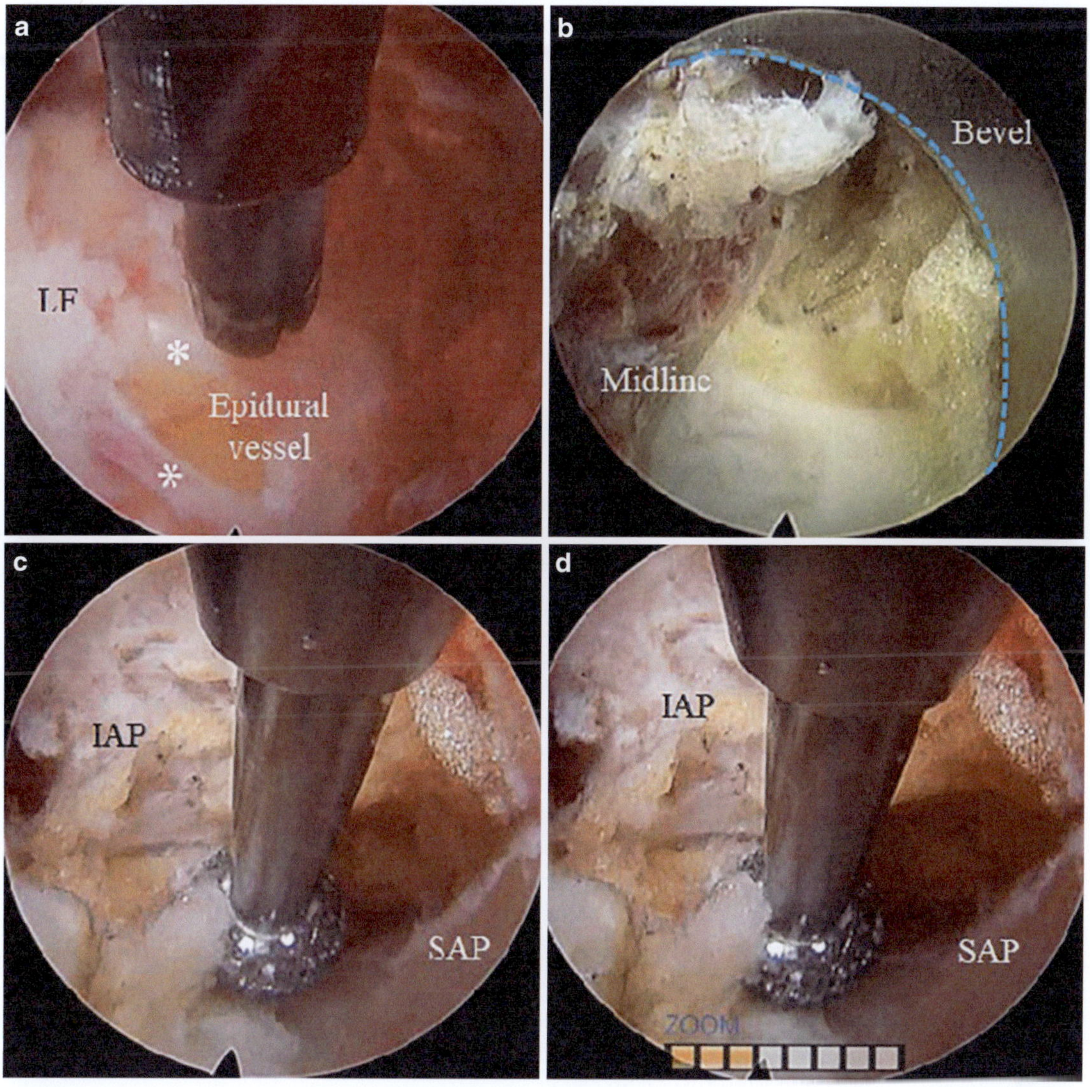


**Fig. 13** Prevention of complications. (**a**) Coagulation of the epidural vessels using the radiofrequency probe. (**b**) A tip of the bevel was maintained away from the spinal cord. (**c**, **d**) Zoomed endoscopic view offers a clear vision to the contralateral corner

## 11 Discussion (Surgical Tips and Pitfalls)

The compressed spinal cord is vulnerable and may be injured with even a slight pressure exerted by the instruments. If contralateral laminar drilling is performed after exposing the dura, the risk of dural tear and direct spinal cord injury might increase even during the careful drilling procedure. Furthermore, continuous saline infusion pressure to the exposed dura may cause spinal cord injury. Therefore, it would be better to use over-the-top decompression, removing the ligamentum flavum as the last surgical step after finishing the circumferential laminotomy instead of inside-out decompression [6, 9, 10]. In this context, if the patient has combined pathologies of symptomatic cervical foraminal stenosis with canal stenosis, we recommend performing foraminotomy before removing the ligamentum flavum to avoid spinal cord injury caused by continued infusion of saline and passing instruments.

Contralateral sublaminar drilling should be extended to the medial border of the contralateral facet joint for successful bilateral canal decompression. The anatomical endpoint of contralateral bony drilling was the medial border of the contralateral SAP (Fig. 14).

Blurred endoscopic view due to diffuse bleeding prohibits intimate bone drilling over the ligamentum flavum. Meticulous bone bleeding control using RF and the maintenance of adequate blood pressure are essential for safe instrument handling in a narrow working space.

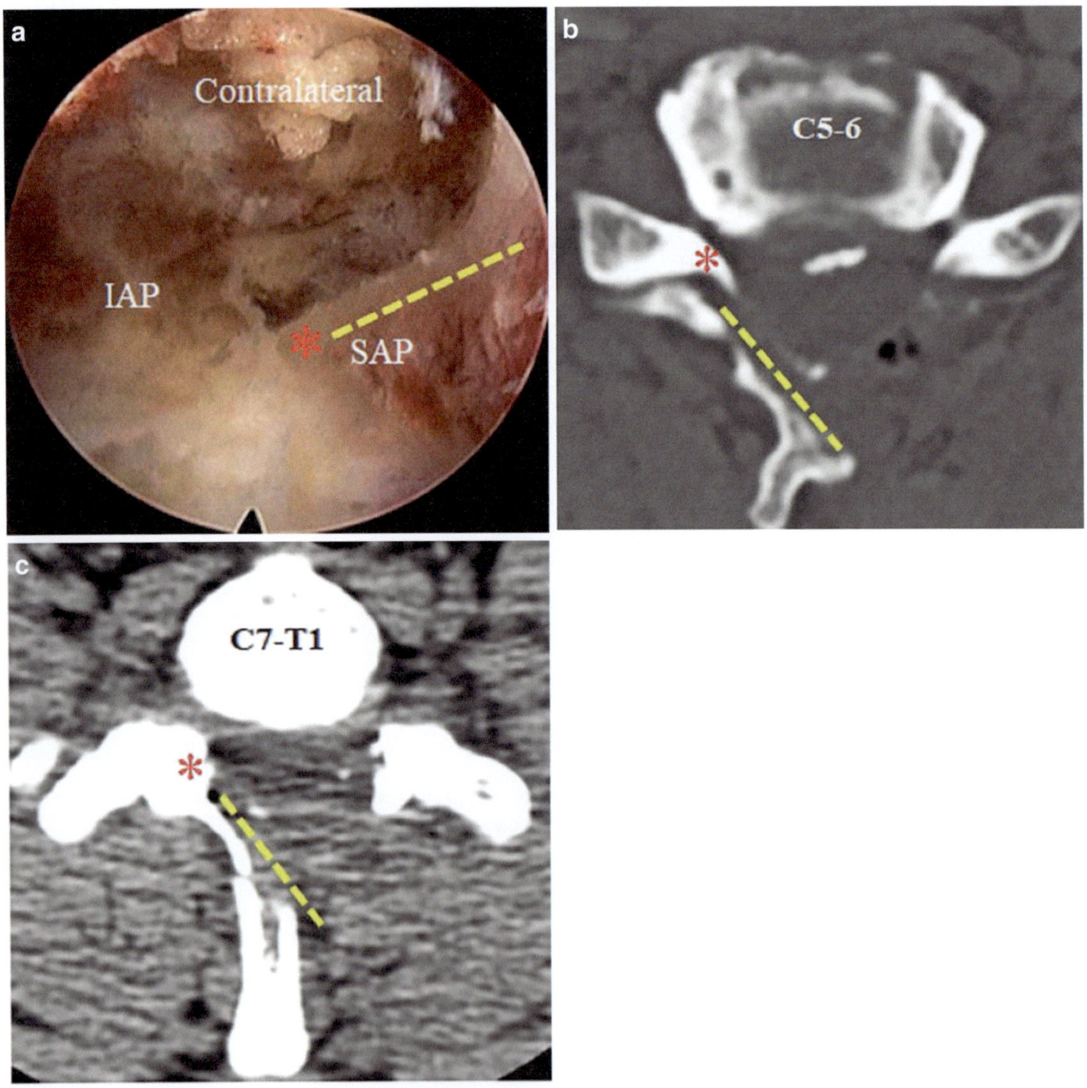


**Fig. 14** Landmark of the complete contralateral decompression. (**a**) Intraoperative endoscopic view after completing the contralateral bony drilling. Drilled medial border of the contralateral superior articular process (SAP, *: tip part) and inferior articular process (IAP) were exposed. (**b**, **c**) Postoperative axial CT images show the left unilateral laminotomy and tract of the contralateral sublaminar drilling (yellow dotted line). Medial border of the contralateral SAP (*) was partially drilled, and the bilateral spinal canal was sufficiently expanded

**Conflict of Interest** None

**Disclosure of Funding** None

## References

1. Shiraishi T, Kato M, Yato Y, Ueda S, Aoyama R, Yamane J, et al. New techniques for exposure of posterior cervical spine through intermuscular planes and their surgical application. Spine (Phila Pa 1976). 2012;37(5):E286–96.
2. Lee BJ, Park JH, Jeon SR, Roh SW, Rhim SC, Jung SK. Posterior cervical muscle-preserving Interspinous process approach and decompression: more minimally invasive and modified Shiraishi's selective laminectomy. World Neurosurg. 2020;133:e412–e20.
3. Zhang C, Li D, Wang C, Yan X. Cervical endoscopic Laminoplasty for cervical myelopathy. Spine (Phila Pa 1976). 2016;41(Suppl 19):B44–51.
4. Carr DA, Abecassis IJ, Hofstetter CP. Full endoscopic unilateral laminotomy for bilateral decompression of the cervical spine: surgical technique and early experience. J Spine Surg. 2020;6(2):447–56.
5. Shen J, Telfeian AE, Shaaya E, Oyelese A, Fridley J, Gokaslan ZL. Full endoscopic cervical spine surgery. J Spine Surg. 2020;6(2):383–90.
6. Kim J, Heo DH, Lee DC, Chung HT. Biportal endoscopic unilateral laminotomy with bilateral decompression for the treatment of cervical spondylotic myelopathy. Acta Neurochir. 2021;163(9):2537–43.
7. Kim HS, Wu PH, Lee YJ, Kim DH, Kim JY, Lee JH, et al. Reprint of: safe route for cervical approach: partial Pediculotomy, partial Vertebrotomy approach for posterior endoscopic cervical Foraminotomy and discectomy. World Neurosurg. 2021;145:621–30.
8. Hwa Eum J, Hwa Heo D, Son SK, Park CK. Percutaneous biportal endoscopic decompression for lumbar spinal stenosis: a technical note and preliminary clinical results. J Neurosurg Spine. 2016;24(4):602–7.
9. Kim HS, Wu PH, Jang IT. Lumbar endoscopic unilateral Laminotomy for bilateral decompression outside-in approach: a proctorship guideline with 12 steps of effectiveness and safety. Neurospine. 2020;17(Suppl 1):S99–s109.
10. Lim KT, Meceda EJA, Park CK. Inside-out approach of lumbar endoscopic unilateral Laminotomy for bilateral decompression: a detailed technical description, rationale and outcomes. Neurospine. 2020;17(Suppl 1):S88–s98.

# Full Endoscopic Anterior Cervical Discectomy and Fusion (ACDF) and Arthroplasty

Kangtaek Lim, Chun-Kun Park,
and Han Ga Wi Nam

**Abstract**

Cervical spondylosis and disc degeneration can lead to radiculopathy and myelopathy from progressive foraminal or central stenosis. For the surgical treatment of cervical spondylosis and disc degeneration, direct anterior decompression with fusion or indirect posterior decompression using microscopy has been used widely as the standard procedure depends on the location of pathology as well as the surgeon's own preference. Anterior cervical discectomy and fusion (ACDF) can be performed for a variety of pathologies. The procedure involves an anterior decompression of the disc space followed by interbody grafting and fusion. It provides excellent visualization for central and bilateral foraminal decompression without manipulation of neural structures. ACDF using 8 mm endoscopy is a new technology for cervical spondylosis and disc degeneration. Optimized endoscopic system for cervical anterior approach has a 5.5-mm working channel that allows full decompression of spinal canal by removing the intervertebral disc, posterior osteophyte and posterior longitudinal ligament by using 3 mm drill and Kerrison punch, and allows the implantation of cage through the endoscopy. In this chapter, we describe the surgical technique and summarize the endoscopic process to discuss its operative pitfalls.

**Keywords**

Cervical spondylotic myelopathy · Anterior cervical discectomy and fixation · Endoscopic Spine surgery · Stenoscope

## 1 Advantages of this Approach (Introduction)

The potential of endoscopy for ACDF has become the center of attention. There have been only a few articles published dealing with the full endoscopic anterior approach in cervical degenerative pathology. This new technology and high-definitive resolution of E-ACDF allow better visualization of the anatomical structure of anterior cervical vertebrae [1]. Also, using continu-

**Supplementary Information** The online version contains supplementary material available at https://doi.org/10.1007/978-981-99-1133-2_7.

K. Lim
Department of Neurosurgery, Seoul Segyero Hospital, Hanam, South Korea

C.-K. Park
Department of Neurosurgery, Seoul St. Mary's Hospital, The Catholic University of Korea, Seoul, South Korea

H. G. W. Nam (✉)
Department of Neurosurgery, Suncheon Chuck Hospital, Suncheon, South Korea



H. S. Kim et al. (eds.), *Advanced Technique of Endoscopic Cervical and Thoracic Spine Surgery*,
https://doi.org/10.1007/978-981-99-1133-2_7

ous water irrigation during procedures provides the surgeon with a clearer operation field and the ability to get the endoscope close to the pathology, normal anatomy, and less bloody surgical view, and can reduce surrounding organ damage and surgical infection. As a result, an operated patient can minimize pain medication and antibiotics usage.

## 2 Indications and Contraindications

- The possible indications for the procedure include.
    1. Intractable or progressive cervical radiculopathy or myelopathy refractory to conservative management with evidence of spondylosis or disc herniation causing foraminal or central stenosis at the corresponding level on imaging evidence of stenosis on magnetic resonance imaging and/or computed tomography correlating with clinical presentation.
- The possible contraindications include.
    1. Prior neck irradiation.
    2. Prior anterior neck surgery.
    3. Tracheostomy.
    4. Primary posterior pathology.
    5. Ossification of the posterior longitudinal ligament.
    6. Severe osteoporosis.

## 3 Anesthesia and Position

- The operation is performed under the general anesthesia in a supine position with neck slightly extended. Both shoulders are gently pulled down caudally with sticking plaster to ensure the surgical index visible on C-arm during operation.
- Insertion of a radiographically visible Levin tube would be more helpful to a surgeon to keep a safe distance from the esophagus to avoid any possibility of esophagus injury.

## 4 Special Instrument

- All operative procedures were performed with a complete uniportal endoscopic instrument system: Techcord Endoscopic System (Techcord, Daejeon, Korea) (Fig. 1). Uniportal endoscopes are used in a different fashion as an operating microscope employed for open spinal surgery in aspects of 360 degree operating field rotation.
- Surgical instruments can be categorized into four groups (Fig. 2):
    1. Mechanical instruments: Kerrison punches, long pituitary forceps (small/middle/large), dissectors (small/large), blunt-angled probe, ball-tipped probe.
    2. Special instruments: obturator, working sleeve, endoscopic customized root retractor.

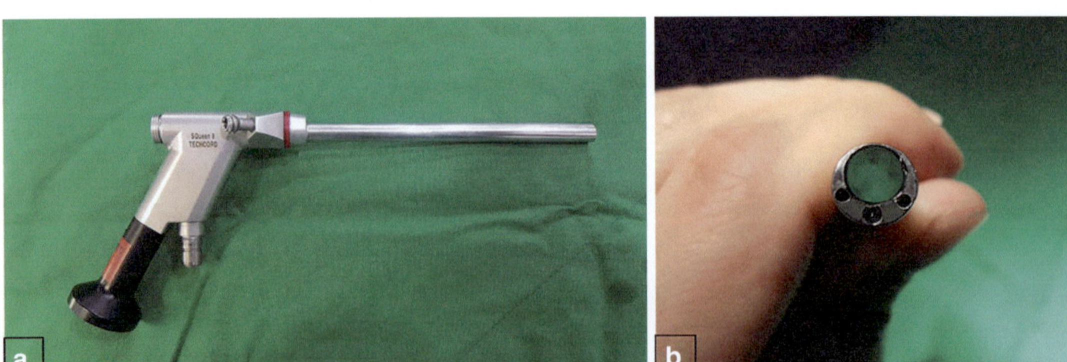


**Fig. 1** The modified large working channel endoscopic system (**a**). A 8.4-mm outer diameter, 5.7-mm working channel (**b**) and 12 degree direction of view, 80 degree field of view)

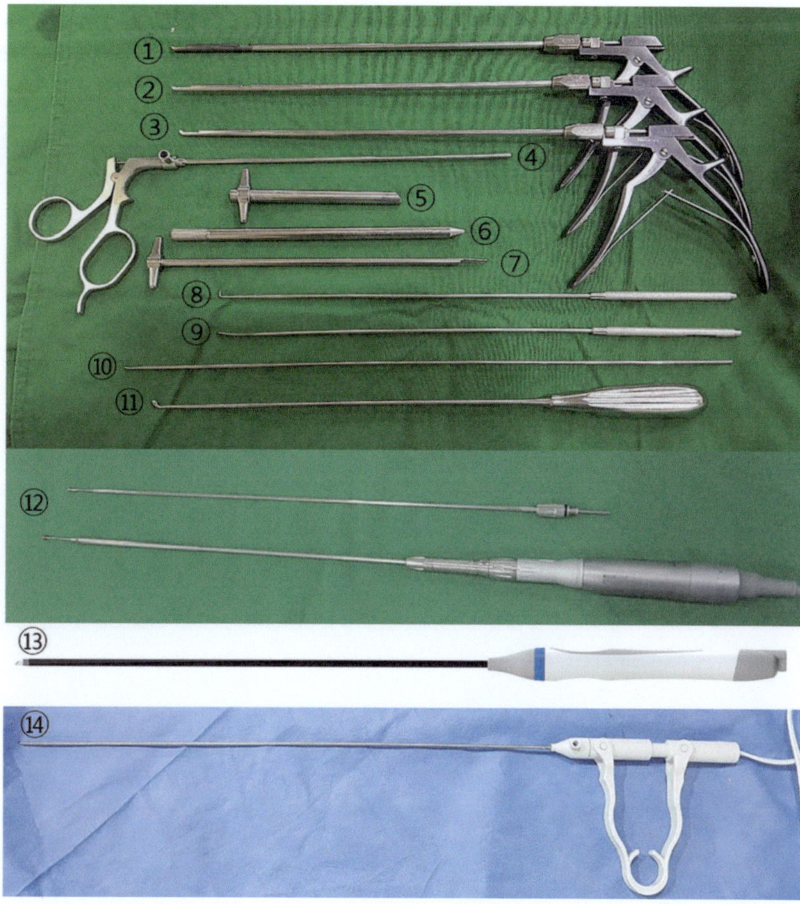


**Fig. 2** Essential unit for uniportal endoscopic decompression: (1–3) Kerrison punches, (4) pituitary forceps (large), (5) working sleeve, (6) obturator, (7) endoscopic customized root retractor, (8) ball-tipped probe, (9–10) dissectors (small/large), (11) up-angled curette, (12) LDRON endoscopic drill system (3 mm, 4-mm-sized burr) (SAESHIN, Daegu, Korea), (13) DELPHI radiofrequency electrode, and (14) bipolar radiofrequency electro-coagulator

3. Electrosurgical instruments: bipolar radiofrequency electro-coagulator (OK MedinetKorea, Seoul, Korea), DELPHI radiofrequency electrode (C&S Medical, Pocheon, Korea).
4. Motorized instruments: LDRON endoscopic drill system (SAESHIN, Daegu, Korea).

## 5 Procedures (Video 1)

- Step 1: skin entry point.
  1. In this approach, a route between the medial border of the common carotid artery and lateral border of the thyroid is usually recommendable.
  2. A surgeon confirms the index level with a C-arm image intensifier.
  3. Approaching the pathology, a surgeon passes a thin needle through the disc space, which a surgeon makes with the index and middle fingers. A surgeon firmly presses and separates the anterior neck complexes with these two fingers: one finger medially on the thyroid, trachea, and esophagus complex, and the other one laterally on the pulsatile carotid sheath complex.
  4. The two fingers should touch and be placed just on the anterior disc leading to the midline of disc space gently after confirming the correct placement of the needle in the operational level using C-arm. This procedure must be a way to make enough working space for endoscopic procedures.
- Step 2: dilation and endoscope insertion (Fig. 3).
  1. A 15-mm transverse skin incision deep to the platysma was built around the thin needle to allow the passage of serial working dilators (2–13 mm outer diameter serial dilator.

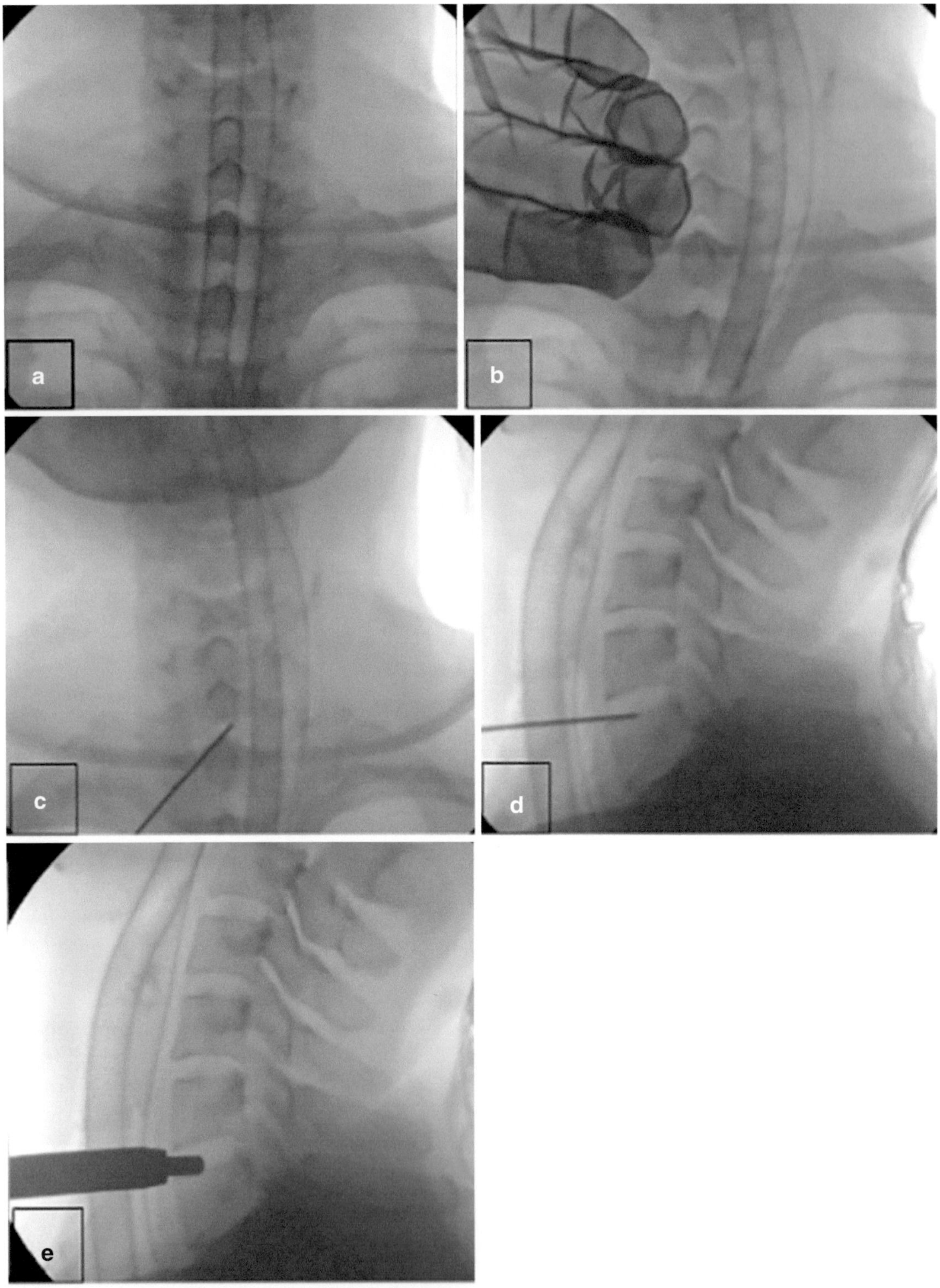


**Fig. 3** C-arm images show that trachea and esophagus are located on the contralateral side by pressing anterior neck firmly using the left index and middle finger (**a**, **b**). Insertion of a thin needle into the midline of disc space gently under the C-arm confirmation (**c**–**e**)

2. A surgeon puts the 9.5-mm outer diameter of the working sleeve and 8-mm outer diameter of the endoscope into the anterior part of the disc through the 15-mm skin incision.
3. Then, the surgeon places the working sleeve and endoscopy in the midline (in between ipsilateral and contralateral longus coli muscles) of the disc and not advancing over the contralateral longus coli muscle on C-arm AP view to prevent injury of the esophagus.
4. A surgeon docks an endoscopic system on the anterior neck and must maintain the system upright and perpendicular to the disc space to put a fusion cage into the disc space properly.

- Step 3: exposure of the vertebra.
  1. The prevertebral fascia at the index segment is sacrificed using a steerable RF device to make enough safe zone on the anterior annulus surface of the vertebral body to be removed (Fig. 4a).
  2. The endoscopy can provide a clear vision with a 12° lens angle. The reason for the 12° lens in the cervical endoscope is that a surgeon watches the whole length of the disc space from the anterior to the posterior margin and from ipsilateral uncovertebral joint to contralateral side in one view.

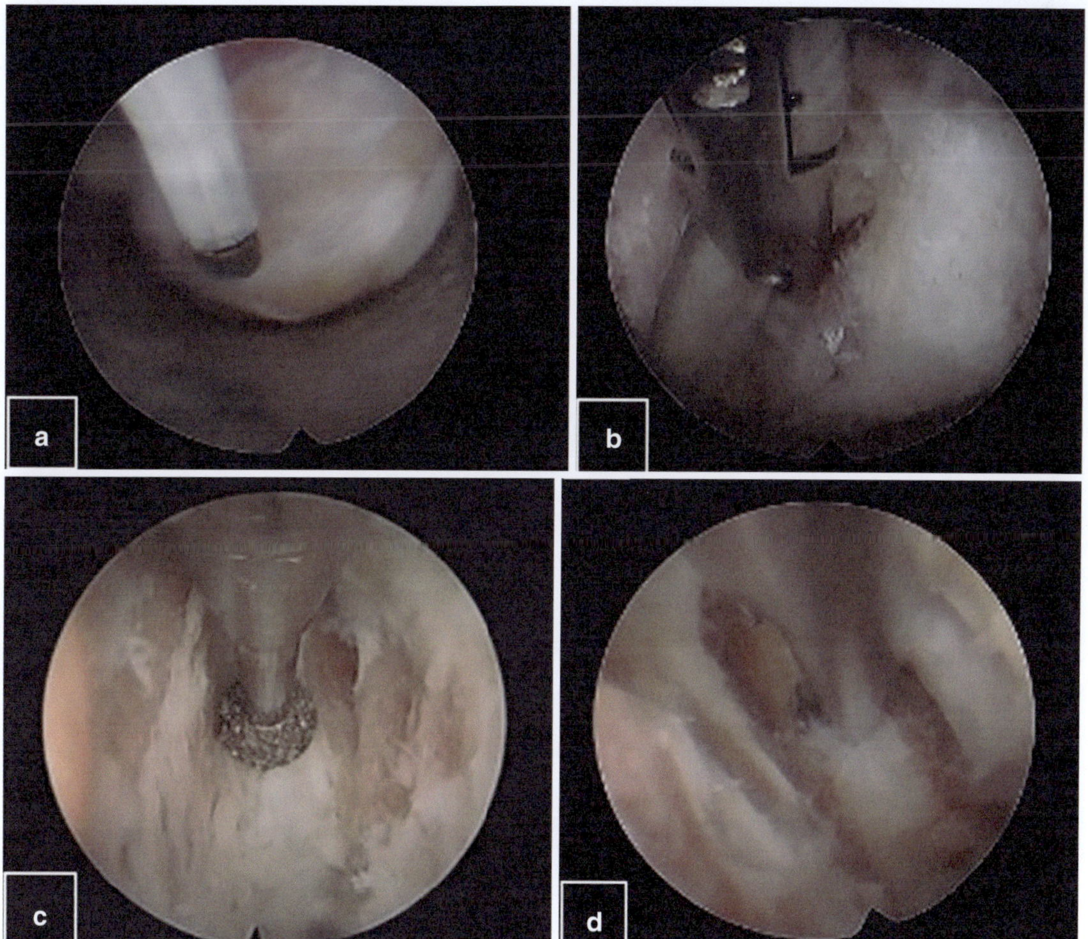


**Fig. 4** Process of endoscopic decompression. Ablation of prevertebral fascia by radiofrequency (**a**). Forceps and drilling for endplate preparation after discectomy (**b**, **c**). The removal of the uncovertebral joint (**d**). The removal of posterior osteophyte (**e**). Dura exposure after posterior longitudinal ligament removal (**f**). The final view of endplate preparation (**g**)

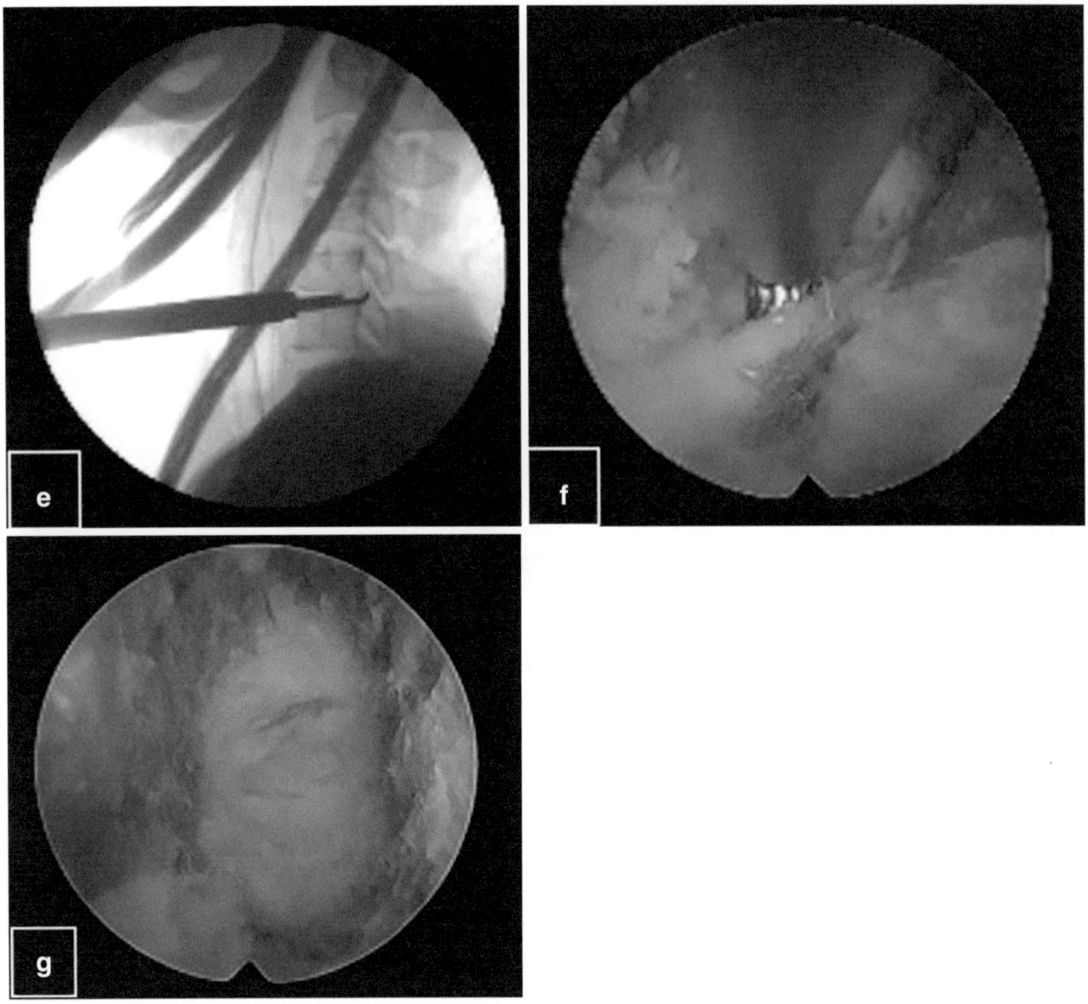


**Fig. 4** (continued)

   3. We did not use the Casper distractor in order to open up the disc space for subsequent decompression and allow implant insertion in this endoscopic procedure.
   4. Ablation on the medial portion of the ipsilateral longus coli muscle by RF is essential to expose the medial parts of the uncovertebral joint to remove at the end stage of the procedure.
   5. Once the medial portion of the longus coli is detected, it is clearer to see the surrounding structures.
- Step 4: discectomy and foraminotomy.
   1. The annulus is removed, then careful discectomy and removal of the endplate are done using RF and 1-mm Kerrison punch first and then using the 2-mm forceps, curette, and drill (Fig. 4b, c).
   2. The bilateral uncovertebral joints are removed to decompress the spinal cord and the underlying root entirely is the third step (Fig. 4d–f). It is necessary to proceed cautiously with drilling at the base of the uncinate process because the nerve root lies just behind it.
   3. When decortication and detaching the endplate cartilage using 3-mm high-speed burr and angled curette, make adequate fusion bed and enlarge the disc space to secure a proper working space.

4. The removal of posterior osteophyte and the posterior longitudinal ligament (PLL) should be careful so as not to put the Kerrison punch too profoundly into the epidural space to prevent spinal cord injury (Fig. 4e).

- Step 5: intervertebral graft.
  1. All procedures of implantation using a Poly Ether Ketone (PEEK) cage is like that of conventional open cervical fusion surgery (Fig. 5a).
  2. After the height of empty disc space is determined, a cage is selected, 1-mm larger size than the measured result, to increase the disc space height, followed by filling up the cage with demineralized bone matrix (DNM) as a bone graft before implantation (Fig. 5b).
  3. To insert the cage into the disc space, a 4-mm cage holder is introduced into the 5.5-mm endoscopic working channel to hold PEEK cage selected.
  4. In order to insert the fusion cage under the endoscopic view, we use 80-mm width two blade retractor system through 1.5-cm skin incision, which allows inspection of relevant anatomical structure while providing sufficient space for implantation with

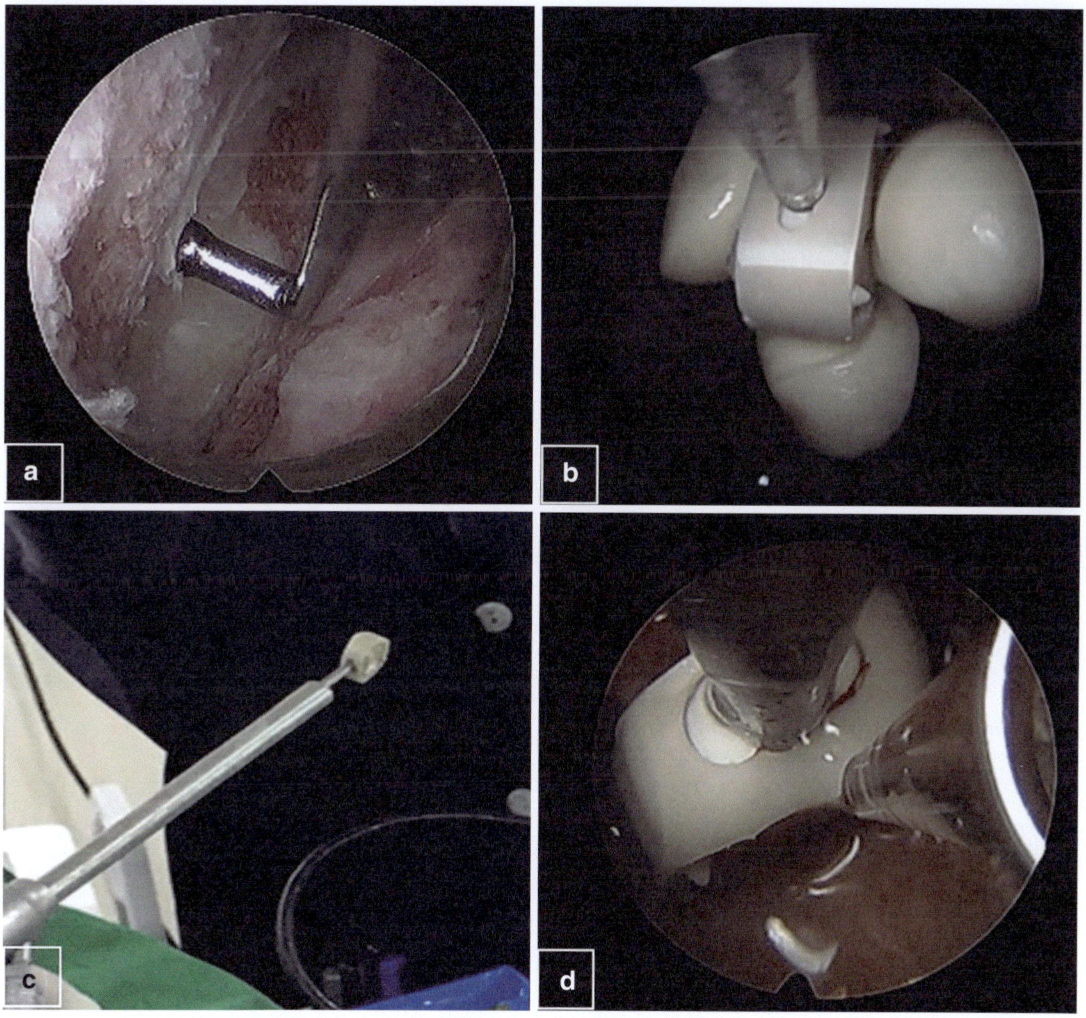

**Fig. 5** Measurement of disc height (**a**). The assembly of the cage through endoscopy (**b, c**). Implantation of cage into disc space (**d**)

safety, also including drainage of irrigation water and blood at the final stage, which would cause the soft tissue swelling, postoperatively.

5. The implantation undergoes the process of holding the ends of the cage and inserting an implant into the surgical field under the endoscopic visualization (Fig. 5c, d). The C-arm is then used to confirm the appropriate position and alignment of the cage.

- Step 6: closure.
  1. In the final stage, bleeding control in the prevertebral space by bipolar cautery meticulously, placement of suction drain under the endoscopic view, and confirmation of the correct installation of a drain in surgical field by the C-arm are essential to prevent postoperative hematoma, which can lead a patient into critical status (Fig. 6).

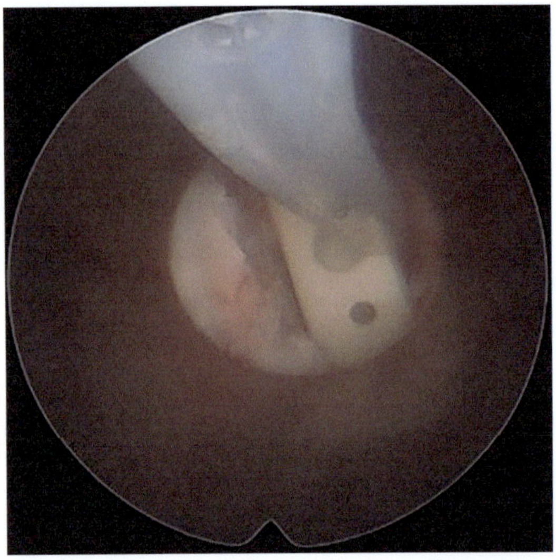

**Fig. 6** End stage of ACDF, keeping drain in the operated site, is essential to prevent postoperative hematoma

  2. Closing the fascia and skin in the usual fashion is followed by the removal of the working sleeve. The suction drain is taken off after one day postoperatively based on the total amount of drainage measured and confirmation of postoperative MRI.
  3. The patient leaves the hospital within the next 24 hours after surgery. All patients need to wear the Philadelphia brace for at least four weeks after surgery.

## 6 Illustrated Cases

- Case 1.
  – A 36-year-old male with radicular pain in the left C6 dermatome and weakness in both arms with myelopathy in C6–7. The postoperative MRI shows increased anterior–posterior diameter of spinal canal. Postoperative X-ray shows the correct placement of the cervical cages (Fig. 7).
- Case 2.
  – The second patient reviewed was a 46-year-old female with symptoms of significant radicular pain in the right arm and upper extremity weakness. MRI demonstrated signal change in the C3–4 spinal cord (Fig. 8).

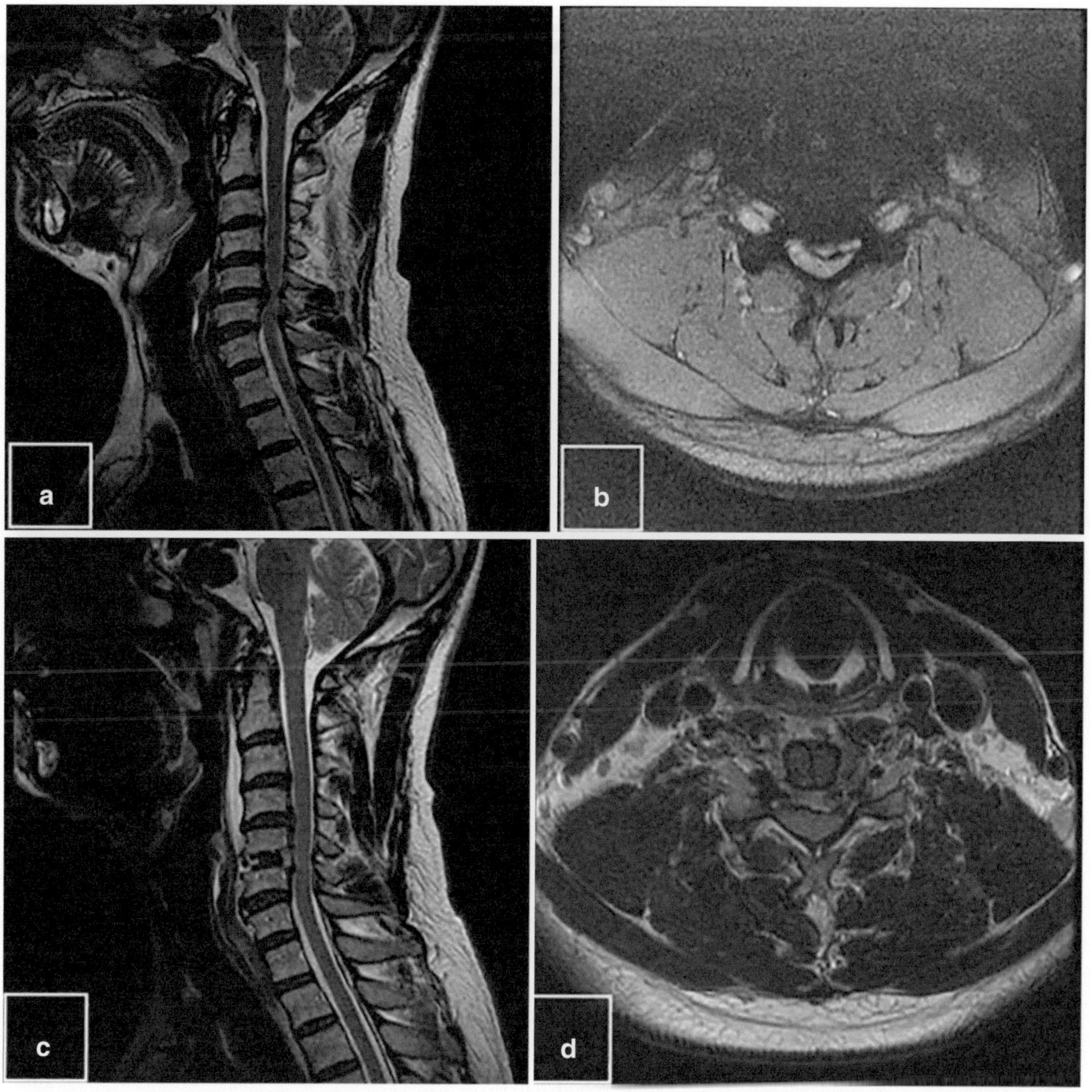


**Fig. 7** Case 1 images. Preoperative MRI, C5/6 myelopathy (**a**, **b**). Postoperative MRI (**c**, **d**). Postoperative X-ray showing the correct placement of the cervical cages (**e**, **f**). Skin scar postoperative 1 week (**g**)

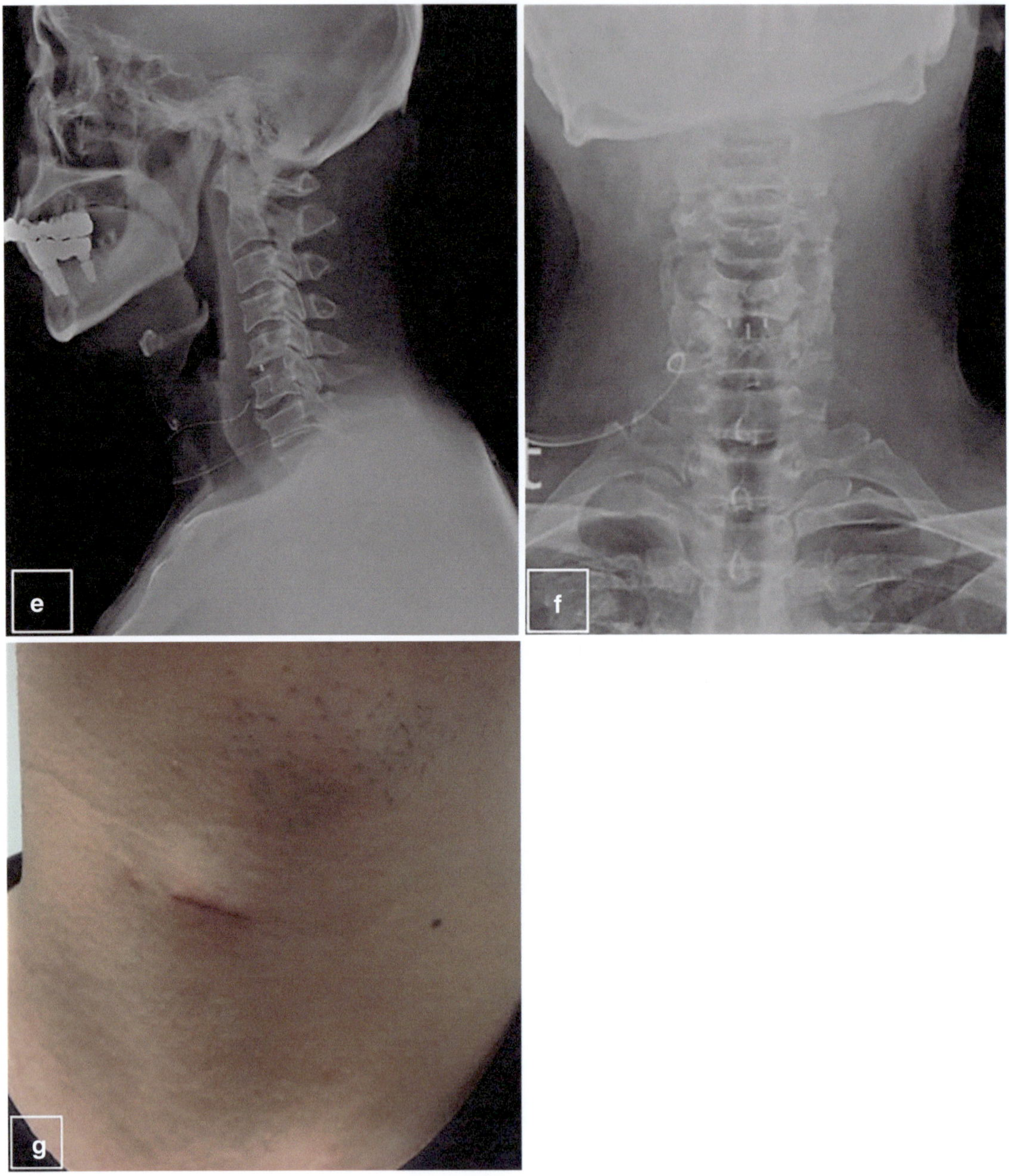


**Fig. 7** (continued)

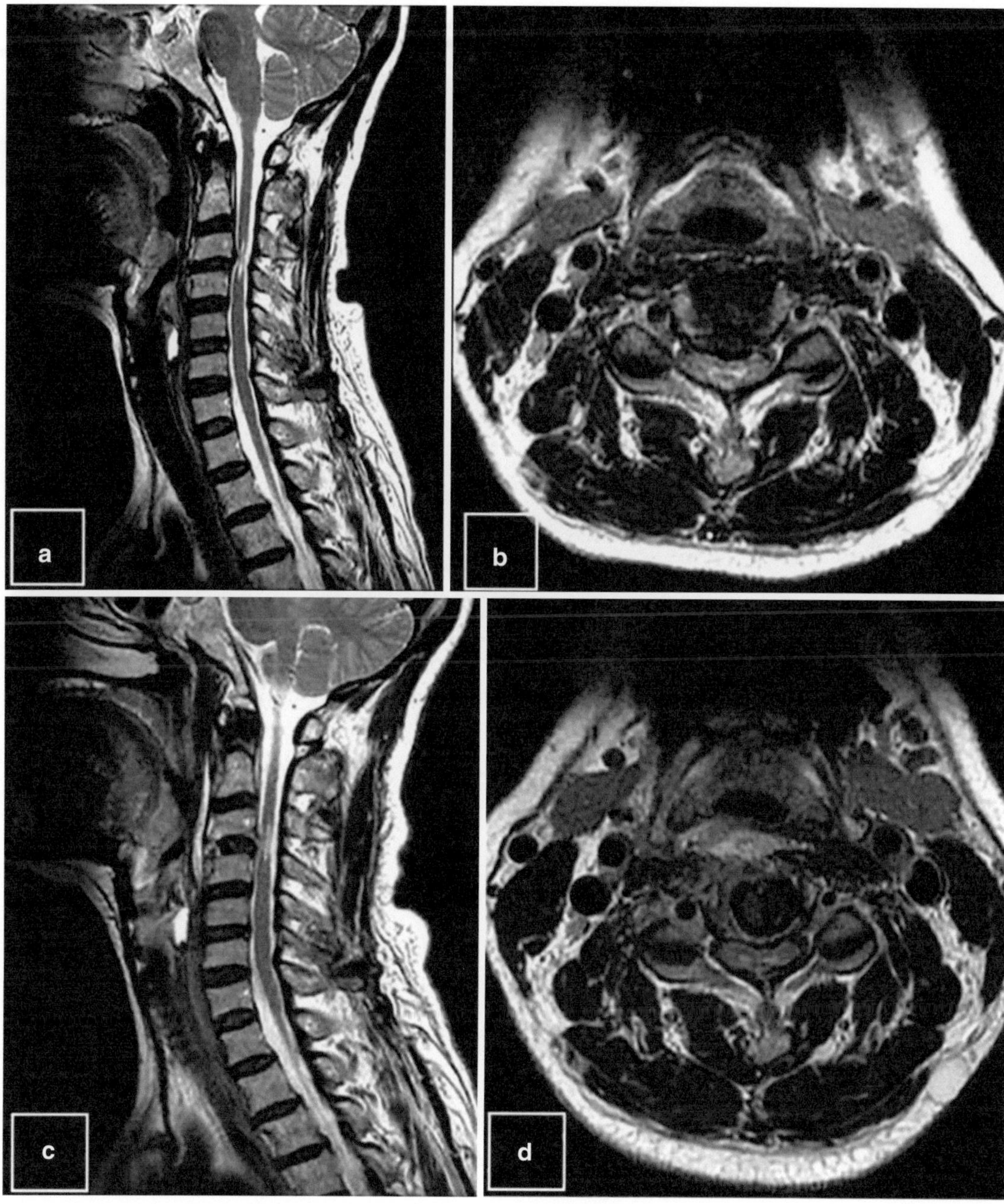


**Fig. 8** Case 2 images. Preoperative MRI shows signal change on C3/4 (**a**, **b**). Postoperative MRI (**c**, **d**). Postoperative 1-day X-ray (**e**, **f**). Postoperative 1-week skin wound (**g**)

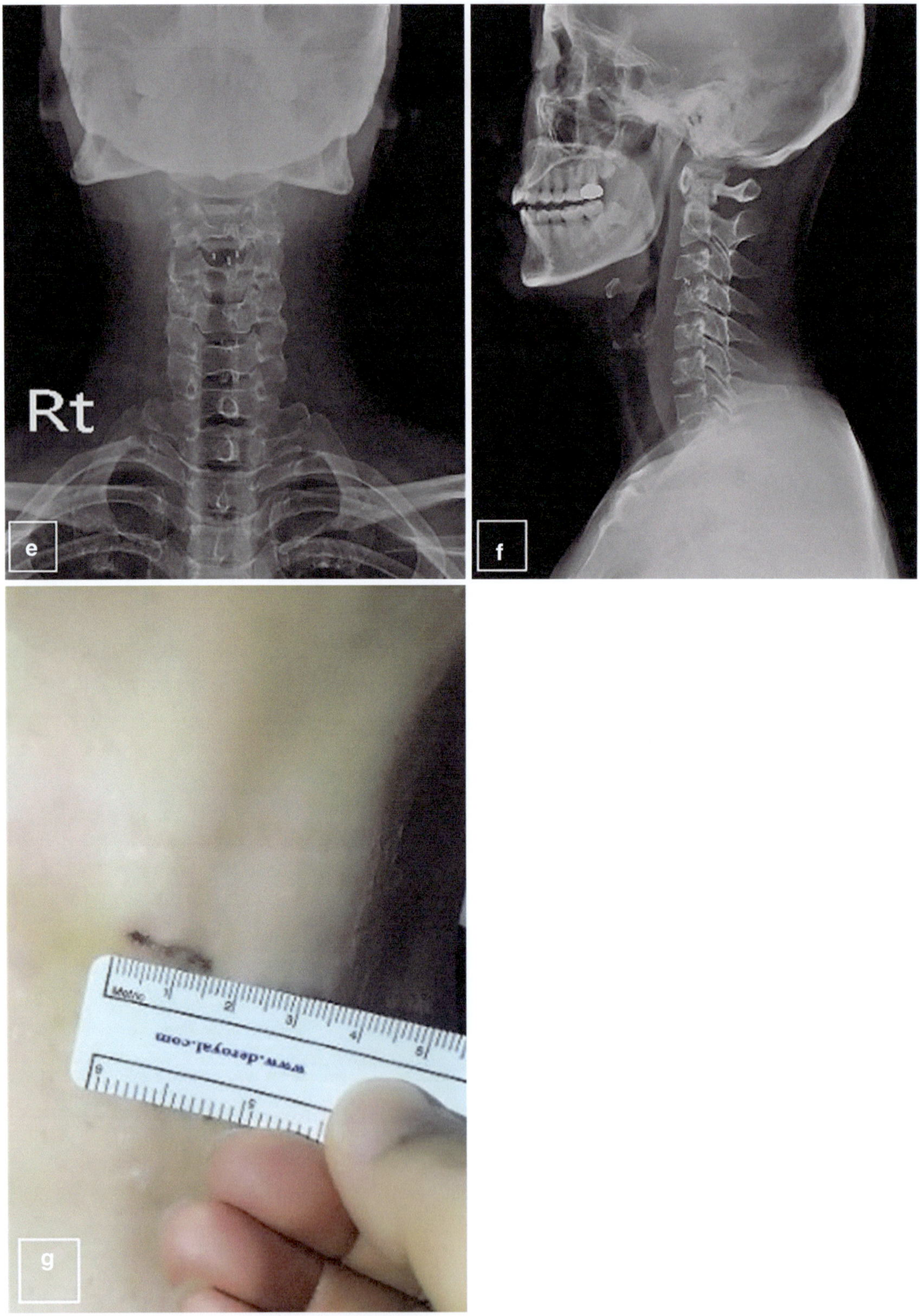


**Fig. 8** (continued)

## 7 Prevention and Management of Complications

The authors have experienced one case of surgery-related complication: surface hematoma at the very beginning of this trial. The patient needed revision surgery for this complication.

5.6% of the complication was comparable to the published other data [2]. The hematoma might form immediately after the surgery and should be inevitable because of, in fact, no significant blood or active bleeding while closing the surgical wound. Almost bloodless operation field is one of the advantages of endoscopic spinal surgery (ESS) [3], but sometimes a surgeon encounters bleeding that is not expected and not controlled well after all the control of intraoperative bleeding should be a potential challenge.

Commonly, surgeons achieve hemostasis in such ways as lavaging the operation field, with cold saline adding adrenalin, or inserting saline-soaked cottonoids and gelatin sponge admixing thrombin [1]. Meanwhile, the authors additionally apply other countermeasures against bleeding during ESS as follows: first, decreasing blood pressure (down to 30–40% of mean BP) and maintaining it, and second, increasing the pumping pressure (up to 60 mm Hg) of continuous saline irrigation.

## 8 Discussion

The goal of ESS in cervical disc diseases is to achieve appropriate decompression with efficient interbody fusion and avoid collateral injury at once and related complications [4]. The development of endoscopic systems has brought about the improvement of the resolution and clearness of endoscopy, and a surgeon can explore the intradiscal and spinal canal anatomy in detail.

ESS surgeons may expect that E-ACDF would have the merit of endoscopic surgery and the familiarity of conventional ACDF surgical technique. If speaking of the curative advantages of ESS, their enumeration includes less collateral tissue damage and maintenance of clean surgical field by less bleeding and constant saline irrigation under high pressure. Furthermore, the census of postoperative clinical benefits includes less need for analgesics, early recovery followed by a rapid return to the workplace, and high satisfaction. E-ACDF possesses almost all these surgical and clinical merits listed above.

On the other hand, full E-ACDF has a few shortcomings but mostly not so frequent. If the specific procedures may classify these shortcomings according to a source, there are two kinds of sources; ACDF-related and endoscopy-related. ACDF-related stands for the deficiencies caused by the ACDF surgical procedure and postoperative graft-related complications, and follow-up results include displacement, migration, and esophageal injury, surgical wound hematoma, immediate postoperatively, and adjacent segment disease (ASD) in long-term follow-up and subsidence of graft and pseudoarthrosis [5, 6].

The endoscopy-related shortcomings that occur during the operation and postoperative follow-up are a limitation of the distraction of upper and lower bodies to put a graft cage larger than the diameter of the working channel into the disc space, and more importantly, limited visibility is restricting the use of specific surgical tools and implants.

## References

1. Yao N, Wang C, Wang W, Wang L. Full-endoscopic technique for anterior cervical discectomy and interbody fusion. 5-year follow-up results of 67 cases. Eur Spine J. 2011;20(6):899–904.
2. Ruetten S, Komp M, Merk H, Godolias G. Full-endoscopic anterior decompression versus conventional anterior decompression and fusion in cervical disc herniations. Int Orthop. 2009;33(6):1677–82.
3. Lim KT, Nam HGW, Kim SB, Kim HS, Park JS, Park CK. Therapeutic feasibility of full endoscopic decompression in one- to three-level Lumbar Canal stenosis via a single skin port using a new endoscopic system, percutaneous Stenoscopic lumbar decompression. Asian Spine J. 2019;13(2):272–82.
4. Rao RD, Gourab K, David KS. Operative treatment of cervical spondylotic myelopathy. J Bone Joint Surg Am. 2006;88(7):1619–40.
5. Smith ZA, Fessler RG. Paradigm changes in spine surgery: evolution of minimally invasive techniques. Nat Rev Neurol. 2012;8(8):443–50.
6. Lebl DR. Minimally invasive spine surgery. Curr Rev Musculoskelet Med. 2017;10(3):407–8.

# Part III

# Cervical - Biportal

# Biportal Endoscopic Posterior Cervical Foraminotomy and Discectomy

Dong Hwa Heo, Hyun Jin Hong, Don Young Park, and Choon Keun Park

**Abstract**

Posterior cervical foraminotomy or laminoforaminotomy is an effective surgical method for treating cervical radiculopathy caused by foraminal disc herniation or foraminal stenosis. Minimally invasive posterior cervical foraminotomy using a tubular retractor has the advantage of reducing damage to the normal tissues during surgery while maintaining the advantages of posterior foraminotomy. Recently, spinal endoscopy has been used to treat degenerative cervical disease with various types of approaches currently used in cervical endoscopy. In this report, the biportal endoscopic approach was performed using two portals. The first portal was an endoscopic portal for the spinal endoscope, and the other portal was a working portal for surgical instruments. The surgical techniques and related anatomy of the biportal endoscopic posterior cervical approach are similar to those of microsurgery.

**Keywords**

Cervical · Foraminotomy · Discectomy Endoscopy · Biportal

## 1 Introduction

Biportal endoscopic posterior cervical foraminotomy, which is also known as discectomy, has many advantages over endoscopic spine surgery, as well as minimally invasive spine surgery [1, 2]. Biportal endoscopic posterior cervical foraminotomy can minimize trauma to normal muscles and ligamentous structures. Therefore, bleeding and postoperative wound pain may be lower in this approach than in other approaches [3]. Additionally, cervical biportal endoscopic surgery makes use of two portals (endoscopic channel, working channel), which is similar to lumbar biportal endoscopic surgery [1, 2] (Fig. 1). This makes handling spinal instruments easier and more comfortable than microsurgery. The biportal endoscopic posterior cervical approach can also be safely performed in a magnified endoscopic field of view [2–5]. In this view, continuous saline irrigation can be performed to reduce

**Supplementary Information** The online version contains supplementary material available at https://doi.org/10.1007/978-981-99-1133-2_8.

D. H. Heo
Endoscopic Spine Surgery Center, Neurosurgery, Champodonamu Spine Hospital, Seoul, South Korea

H. J. Hong (✉) · C. K. Park
Neurosurgery, Spine Center, Wiltse Memorial Hospital, Anyang, South Korea

D. Y. Park
Orthopedics, David Geffen School of Medicine, UCLA, Los Angeles, CA, USA
e-mail: DYPark@mednet.ucla.edu



H. S. Kim et al. (eds.), *Advanced Technique of Endoscopic Cervical and Thoracic Spine Surgery*,
https://doi.org/10.1007/978-981-99-1133-2_8

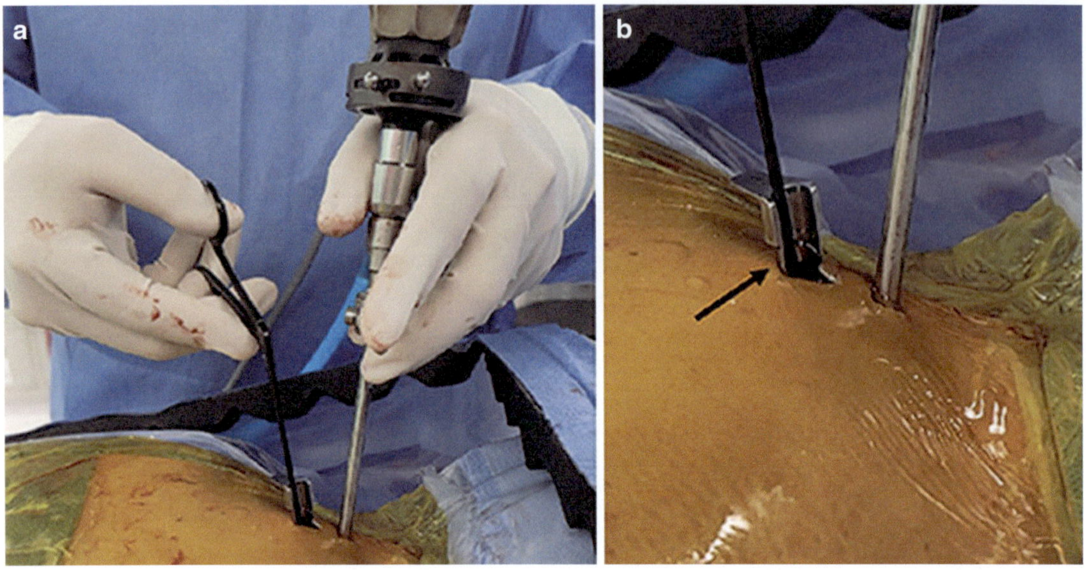


**Fig. 1** Overview of biportal endoscopic posterior cervical foraminotomy (**a**). A working sheath was inserted into a working portal (**b**, arrow)

bleeding during surgery and maintain a clear field of view. Moreover, two levels of posterior cervical foraminotomy can be achieved using a single approach with two portals. Finally, the small skin incisions and small postoperative skin scars of this approach are cosmetically better than those in conventional open posterior cervical surgery.

## 2 Indications and Contraindications

Unilateral cervical radiculopathy caused by single-level foraminal pathologic lesions is the best indication for biportal endoscopic posterior cervical foraminotomy with or without discectomy. Besides these, the approach is also indicated for multilevel cervical foraminal lesions. On the other hand, note that instability and cervical canal stenosis are some contraindications of this approach.

### 2.1 Indications

- Cervical foraminal stenosis.
- Cervical foraminal disc herniation.

### 2.2 Contraindications

- Central disc herniation.
- Cervical myelopathy.
- Cervical central canal stenosis.
- Instability.
- Rheumatoid arthritis.
- Infectious disease.

## 3 Anesthesia and Positioning

General endotracheal anesthesia is recommended for the biportal endoscopic posterior cervical approach [4, 5]. If local anesthesia was to be used, there is a possibility that the patient can move during the operation, resulting in cord injury.

In this report, the biportal endoscopic posterior cervical approach was performed with the patient in the prone position with slight neck flexion (Fig. 2). The patient's face was protected from unwanted pressure during the operation using a polyurethane foam pad. Sometimes, we consider using a Mayfield head fixator for eyeball protection from unwanted pressure in more than three-level posterior cervical foraminotomies.

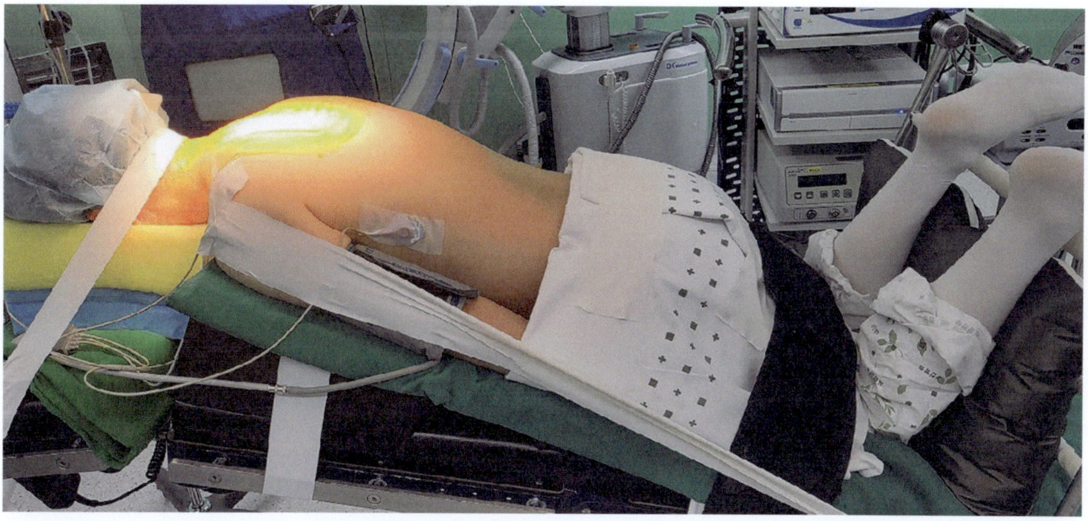

**Fig. 2** Patient positioning in the biportal endoscopic posterior cervical approach

Traction of the shoulder joint using plaster was helpful in demonstrating the lower cervical area via C-arm X-ray monitoring (Fig. 2).

## 4 Special Instrument

We strongly recommend the insertion of a working sheath to maintain continuous irrigation (Fig. 1), provided that interruption of irrigation patency may increase cervical epidural pressure. If a working sheath is inserted, irrigation fluid patency can be well maintained, and surgical instruments can be inserted and used smoothly. Radiofrequency (RF) probes are necessary for soft tissue dissection and bleeding control (Fig. 3). Specifically, the Ellman-type RF probe is useful for fine control of bleeding around the cervical nerve root and dura. The authors recommend using both a small-size RF tip and a 90-degree large-size RF tip. All general instruments for cervical spine surgery can be used for the biportal endoscopic cervical approach.

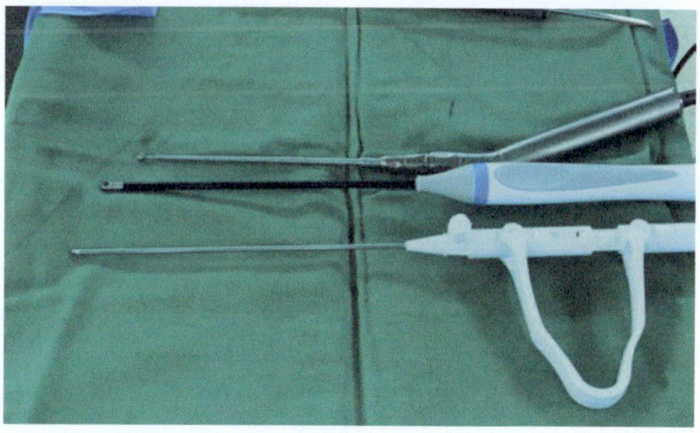

**Fig. 3** Radiofrequency probes and waterproof diamond drill for the biportal endoscopic approach

## 5 Surgical Steps of Posterior Cervical Foraminotomy by Biportal Endoscopy (Video 1)

### 5.1 Making Two Portals

Two portals were created under C-arm fluoroscopic monitoring. Usually, the working portal is made for the dominant hand, and the other endoscopic portal is made for the nondominant hand

[4]. Two portals were created on two pedicle levels. If a right-handed spine surgeon were to perform a left-sided posterior cervical foraminotomy at C6–7, an endoscopic portal was to be made over the left cranial C6 pedicle, and a working portal was to be made over the left caudal C7 pedicle in a lateral X-ray view (Fig. 4a). In an anteroposterior X-ray view, two portals were to be made on the lateral border of the pedicles (Fig. 4b). For our report, we first created a working portal. After incision of the skin and fascia using number 11 or 15 surgical blades, serial dilators were inserted under C-arm monitoring. Finally, a working sheath was inserted. A working sheath was necessary for drainage of the irrigation fluid. An endoscopic trocar was then inserted directly. The trocar should make contact and pass through a working portal in the working space. The endoscope was inserted into the trocar, and continuous saline irrigation was initiated.

## 5.2 Bone Work

Muscle and soft tissue dissection was performed using the RF ablation mode. Point V was first exposed before bone drilling [6]. This point consisted of the upper laminae, lower laminae, and facet joints (Fig. 5). A small ipsilateral laminotomy of both the upper and lower laminae as well as medial

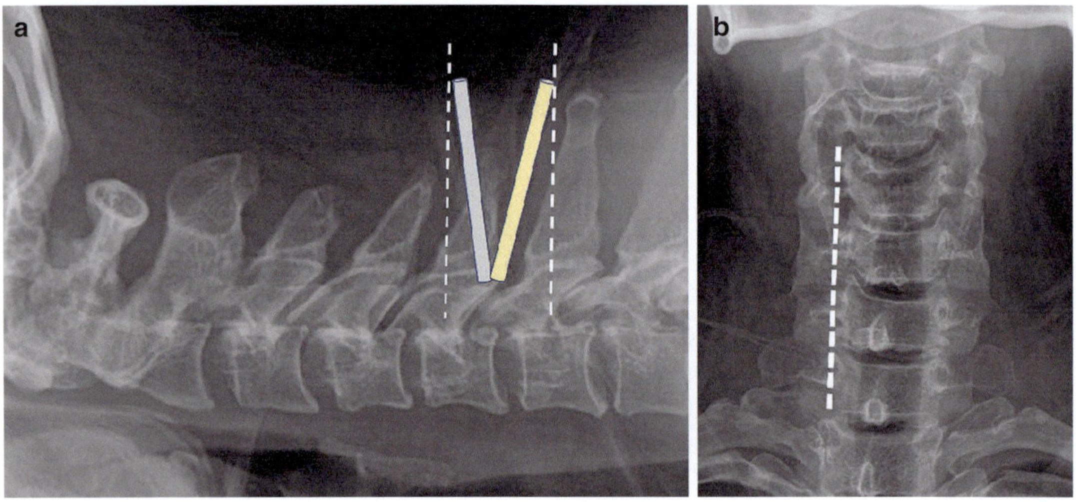


**Fig. 4** The locations of two portals in the biportal endoscopic cervical posterior approach, (**a**) In the lateral view, two portals are made superior to the pedicles. (**b**) In the anteroposterior view, two portals are create at medial border of pedicles

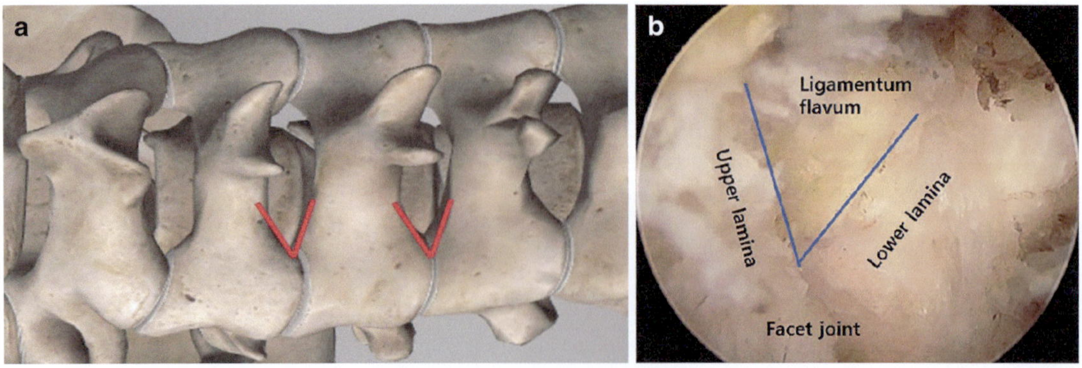


**Fig. 5** Point V of cervical spine. The point was used as the first landmark of biportal endoscopic posterior cervical foraminotomy (**a**). The point consists of the lower margin of the upper lamina, the upper margin of the lower lamina, and the facet joint (**b**)

facetectomy were performed using a diamond drill (Fig. 6). After thinning the bony structures by drilling, bony decompression was meticulously performed with 1- or 2-mm Kerrison rongeurs.

## 5.3 Decompression and Exposure of Dura and Nerve Root

The ligamentum flavum was partially removed to expose the dura and the cervical nerve roots (Fig. 7a). Sometimes, the peridural or adhesive membrane should be removed for clear exposure of the central dura and nerve root (Fig. 7b). If the patients had cervical foraminal stenosis, medial facetectomy was also performed until the medial half of the lateral mass has been removed.

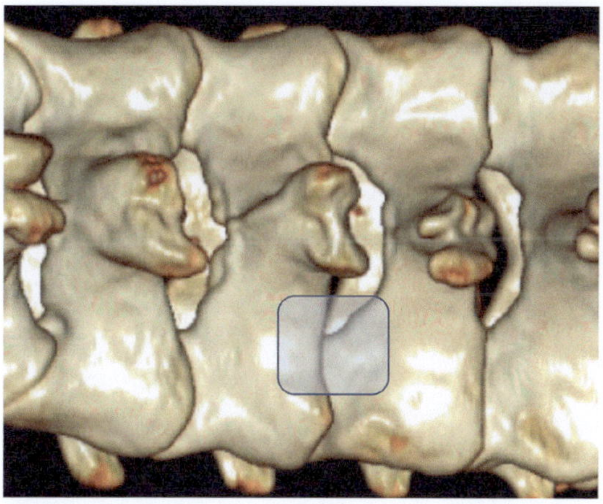

**Fig. 6** The area of cervical laminoforaminotomy. We usually perform small laminotomy with medial facetectomy (box)

## 5.4 Discectomy

After full exposure of the cervical nerve root, ruptured disc particles in the axillary area were explored using small hooks or dissectors (Fig. 8a, b). The cervical nerve root frequently consists of dual nerve roots, which include the sensory and motor nerve roots (Fig. 8c). In this report, the motor nerve root was located under the sensory nerve root. There was a possibility to mistake the motor nerve root as a ruptured disc particle or herniated disc. If the axillary space is very narrow, partial pediculotomy should be considered to reduce nerve retraction and to more easily remove disc particles (Fig. 8a). As such, the shoulder and axillary space of the nerve root were exposed for full decompression (Fig. 8d).

## 5.5 End of Operation

Prior to the removal of the two portals, we routinely infused a gelatin-thrombin matrix (Floseal)

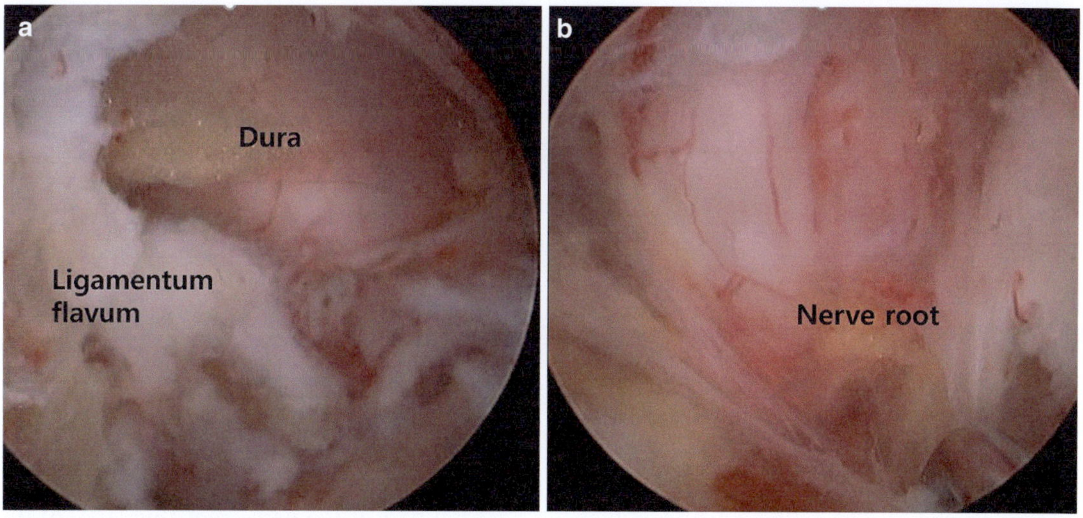


**Fig. 7** After partial removal of ligamentum flavum, dura was exposed (**a**). If the adhesive tissue or peridural membrane is removed, the cervical nerve root will be clearly exposed (**b**)

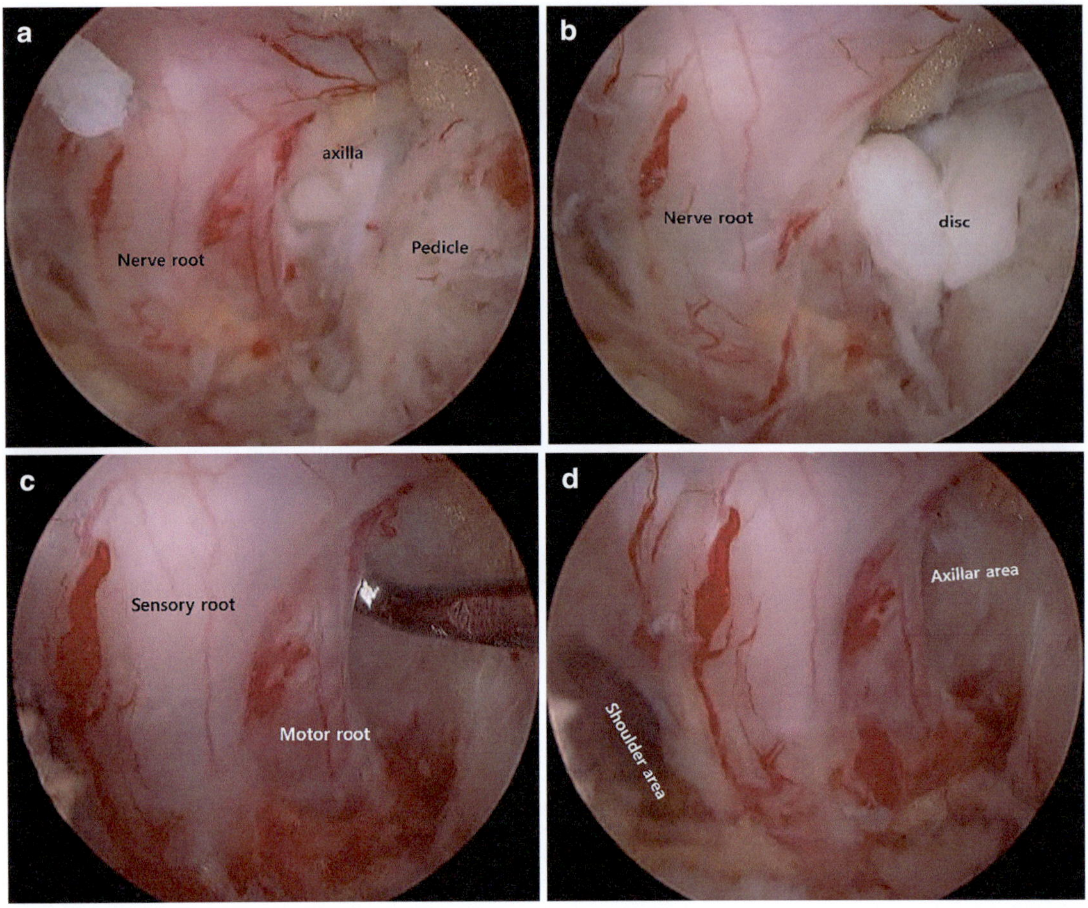


**Fig. 8** Before removal of ruptured disc particles, the nerve root, axillar area, and pedicle should be definitely demonstrated (**a**). Ruptured disc particles are usually located at the axillary area under the nerve root (**b**). The cervical nerve root frequently consists of sensory and motor nerve roots (**c**). After full decompression of the cervical nerve root, we can see the axillary and shoulder areas around the nerve root (**d**)

into the working space. After 2–3 min, the Floseal matrix was irrigated with irrigation fluid. A drainage catheter with a small diameter was then inserted to prevent postoperative epidural hematoma formation.

## 6 Illustrated Cases

1. **Case 1 (Video Clip 1):** A 43-year-old male patient presented with a tingling sensation and radicular pain in his left arm. Preoperative magnetic resonance imaging (MRI) showed foraminal disc herniation at the C6–7, left (Fig. 9a and b). The patient underwent biportal endoscopic posterior cervical foraminotomy with discectomy at C6–7, left (Fig. 9c, d, and e). The foraminal herniated disc was completely removed afterward (Fig. 9c and e). The patient's symptoms significantly improved postoperatively.
2. **Case 2 (Video Clip 2)**: A 67-year-old female patient complained of right arm pain. Preoperative MRI and computed tomography (CT) revealed foraminal stenosis with osteophyte at C6–7, right (Fig. 10a, b). We performed biportal endoscopic posterior cervical foraminotomy of the right C6–7 with partial pediculotomy of C7, right (Fig. 10c, d). We also partially removed the posterior osteophyte and performed decompression of the distal part of the nerve root (Fig. 10c, d). In this case, the C7 nerve root had dual nerve roots, including sensory and motor nerve

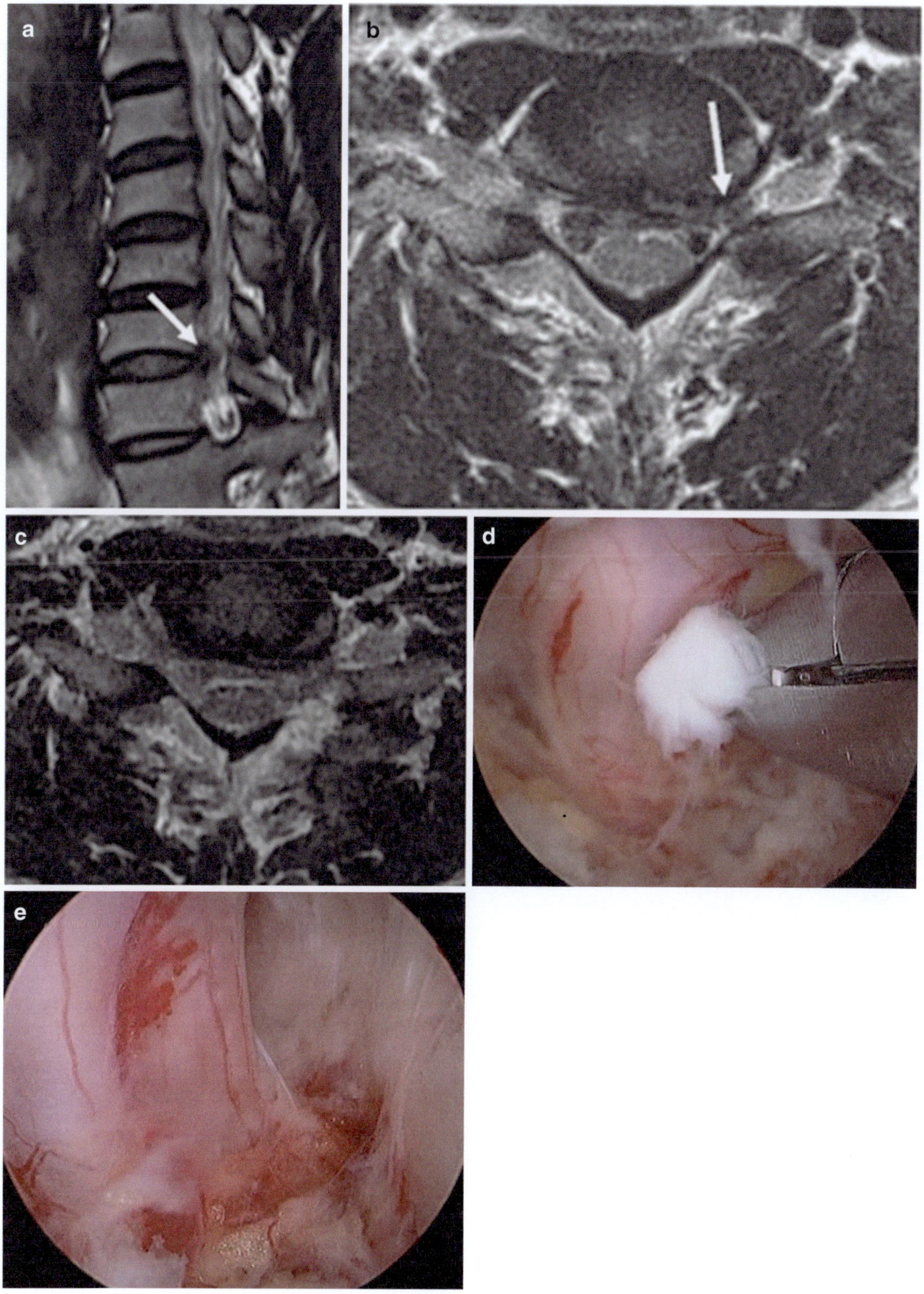


**Fig. 9** Preoperative foraminal (**a**) and axial (**b**) T2-weighted images showed foraminal ruptured disc of C6–7, left (arrow). We performed biportal endoscopic posterior cervical foraminotomy with discectomy (**c**, **d**, and **e**). After biportal endoscopic surgery, the ruptured disc was removed (**c** and **e**)

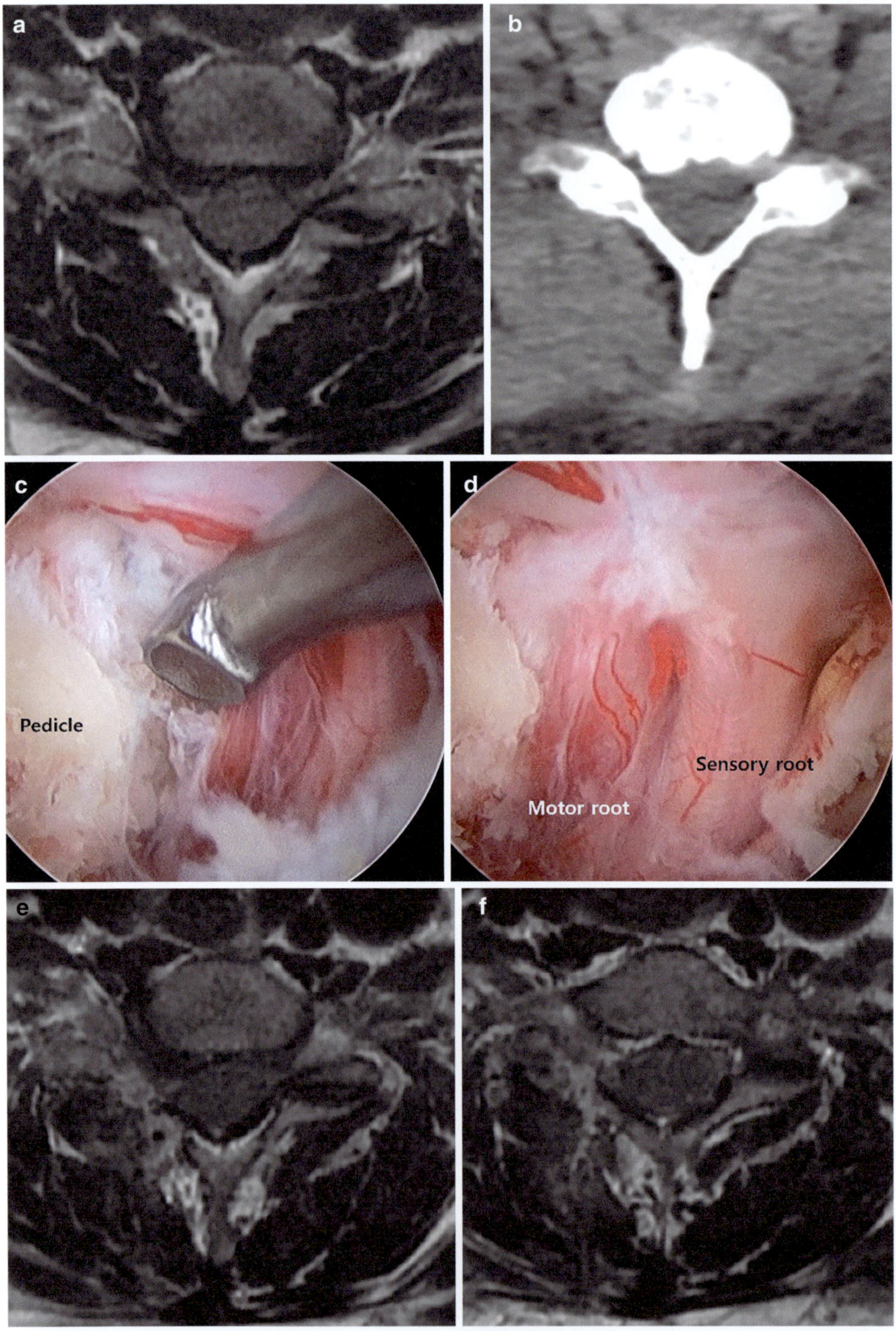


**Fig. 10** Preoperative MRI and CT showed foraminal stenosis of C6–7, right (**a**, **b**). We performed posterior cervical foraminotomy using the biportal endoscopic approach. We also performed partial pediculectomy and removal of osteophyte (**c**, **d**). Postoperative MRI depicted complete decompression of C7 nerve root, right (**e**, **f**)

roots (Fig. 10d). Postoperative MRI revealed complete decompression (Fig. 10e, f), and the patient's pain resolved postoperatively.

3. **Case 3 (Video Clip 3):** A 60-year-old female patient presented with a radiating pain in her right arm and scapular area. Preoperative MRI showed foraminal stenosis with ruptured disc herniation at the C6–7, right (Fig. 11a and b). Also, CT showed foraminal stenosis with endplate bony spur (Fig. 11c). We performed biportal endoscopic posterior cervical foraminotomy with discectomy of C6–7 right (Fig. 11d, e and f). Postoperative MRI revealed complete removal of disc fragment and decompression of nerve root (Fig. 11d).

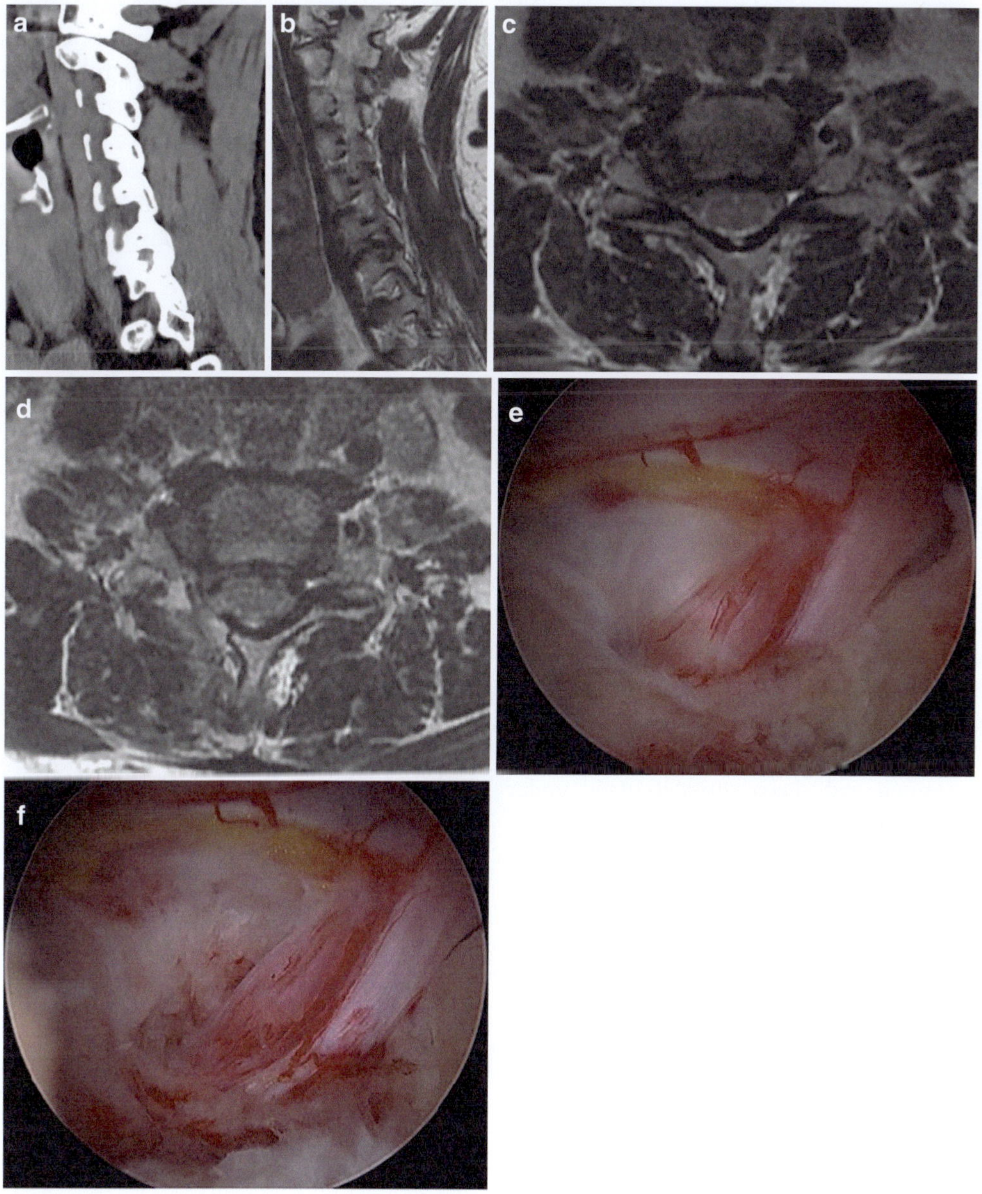

**Fig. 11** Preoperative CT (**a**) and MRI (**b**, **c**) showed foraminal stenosis C6–7 with ruptured disc herniation and endplate bony spur. We performed biportal endoscopic posterior cervical foraminotomy and discectomy with partial pediculotomy C6 and C7. (**d–f**) Endplate bony spur was completely removed by curettage and micro-osteotome (**d**, **f**)

## 7 Prevention and Management of Complications

The patency of continuous saline irrigation should be well maintained to prevent an increase in epidural pressure [4]. The irrigation fluid output must be well maintained, and the use of a working sheath is very helpful in ensuring this.

There is currently a high incidence of dual nerve roots occurring in the cervical spine, with the motor nerve root typically located beneath the sensory nerve root. Occasionally, a motor nerve root located below the sensory nerve root may be mistaken as a ruptured disc particle. Before removing the ruptured disc, the dura and nerve root axes should be clearly exposed.

For clear exposure of the cervical nerve root, the ligamentum flavum and the peridural membrane should be removed [7]. Since the peridural membrane contains an epidural vein, the epidural vein should be coagulated by RF before resection of the peridural membrane and ligamentum flavum.

Note that excessive traction on tvhe cervical nerve root can cause nerve root injury. Therefore, nerve root retraction should be minimized during removal of disc particles. After exposure of the dura, bleeding control was performed using a small-size RF tip. If bleeding control using RF is difficult, it is necessary to control the bleeding using Gelfoam or TachoSil pieces. A Floseal hemostatic matrix can also help control the bleeding. We recommend holding the drainage tube for 1–2 days to prevent postoperative hematoma.

## 8 Discussion (Surgical Tips and Pitfalls)

When creating the two portals of the biportal cervical endoscopic approach, we do not recommend the use of needles. Needling through the cervical interlaminar space may cause dural or cord injuries. Thus, we inserted serial dilators under C-arm real-time monitoring without needling. In the posterior cervical approach, there are several layers of muscle fascia that have to be passed. Therefore, insertion of serial dilators is more difficult than in the lumbar approach. Considering this, a deep fascia incision was made using a small and sharp surgical blade under C-arm monitoring.

Having surgical landmarks is important for safe and complete decompression of the cervical nerve roots. In this report, Point V was the first bony structure landmark that was used for adequate orientation in biportal endoscopic posterior cervical foraminotomy [6]. The medial and superior borders of the lower pedicle were used as surgical landmarks for optimal exposure of the cervical nerve root and axillary space. Sometimes, the pedicle is partially removed to ensure sufficient space in the axillary area for optimal decompression and ruptured disc removal.

## References


1. Heo DH, Lee DC, Kim HS, Park CK, Chung H. Clinical results and complications of endoscopic lumbar interbody fusion for lumbar degenerative disease: a meta-analysis. World Neurosurg. 2021;145:396–404.
2. Kim JY, Hong HJ, Lee DC, Kim TH, Hwang JS, Park CK. Comparative analysis of three types of minimally invasive posterior cervical foraminotomy for foraminal stenosis, uniportal endoscopy, biportal endoscopy, and microsurgery: radiologic and mid-term clinical outcomes. Neurospine. 2022;19:603.
3. Heo DH, Lee DC, Park CK. Comparative analysis of three types of minimally invasive decompressive surgery for lumbar central stenosis: biportal endoscopy, uniportal endoscopy, and microsurgery. Neurosurg Focus. 2019;46(5):E9.
4. Kim J, Heo DH, Lee DC, Chung HT. Biportal endoscopic unilateral laminotomy with bilateral decompression for the treatment of cervical spondylotic myelopathy. Acta Neurochir. 2021;163(9):2537–43.
5. Song KS, Lee CW. The Biportal endoscopic posterior cervical inclinatory Foraminotomy for cervical radiculopathy: technical report and preliminary results. Neurospine. 2020;17(Suppl 1):S145–s53.
6. Kim JY, Kim DH, Lee YJ, Jeon JB, Choi SY, Kim HS, et al. Anatomical importance between neural structure and bony landmark: clinical importance for posterior endoscopic cervical Foraminotomy. Neurospine. 2021;18(1):139–46.
7. Bosscher HA, Grozdanov PN, Warraich II, MacDonald CC, Day MR. The anatomy of the peridural membrane of the human spine. Anat Rec (Hoboken). 2021;304(4):677–91.

# Biportal Endoscopic Posterior Cervical Inclinatory Foraminotomy and Discectomy

Kwan Su Song and Cheol Woong Park

**Abstract**

The minimally invasive posterior cervical foraminotomy procedure has the advantage of maintaining cervical range of motion and minimizing adjacent segment degeneration. The posterior cervical approach has commonly treated cervical spondylotic radiculopathy using a tubular retractor or endoscopic systems. The posterior endoscopic cervical foraminotomy (PECF) has shown the benefits of minimal invasiveness and favorable surgical outcomes. Facet joint preservation during the posterior cervical foraminotomy is critical for postoperative segmental stability. However, excessive facet joint resection is inevitable for sufficient neural decompression in patients who have severe osseous foraminal stenosis. Recently, the advanced technique of biportal endoscopic posterior cervical inclinatory foraminotomy (PCIF) was reported and showed feasible surgical procedures and favorable clinical outcomes. This technique may be an excellent surgical option for treating severe osseous foraminal stenosis while preserving the facet joint.

**Keywords**

Inclinatory · Foraminotomy · Biportal Endoscopy · Radiculopathy · Cervical spine

## 1 Introduction

The cervical nerve roots pass the neuroforamen and curve downward after exiting the neuroforamen near the vertebral artery. Any spondylotic lesions can cause cervical radiculopathy in the neuroforamen, such as hypertrophied uncinate process, superior articular process (SAP), and herniated disc. Therefore, foraminotomy should be extended until the nerve root exits the neuroforamen for sufficient nerve root decompression [1].

During PCIF surgery, the surgeon stands on the contralateral side of the target lesion to make an inclinatory surgical route. This inclined angle enables successful distal foraminal decompression under magnified endoscopic view because surgical instruments and the endoscopic drill access the foramen parallel to the exiting nerve root. Therefore, more safe and comfortable bony decompression is possible without neural compression commonly caused by the repetitive punching of the facet joint. Furthermore, during biportal endoscopic PCIF, the inclined surgical

**Supplementary Information** The online version contains supplementary material available at https://doi.org/10.1007/978-981-99-1133-2_9.

K. S. Song
Department of Neurosurgery, Him-Plus Hospital, Suncheon, South Korea

C. W. Park (✉)
Department of Neurosurgery, Daejeon Woori Hospital, Daejeon, South Korea



H. S. Kim et al. (eds.), *Advanced Technique of Endoscopic Cervical and Thoracic Spine Surgery*,
https://doi.org/10.1007/978-981-99-1133-2_9

route enables facet undercutting to preserve the facet joint and joint capsule as much as we can. Since facet joint plays an important role in cervical stability, decompression of the cervical nerve root while preserving facet joint as much as possible has a significant impact on postoperative prognosis [2, 3]. This advanced technology provides sufficient neural decompression of the entire neuroforamen while preserving the facet joint [4].

This chapter describes the step-by-step PCIF surgical procedure using video and pictures.

## 2 Indications and Contraindications

The indications for biportal endoscopic PCIF are similar to those for PECF. The unilateral cervical radiculopathy due to foraminal stenosis with or without herniated disc that failed conservative treatments [5]. Biportal endoscopic PCIF can treat severe osseous foraminal stenosis, including distal foraminal lesions, even with a high risk of excess facet violation during PECF [6].

The exclusion criteria are central lesions, segmental instability, and severe kyphotic deformity. Infection, tumor, or fracture in the region of the cervical segment is also considered a contraindication.

This contralateral approach is affected by the anatomical variation of the spinous process. If the spinous process is deviated to the target lesion or has a broad base, instruments' access to the contralateral side is limited by the deformed spinous process (Fig. 1a, b).

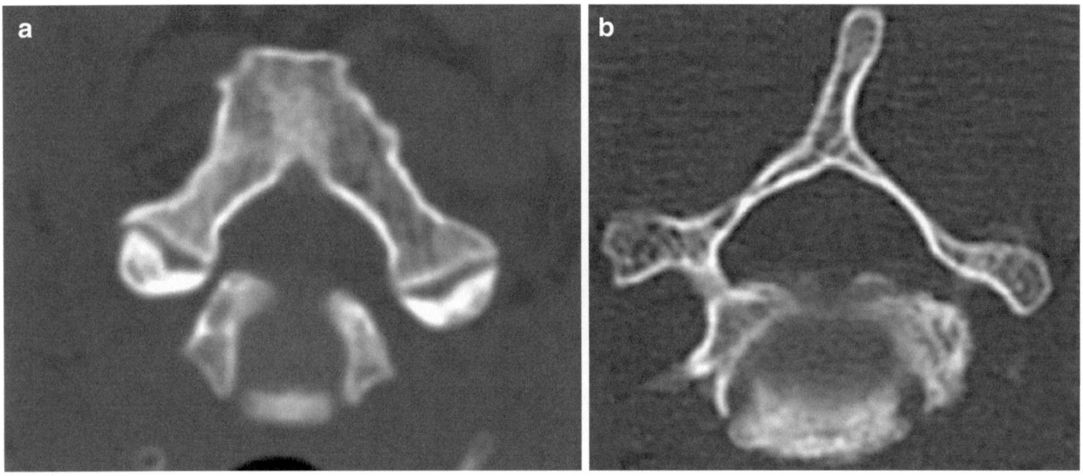


**Fig. 1** Anatomical variation of the spinous process. A broad base of the spinous process (**a**) and deviation to the target lesion (**b**) limit the biportal endoscopic PICF surgery

## 3 Special Instruments

(a) Endoscopic diamond drill (Fig. 2a, b)
   - 3.5-mm diamond burr (ELNA 4 Aesculap, B Braun, Germany)
   - 3-mm bendable diamond burr (All Care, Korea)

(b) Scope retractor (MD & Company, South Korea) (Fig. 2c)

(c) Indian knife (Fig. 2d)

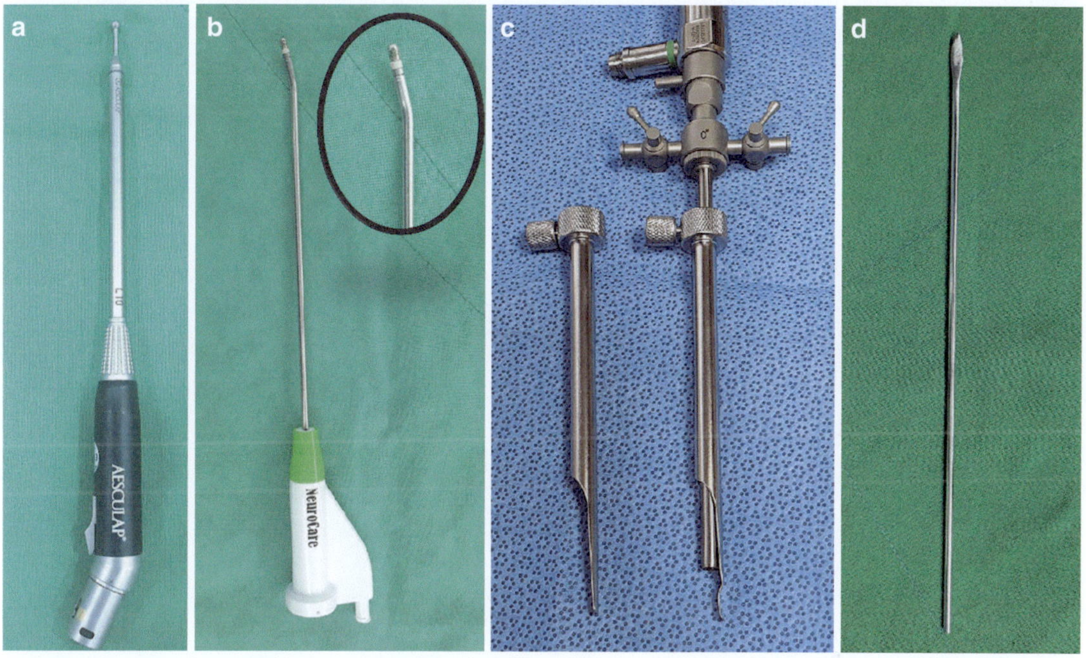


**Fig. 2** The special equipment for biportal endoscopic PCIF. (**a**) The 3.5-mm spherical diamond burr, (**b**) 3.0-mm conical diameter bendable diamond burr, (**c**) scope retractor, and (**d**) Indian knife for annulotomy

## 4 Anesthesia and Position

The patient underwent surgery under general anesthesia in the prone position on an H-shaped pillow, preventing high abdominal pressure. A compression-free sponge device was placed under the face of the patient, and the neck was slightly flexed (Fig. 3a). Without skull fixation, the slightly flexed neck position can be maintained using skin tape. The bilateral shoulder was obliquely pulled downward and fixed on the surgical table using the skin tape to confirm the lower cervical levels on the C-arm lateral images. The upper trunk was elevated by tiling the table for proper venous return during surgery (Fig. 3b).

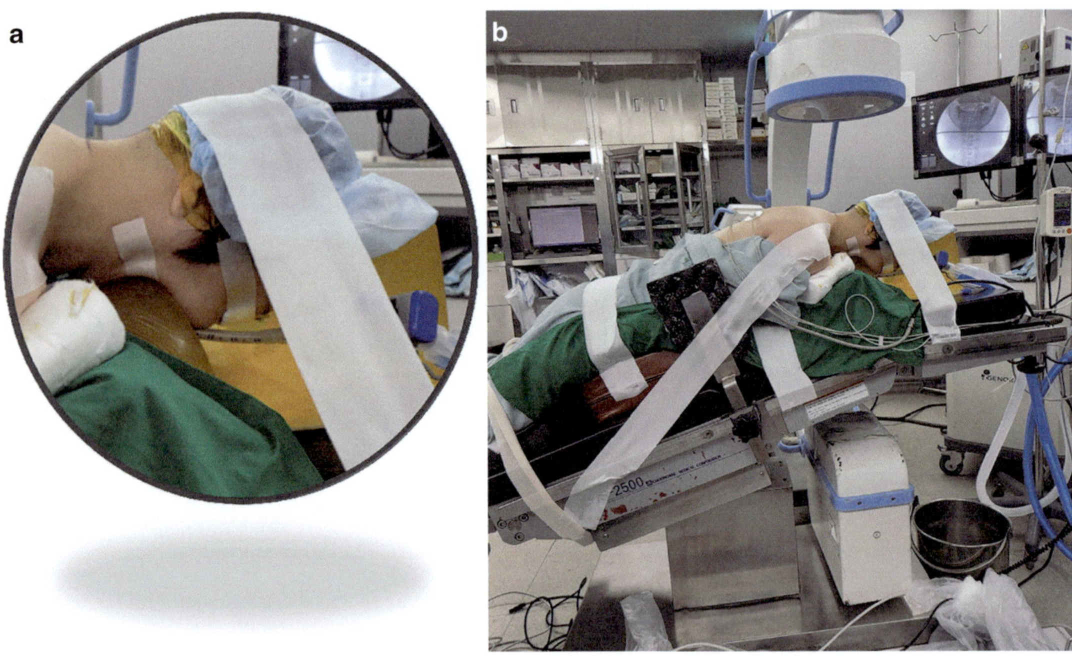


**Fig. 3** The surgical position and setting. (**a**) The eyeball and chin must be protected by corneal ointment and a facial gel pad, respectively. (**b**) Neck and bilateral shoulders are fixed with skin tape. The upper trunk is elevated for proper venous return

## 5 Surgical Steps of Biportal Endoscopic PCIF

- **Skin Incision and Making Two Portals**

  The surgeon stands on the opposite side of the target lesion. Under the guidance of C-arm fluoroscopy, two vertical skin incisions are made in the midline tip part of the adjacent upper and lower spinous process (Fig. 4a). The 18-gauge needles are used to confirm the proper location of two portals and surgical route for the target lesion before skin incision (Fig. 4b, c). Vertical fascia incisions were made along the lateral border of the spinous process through the free space made after subcutaneous dissection. The distance between the two portals is about 2–3 cm. Serial dilators were inserted at the working portal, and then a working cannula was inserted along the serial dilator.
- **Laminotomy (Video 1)**

  The docking point of the endoscope and instrument is the confluence of the cranial laminar, caudal laminar, and medial border of the facet joint, which is called anatomical "V-point" [7]. After soft tissue dissection using the forceps and radiofrequency (RF) probe, the distal end of the endoscope and instruments was met on the V-point with an inclined surgical route of 20–25° (Fig. 5a, b, and c).

  Firstly, the inferior border of the upper-level lamina is drilled around V-point until exposing the proximal end of the ligamentum flavum (Fig. 5c). Drilling the superior edge of the lower-level lamina is then performed until confirming the distal end of the ligamentum flavum (Video 1, Fig. 6a, b).
- **Foraminotomy (Video 2)**

  After initial laminotomy, sufficient space is created for free accessing of the instruments and endoscope to the foraminal area. Subsequently, bony drilling was laterally extended for distal foraminal decompression by undercutting the facet joint while preserving the outer part of the facet joint using a cone-shaped 3-mm diamond drill (Fig. 6c). The medial part of the facet joint was drilled

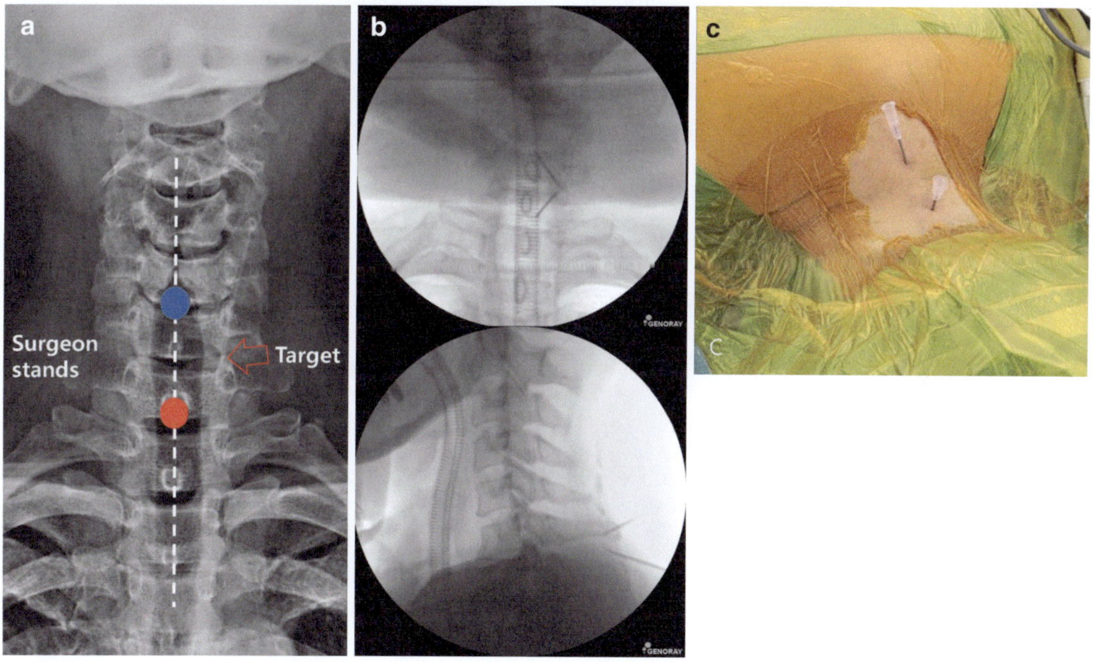


**Fig. 4** Skin incision sites for making two portals. (**a**) The two-skin incisions are made in the midline tip parts of one level upper and lower spinous process (blue circle: endoscopic portal; red circle: working portal). (**b**, **c**) The 18-gauge needles are used to confirm the proper location of two portals and surgical route for the target lesion before skin incision

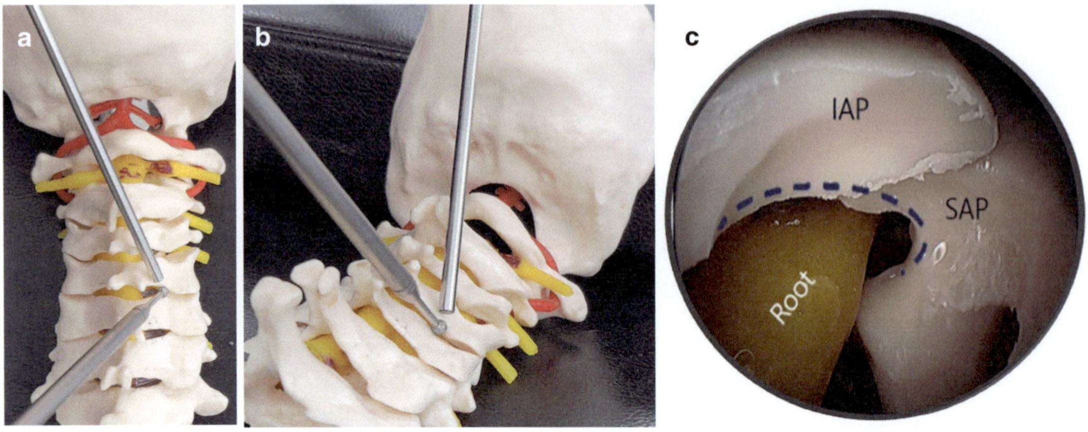


**Fig. 5** Docking of endoscope and instruments with triangulation. (**a**, **b**) The endoscope and instruments are initially docked on the V-point. The inclined approach angle from the midline entry points to the target lesion is approximately 20–25°. (**c**) Endoscopic view from the inclined surgical route is represented by undercutting the facet joint

similar to thin paper so that contour of the nerve root can be seen through the thinned inner cortical bone. Bony drilling is extended to the distal foraminal part until exposing the lateral border of the caudal lamina's pedicle. Circumferential bony drilling was completed along the contour of the exiting nerve root. Remained thinned inner cortical bone can be easily removed with 1-mm punches, chisel, and curettes without excessive neural manipulation (Video 2, Fig. 6d). Bony drilling should be performed before removing the ligamentum flavum to prevent neural structures.

- **Flavectomy (Video 3)**

  The ligamentum flavum is detached from the drilled bony margin using the dissectors and then removed with forceps as the last surgical step (Fig. 6e). The epidural vessel is coagulated using the RF probe at the time of bleeding is found. It is difficult to coagulate the floating epidural vessel close to the spinal cord due to the risk of neural heating injury. The RF probe elevates the epidural vessel away from the spinal cord and coagulation is then performed (Video 3, Fig. 6f).

- **Discectomy (Video 4)**

  After the flavectomy, we explore the disc space under the nerve root and thecal sac using the hook and dissectors. Annulotomy is performed using the RF probe or endoscopic knife named "Indian knife" while protecting neural structures with a scope retractor. Subsequently, the discectomy was performed using the hook and forceps (Fig. 7a–e). If thick peridural adhesions still entrap the nerve root and limit the restoration of the natural downward course, the adhesion band should be removed using forceps and dissectors. The lateral endpoint of foraminal decompression can be confirmed using the intraoperative C-arm AP view (Fig. 7f). The vertebral artery is occasionally seen beside the exiting nerve root due to the inclined endoscopic view of the extraforaminal area (Fig. 7g). A closed drainage tube is inserted to prevent the surgical site hematoma and is usually removed one day after surgery. The wound is closed with suture materials or skin tape. The patients wear the soft neck collar for one or two weeks.

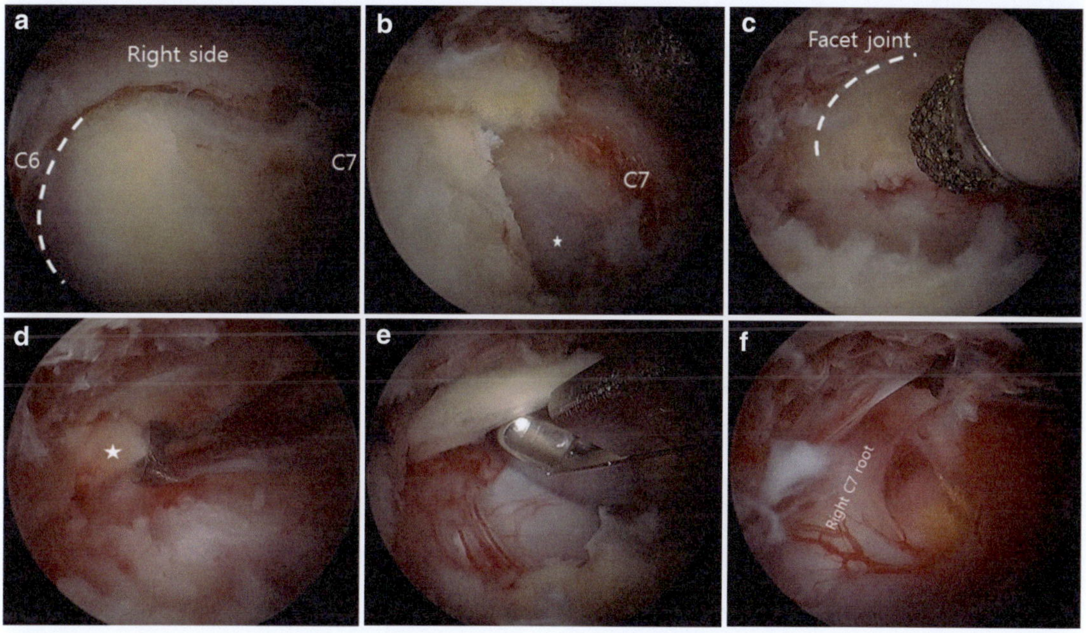


**Fig. 6** Intraoperative endoscopic views of biportal endoscopic PCIF at the right C5–6 level. (**a**) Drilling the inferior border of the upper-level (C6) lamina. The proximal end of the ligamentum flavum (white dotted line) was exposed. (**b**) Lower level laminotomy was extended more caudally pass through the distal end of ligamentum flavum until the dura and nerve root can be seen through the thinned lamina (asterisk). (**c**) Drilling the medial part of the facet joint along the facet joint line (white dotted line). (**d**) Tip of SAP is removed using a small curette. (**e**) Flavectomy. (**f**) RF probe was used for epidural vessel coagulation and epidural dissection

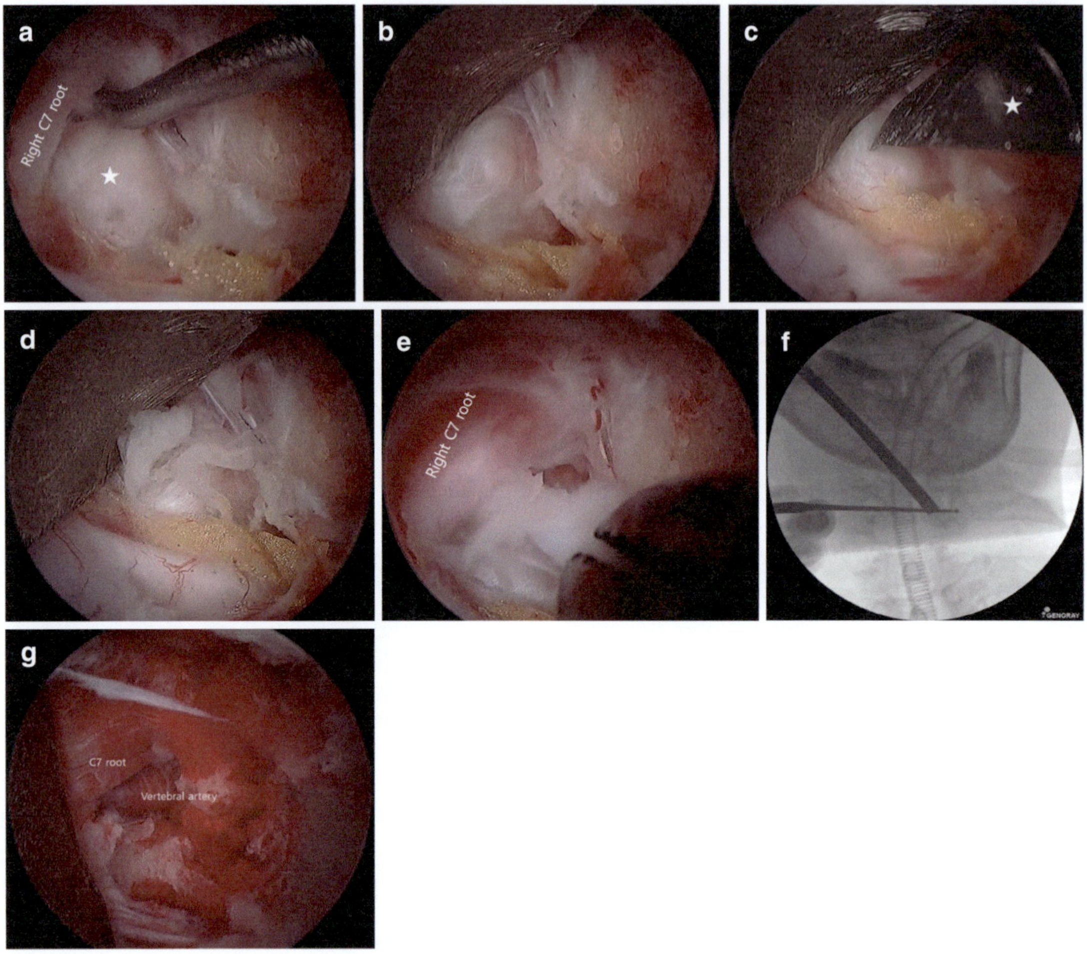


**Fig. 7** Intraoperative endoscopic view of discectomy at the right C5-6 level. (**a**) Herniated disc (asterisk) was found at the axillary area of the right C5 nerve root. Pediculotomy was performed to make space for instruments (blue asterisk). (**b**) Nerve root retraction using the scope retractor. (**c**) Annulotomy using the Indian Kinfe (asterisk). (**d**) The scope retractor was used for squeezing the herniated disc particle. (**e**) Discectomy was performed through the space made by partial pediculotomy (blue asterisk). (**f**) Extent of foraminotomy was confirmed with intraoperative C-arm image. (**g**) Occasionally, the vertebral artery is found

## 6 Illustrated Cases

### 6.1 Case 1: Biportal Endoscopic PCIF on the Right Side of the C5-6 and C6-7 Levels

A 43-year-old woman presented with right shoulder pain, right scapular pain, and numbness of the right upper extremity about one year ago. The patient complained the radiating pain in the right arm through the C6 and C7 dermatomes. Motor power of right elbow flexion was decreased to grade 4 (out of grade 5). Spurling's test was positive. Preoperative magnetic resonance imaging (MRI) and computed tomography (CT) showed foraminal stenosis with herniated disc on the right side of the C5-6 and C6-7 levels (Fig. 8a–e). We performed the biportal endoscopic PCIF and discectomy at the C5-6 and C6-7 levels from the patient's left side. Postoperative MRI showed the sufficiently decompressed nerve root after foraminotomy and discectomy in both cervical levels (Fig. 8f–h). Postoperative CT images revealed the extent of bony decompression and well-preserved facet joints (Fig. 8i–k). The herniated disc was found in the axillary part of the nerve root and successfully removed (Fig. 8l, m). Postoperatively, symptoms of neurological deficits and radicular pain were significantly improved.

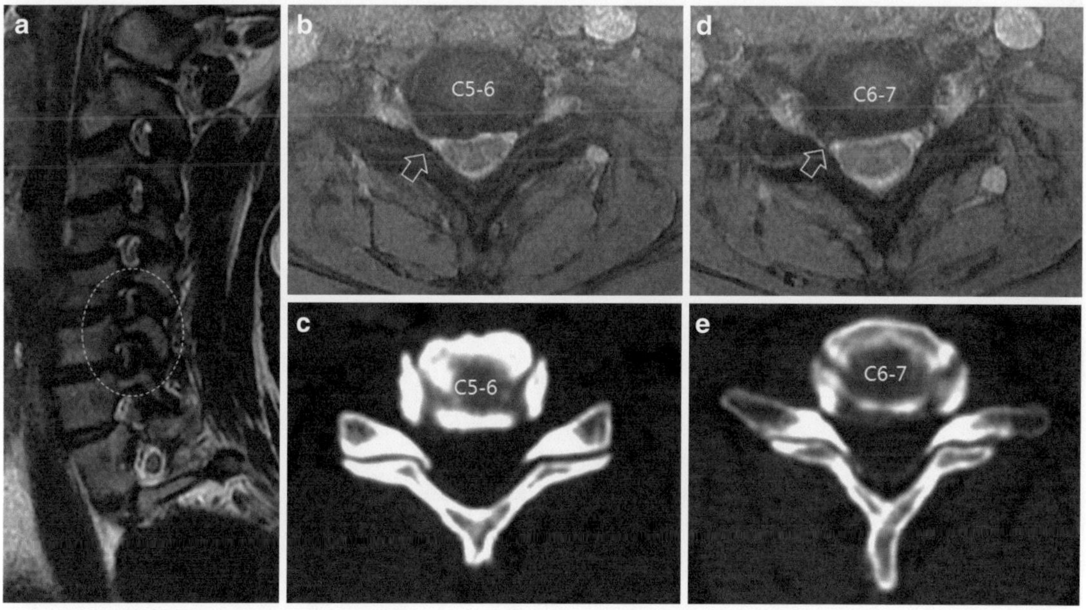


**Fig. 8** An illustrated case of biportal endoscopic PCIF at the C5-6 and C6-7 levels. (**a**) The preoperative right foraminal MRI shows foraminal stenosis and herniated disc (white dashed circle) at the C5-6 and C6-7 levels. (**b**, **c**) The preoperative T2-weighted axial MRI showed foraminal stenosis with herniated disc (open white arrow). (**d**, **e**) Preoperative CT image revealed osseous foraminal stenosis. (**f**–**h**) Postoperative MRI show sufficient foraminal decompression at the right C5-6 and C6-7 level (yellow dotted circle). (**i**–**k**) Postoperative CT images revealed the extent of bony decompression (open arrows) and well-preserved facet joints. (**l**) The intraoperative endoscopic view showed herniated disc with a compressed C5 nerve root (asterisk). (**m**) After discectomy, nerve root compression was resolved, and the downward course of the nerve root was restored. The facet joint was illustrated with a white dashed line

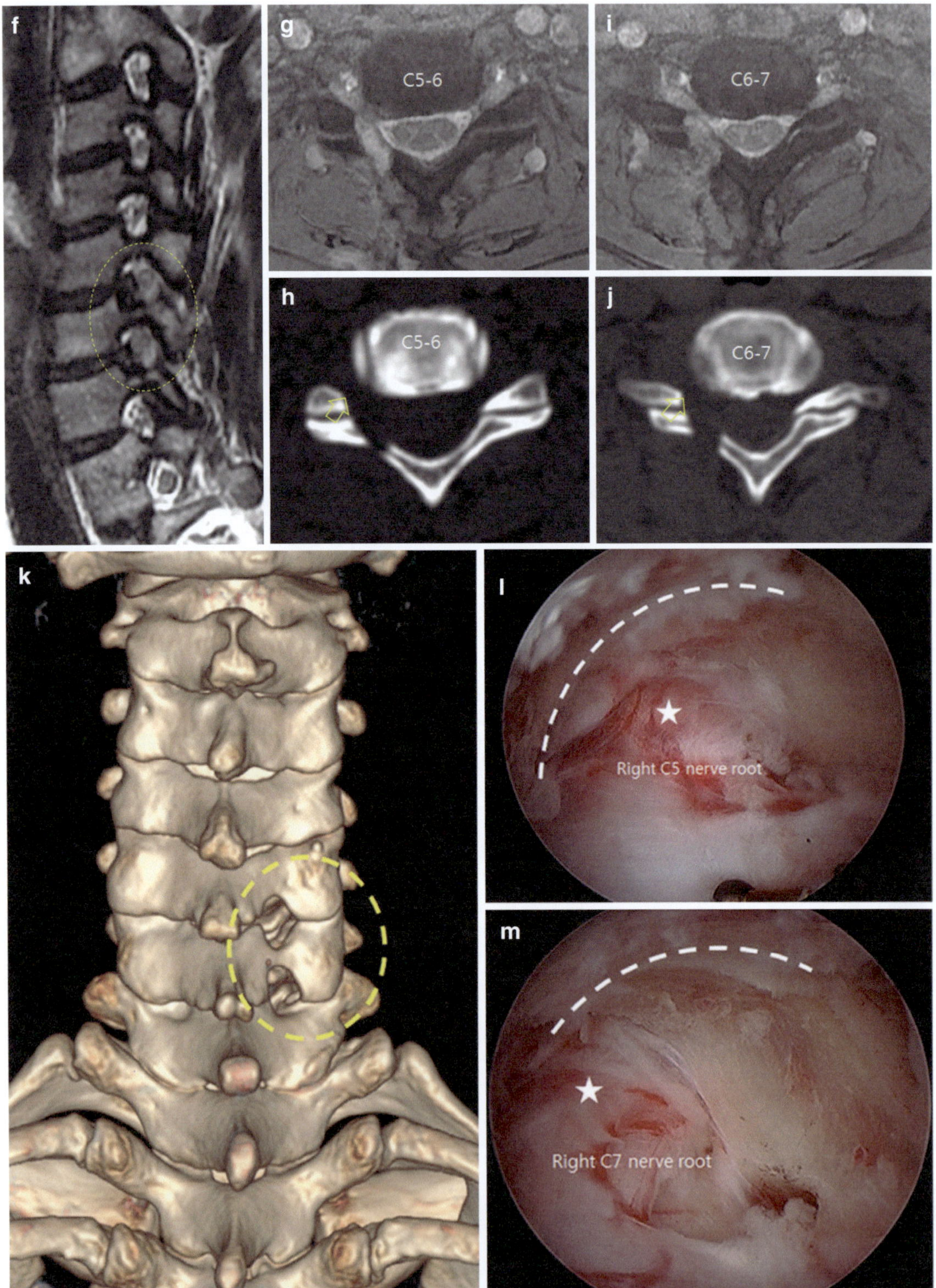


**Fig. 8** (continued)

### 6.2 Case 2: Biportal Endoscopic PCIF on the Left Side of the C5-6 Level

A 47-year-old woman presented with left upper back and radiating pain in the right arm for two years. The patient had a motor weakness (grade 4 out of 5) of left elbow flexion and radiating arm pain through the left C6 dermatome. Preoperative MRI and CT images showed osseous foraminal stenosis at the left C5-6 level (Fig. 9a–c). We performed the biportal endo-

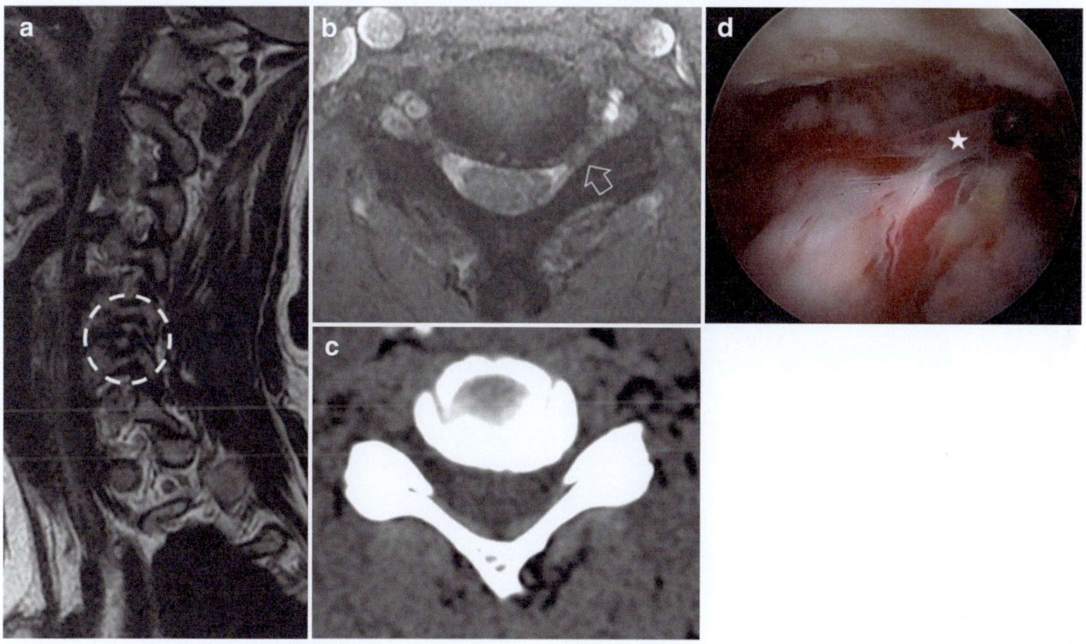


**Fig. 9** An illustrated case of biportal endoscopic PCIF at the left C5-6 level. (**a**) The preoperative left foraminal MRI shows foraminal stenosis at the C5-6 level. (**b**, **c**) Preoperative axial MRI and CT image reveals the foraminal stenosis with bony spur (open white arrow). (**d**, **e**) Postoperative MRI shows sufficient foraminal decompression at the left C5-6 level (white circle). (**f**) Postoperative CT images revealed the inclined surgical route made by undercutting the facet joint (white dotted line). (**g**) The RF probe removed a thick peridural adhesion band (white asterisk) to release the nerve root

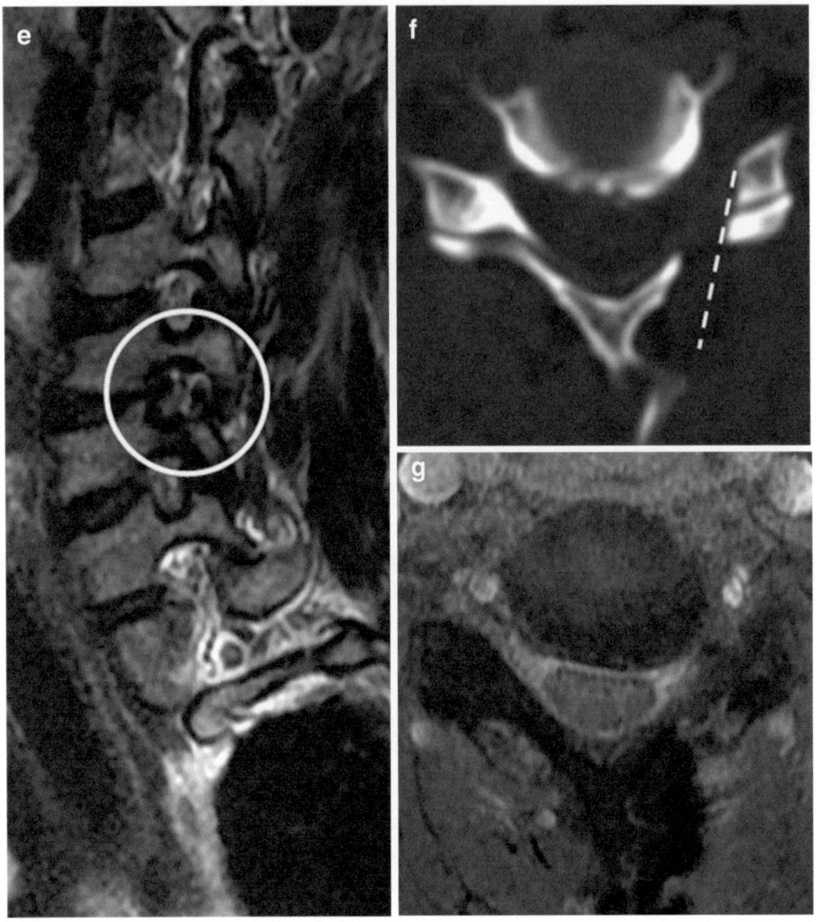


**Fig. 9** (continued)

scopic PCIF and discectomy at the C5-6 level from the patient's right side. Postoperative MRI and CT images revealed adequately decompressed foraminal space and well-preserved facet joint (Fig. 9d–f). A severe peridural adhesion band that entrapped the C6 nerve root was found (Fig. 9g). Motor weakness and radicular pain were improved after surgery.

# 7 Prevention and Management of Complications

## 7.1 Bleeding

Hemostasis is essential to maintain a clear endoscopic vision for safe procedures intimate with neural structures. If the bleeding focus is found, we should stop the bleeding immediately using the RF probe (Fig. 10) or bone wax. The massive use of RF on the epidural vessels may induce spinal cord injury, and we recommend the foamy hemostatic agent for diffuse and multifocal bleeding.

Proper venous return decreases epidural venous congestion, reducing the epidural bleeding from the vein and cancellus bone. We recommend using the H-shape pillow to lower the abdominal pressure and elevate the upper trunk for proper venous flow.

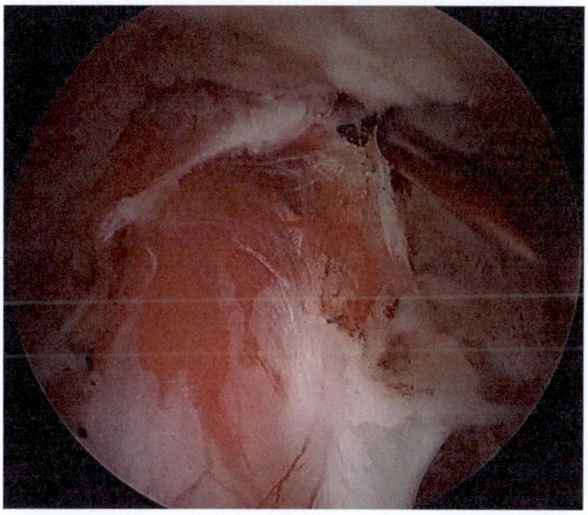

**Fig. 10** Coagulation of the epidural vessel. The epidural vessels are elevated away from the neural structure using the RF probe and then coagulated to prevent thermal injury

## 7.2 Dural Tear

Most of the dural tears occur during bony drilling intimate with neural structures. Therefore, we recommend removing the ligamentum flavum after finishing the bony drilling to protect the neural structures.

Incidental durotomy sites may not be identified because infused saline presses the dura and conceal the durotomy site. If durotomy is suspected during procedure, we should explore the neural structures to find the durotomy site.

Small dural tear can be repaired using a fibrin sealant patch (Fig. 11) or nonpenetrating clips. If the primary dura repair fails, endoscopic surgery should be converted to open microscopic surgery for successful dural repair.

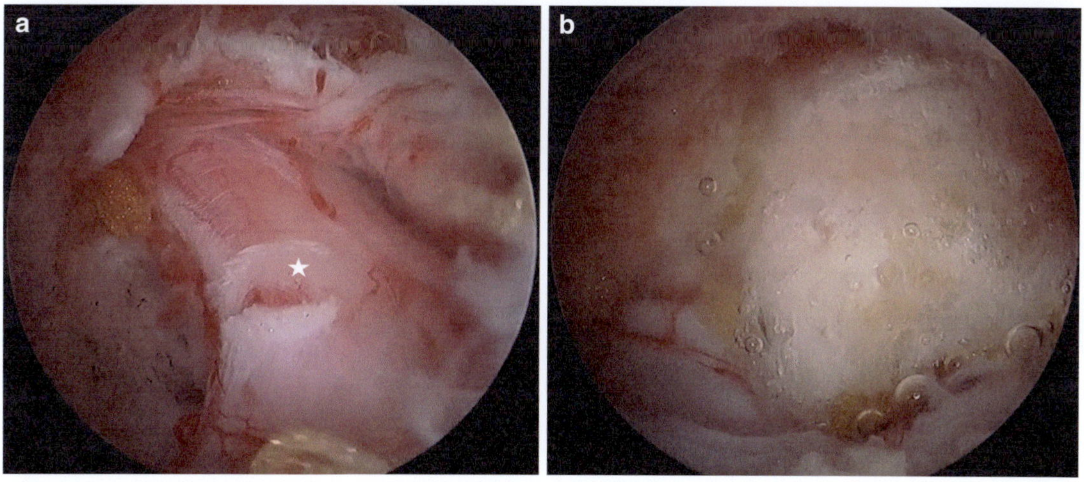

**Fig. 11** Sealing the dural tear. Durotomy occurred during bony drilling (asterisk) (**a**). The durotomy site was repaired using a fibrin sealant patch (**b**)

## 7.3 Nerve Root Retraction Injury

If the prominent bony spur and herniate disc compress the nerve root, neural retraction can induce the neural root injury in the vulnerable state.

We recommend performing the partial pediculotomy of the superior-medial part and continued vertebrotomy using the 3-mm diamond drill to create space for safe instrument use. Bony spur and herniated disc can be removed through the constructed space using forceps and small curettes with minimal neural manipulation [7].

## 7.4 Insufficient Neural Decompression

The ideal goal of the posterior cervical foraminotomy is to achieve sufficient neural decompression while preserving the facet joint as much as we can. In this context, biportal endoscopic PCIF can be an excellent surgical option. However, if we focus on facet preservation, insufficient neural decompression may occur, and preoperative symptoms may not be resolved. Therefore, we recommend prioritizing sufficient bony decompression over facet preservation for complete neural decompression, even in the biportal endoscopic PCIF.

# 8 Surgical Tips and Pitfalls

The anatomical orientation of this technique is different a lot from ipsilateral posterior cervical foraminotomy. Therefore, identifying the V-point is critical to the success of the operation. We should consider the variation of the V-point depending on the degree of the patient's neck flexion.

Using conventional punches and straight instruments in the narrow inclined operating space is not easy. Small curved curettes and chisel are efficiently utilized for bony decompression in the distal foraminal area.

This technique is technically demanding and has limitations depending on the anatomical variations. Therefore, we should determine the indication with preoperative MRI and CT images.

**Conflict of Interest** None

**Disclosure of Funding** None

# References

1. Demondion X, Lefebvre G, Fisch O, Vandenbussche L, Cepparo J, Balbi V. Radiographic anatomy of the intervertebral cervical and lumbar foramina (vessels and variants). Diagn Interv Imaging. 2012;93(9):690–7.
2. Voo LM, Kumaresan S, Yoganandan N, Pintar FA, Cusick JF. Finite element analysis of cervical facetectomy. Spine. 1997;22(9):964–9.
3. Zdeblick TA, Zou D, Warden KE, McCabe R, Kunz D, Vanderby R. Cervical stability after foraminotomy. A biomechanical in vitro analysis. J Bone Joint Surg Am. 1992;74(1):22–7.
4. Heo J, Chang JC, Park HK. Long-term outcome of posterior cervical inclinatory foraminotomy. J Korean Neurosurg Soc. 2016;59(4):374–8.
5. Leheta F, Kazner E, Kollmannsberger A. Therapy of cervical nerve root compression syndromes. Indication, technic and results of foraminotomy. Fortschr Med. 1973;91(17):725–31.
6. Song KS, Lee CW. The biportal endoscopic posterior cervical inclinatory foraminotomy for cervical radiculopathy: technical report and preliminary results. Neurospine. 2020;17(Suppl 1):S145–s53.
7. Kim HS, Wu PH, Lee YJ, Kim DH, Kim JY, Lee JH, et al. Safe route for cervical approach: partial pediculotomy, partial vertebrotomy approach for posterior endoscopic cervical foraminotomy and discectomy. World Neurosurg. 2020;140:e273–e82.

# Cervical Laminectomy via Interspinous Approach by Unilateral Biportal Endoscopy

Man Kyu Park and Sang-Kyu Son

**Abstract**

The conventional posterior approach for cervical spondylotic myelopathy has several disadvantages caused by posterior cervical muscle and ligament injury. Compared with the conventional posterior approach, cervical laminectomy by unilateral biportal endoscopy (UBE) is advantageous because it involves smaller skin incisions, preserved paraspinal muscle and ligamentous complex, and a better high-resolution magnification. Cervical laminectomy by UBE comprises bilateral decompression using the unilateral approach. However, contralateral decompression performed using the sublaminar approach such as lumbar unilateral laminotomy for bilateral decompression is associated with a risk of cord injury in cervical spine. Therefore, bilateral subtotal laminectomy via the interspinous approach is recommended. In this chapter, we presented the general indications for cervical laminectomy by UBE and its correlated surgical techniques. Moreover, whether the procedure is safe and can prevent cord injury was investigated.

**Keywords**

Biportal · Cervical myelopathy · Cervical Endoscopy · Minimally invasive surgery

## 1 Advantages of this Approach

Cervical spondylotic myelopathy (CSM) is the most common type of cervical spinal stenosis and often requires surgical procedure [1]. Traditionally, CSM is managed with cervical laminectomy or laminoplasty [2]. However, the conventional posterior approach has several disadvantages caused by posterior cervical muscle and ligament injury. The complications of this approach may include persistent neck pain and loss of cervical lordosis [3]. To address these issues, less invasive techniques such as muscle-preserving selective laminectomy, microendoscopic laminectomy, and posterior cervical percutaneous channel endoscopic decompression are used, and they are associated with good outcomes [1, 4, 5].

The indications for unilateral biportal endoscopy (UBE) techniques have expanded to conditions including lumbar or thoracic degenerative disease and, more recently, cervical spondylosis causing myelopathy [6–9]. Compared with the

**Supplementary Information** The online version contains supplementary material available at https://doi.org/10.1007/978-981-99-1133-2_10.

M. K. Park · S.-K. Son (✉)
Department of Neurosurgery, Good Moonhwa Hospital, Busan, South Korea
e-mail: jihak3@hanmail.net


H. S. Kim et al. (eds.), *Advanced Technique of Endoscopic Cervical and Thoracic Spine Surgery*, https://doi.org/10.1007/978-981-99-1133-2_10

conventional posterior approach, cervical laminectomy by UBE is advantageous because it involves smaller skin incisions, preserved paraspinal muscle and ligamentous complex, and a better high-resolution magnification. Moreover, the procedure is relatively safe and easy to perform as the endoscope and surgical instruments can be moved independently. This can help achieve sufficient decompression and improve outcomes while preventing complications correlated with the conventional posterior approach.

In this chapter, we presented the general indications for cervical laminectomy by UBE and its correlated surgical techniques. Moreover, whether the procedure is safe and can prevent cord injury was investigated.

## 2 Indications and Contraindications

The application of cervical laminectomy by UBE is relatively limited. Based on our clinical experiences, the indications and contraindications for cervical laminectomy by UBE are presented below.

The indications are as follows:

1. One- to three-segment cervical canal stenosis with associated myelopathy if the major compressive lesion is not located anteriorly
2. Ossification of posterior longitudinal ligament (OPLL) with segmental or localized type
3. Need in combination with the anterior approach such as auxiliary surgical treatment

The contraindications are as follows:

1. Multiple segmental cervical spondylotic myelopathy (> 3 levels)
2. Severe OPLL with continuous type
3. Centrally located cervical disc herniation
4. Cervical spine instability
5. Significant kyphotic deformity

## 3 Anesthesia and Position

After the induction of general anesthesia and intraoperative neurophysiological monitoring (if possible) are performed, the patient is placed in prone position with the cervical spine flexed and the head secured with tape (Fig. 1). The knees are gently flexed, and a pad is placed under the legs. All areas are confirmed and well padded. The posterior neck, which is the area of interest, is shaved, prepped, and draped.

Generally, the left-side approach is suitable for a right-handed surgeon. Further, the left-side portal is used to establish the endoscopic portal

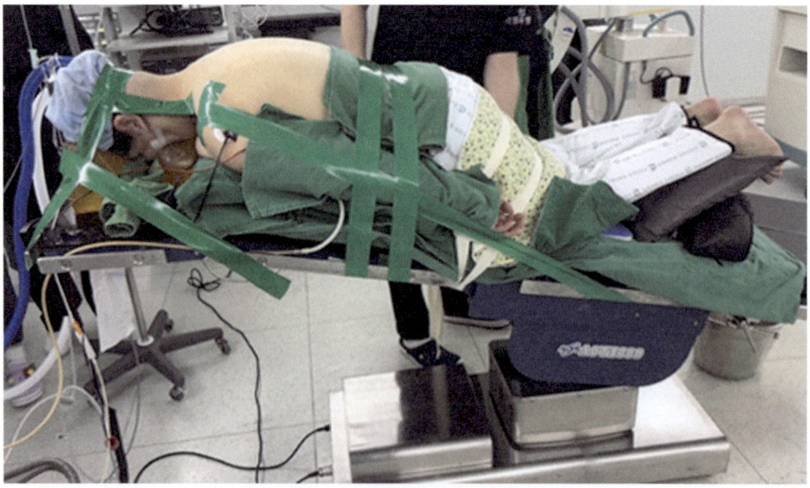

**Fig. 1** Positioning of the patient

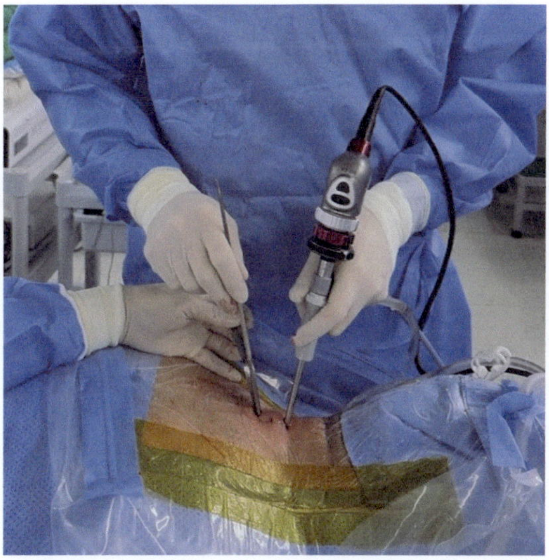

**Fig. 2** Overview of cervical laminectomy by unilateral biportal endoscopy

for the endoscope, and the right-side portal is utilized to construct the working portal for instrument handling. An assistant, who is on the opposite side of the operator, holds the semi-tubular retractor (Fig. 2).

## 4 Special Instruments

The instruments used in cervical laminectomy by UBE are similar to those in other lumbar or thoracic procedures by UBE. Diamond drill, 1-mm Kerrison rongeur, and small-sized double-ended elevator are required to perform cervical laminectomy by UBE.

## 5 Procedures

### 5.1 The Concept of Cervical Laminectomy by UBE

Unilateral laminectomy for bilateral decompression (ULBD) is used for the successful management of lumbar spinal stenosis [10]. Moreover, ULBD by UBE is applied for the treatment of cervical spondylosis. Namely, cervical laminectomy by UBE comprises bilateral decompression using the unilateral approach. However, contralateral decompression performed using the sublaminar approach such as lumbar ULBD is associated with a risk of cord injury in cervical spine. Therefore, bilateral subtotal laminectomy using the interspinous approach is recommended. The docking point to the caudal lamina rather than the cranial lamina is not obstructed by the spinous process (Fig. 3a). Furthermore, a sufficient space for contralateral decompression is achieved by drilling the base of the spinous process and median crest of the upper part of the caudal lamina (Fig. 3b). The base of the spinous process and median crest are resected to reduce spinal cord compression caused by the endoscope or surgical instruments in contralateral decompression.

### 5.2 Skin Marking and Establishment of Portals

C-arm fluoroscopy is required to confirm the level of surgery. The docking point, which is the upper part of the caudal lamina at the ipsilateral side, is assessed using the anteroposterior (AP) view on fluoroscopy. Two skin incisions that are approximately 3 cm apart, with the center at the upper part of the caudal lamina at the midline of the proximal and distal pedicles, are established (Fig. 4a). The cervical fascia should be sufficiently incised in the direction of the docking point, rather than forcing the dilators via the fascia, to prevent risk of spinal cord or lamina fracture injury.

Under fluoroscopy guidance, a series of dilators are inserted sequentially via the working portal, and an endoscopic sheath is inserted into the docking point via the scope portal. The tip of the dilator and the endoscopic sheath make a triangulation above the upper part of the caudal lamina, and AP and lateral fluoroscopic images are

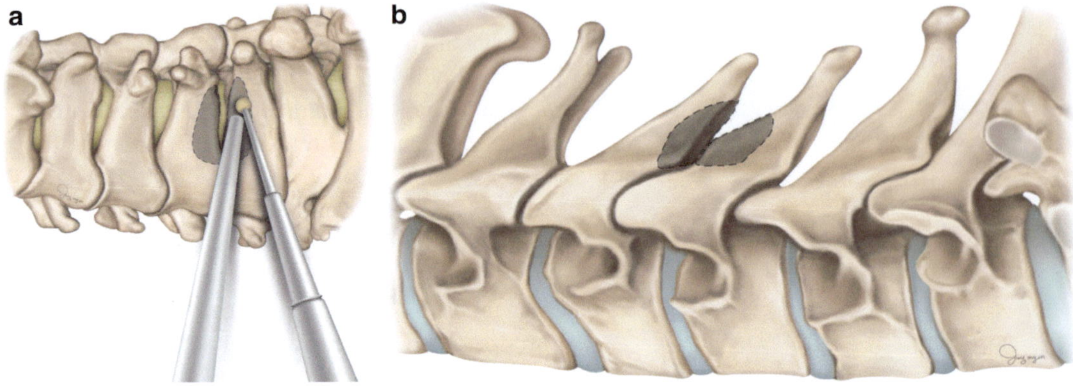


**Fig. 3** Concept of cervical laminectomy by unilateral biportal endoscopy. The docking point to the caudal lamina rather than the cranial lamina is not obstructed by the spinous process (**a**). A sufficient space for contralateral decompression is achieved by drilling the base of the spinous process and median crest of the upper part of the caudal lamina (**b**)

obtained as needed to ensure the proper location (Fig. 4b and c).

After the endoscope and the semi-tubular retractor are inserted, it is ready to start operation under endoscopic guidance. Proper positioning of the semi-tubular retractor is essential to maintain the fluid output and to retract the paraspinal muscles laterally (Fig. 2).

### 5.3 Initial Working Space and Bone Working (Video 1)

After the soft tissues have been cleared off from the level of interest using the radiofrequency (RF) probe, the upper portion of the caudal lamina, interlaminar space, and inferior edge of the cranial lamina are defined (Fig. 5a). If an ipsilateral foraminotomy is not planned, lateral exposure is commonly discontinued at the beginning of the lateral mass. When the endoscope and instruments are disturbed by the bifid or prominent tip of the spinous process, the tip of the spinous process is drilled to establish a working space for decompression. Subsequently, the cranial lamina is resected starting at its inferior edge, thereby identifying the underlining of the ligamentum flavum (LF) and then proceeding to the cranial direction (Fig. 5b). Caution should be taken to prevent LF compression. The base of the spinous process should be resected to provide a better visualization and enough space for a safe decompression at the contralateral side (Fig. 5c). The base of the spinous process is resected to reduce the risk of spinal cord compression caused by the endoscope or surgical instruments in contralateral decompression. After the partial resection of the cranial lamina and base of the spinous process, the median crest of the upper part of the caudal lamina and the contralateral side are identified (Figs. 3b and 5d). Simultaneously, the median crest should be resected with a diamond burr to secure the space for contralateral decompression because the medial crest interferes with the insertion of the endoscope and instruments in contralateral decompression (Fig. 5e and f). Thereafter, we can identify the cranial lamina at the contralateral side (Fig. 5g). Then, to prevent LF compression, subtotal laminectomy, rather than sublaminar drilling of the contralateral cranial lamina, is performed (Fig. 5h).

Next, the midline gap of the LF, which is the anatomical landmark of the midline orientation, is identified (Fig. 5i). Cranial bone working is performed up to the superior attachment of the LF using a diamond drill (Fig. 5j). The superior attachment of the LF is an anatomical landmark of the appropriate cranial bone working (Fig. 5k).

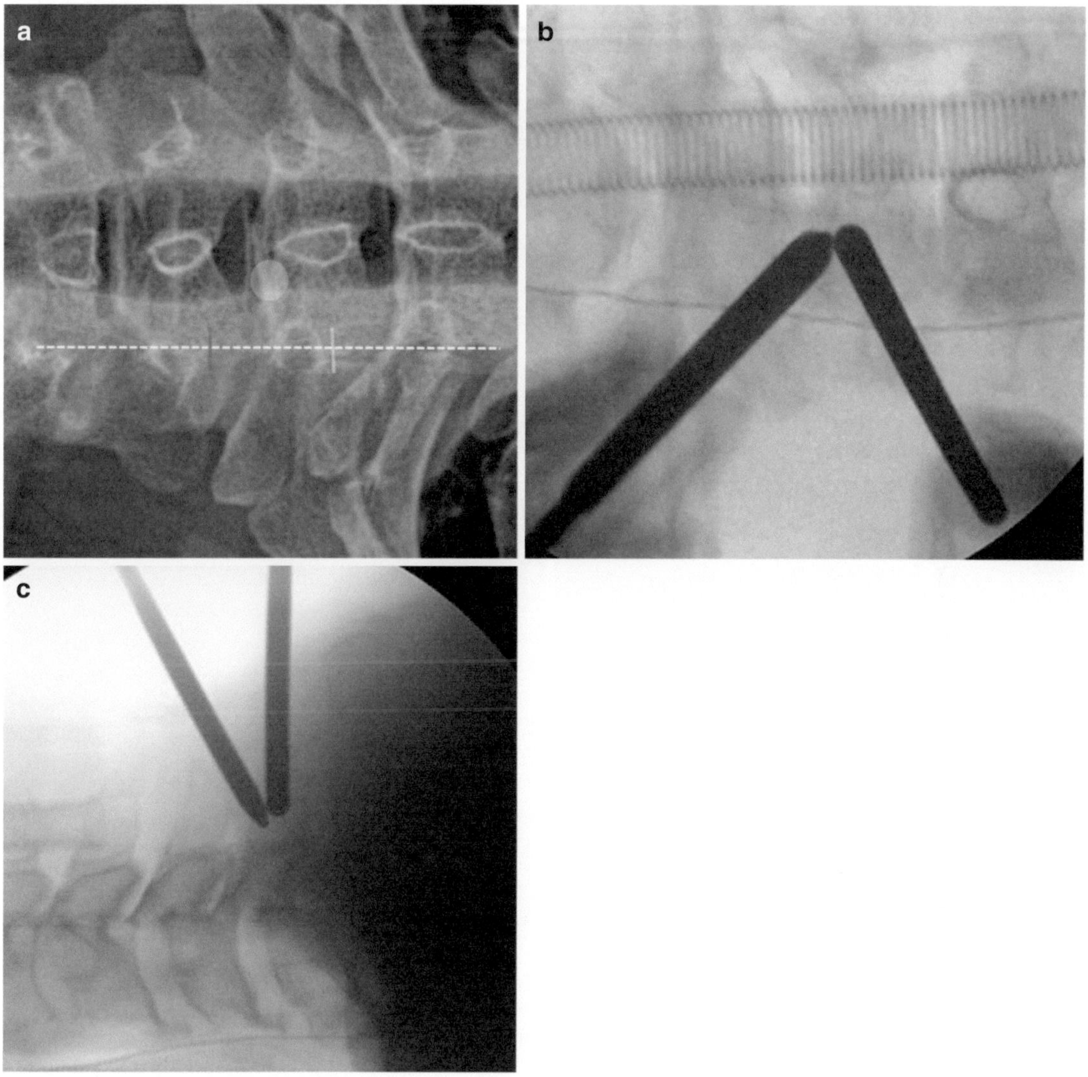


**Fig. 4** Fluoroscopic anteroposterior view (AP) of the skin incision and docking point. The docking point (white circle) is the upper part of the caudal lamina. Two skin incisions (working portal: white line; scopic portal: blue line) are made approximately 3 cm apart, with the center as the upper part of the caudal lamina at the midline of the proximal and distal pedicles (dotted line) (**a**). Triangulation of the tip of the dilator and the endoscopic sheath above the upper part of the caudal lamina. AP (**b**) and lateral fluoroscopic images (**c**)

The superior attachment of the LF is exposed, and partial laminectomy is then continued to the upper portion of the caudal lamina.

Subsequently, the upper portion of the caudal lamina and the medial aspect of the superior articular process (SAP) are grounded into a thin and translucent form using a diamond drill, without the Kerrison rongeur compressing the spinal cord underneath the caudal lamina (Fig. 5l). This technique could prevent the placement of instruments such as the Kerrison rongeur under the lamina if there is significant cord compression, thereby preventing possible cord injury. We preferred using the diamond drill to work through the outer cortical and cancellous bones, leaving a paper-thin inner cortical layer (Fig. 5m). Notably,

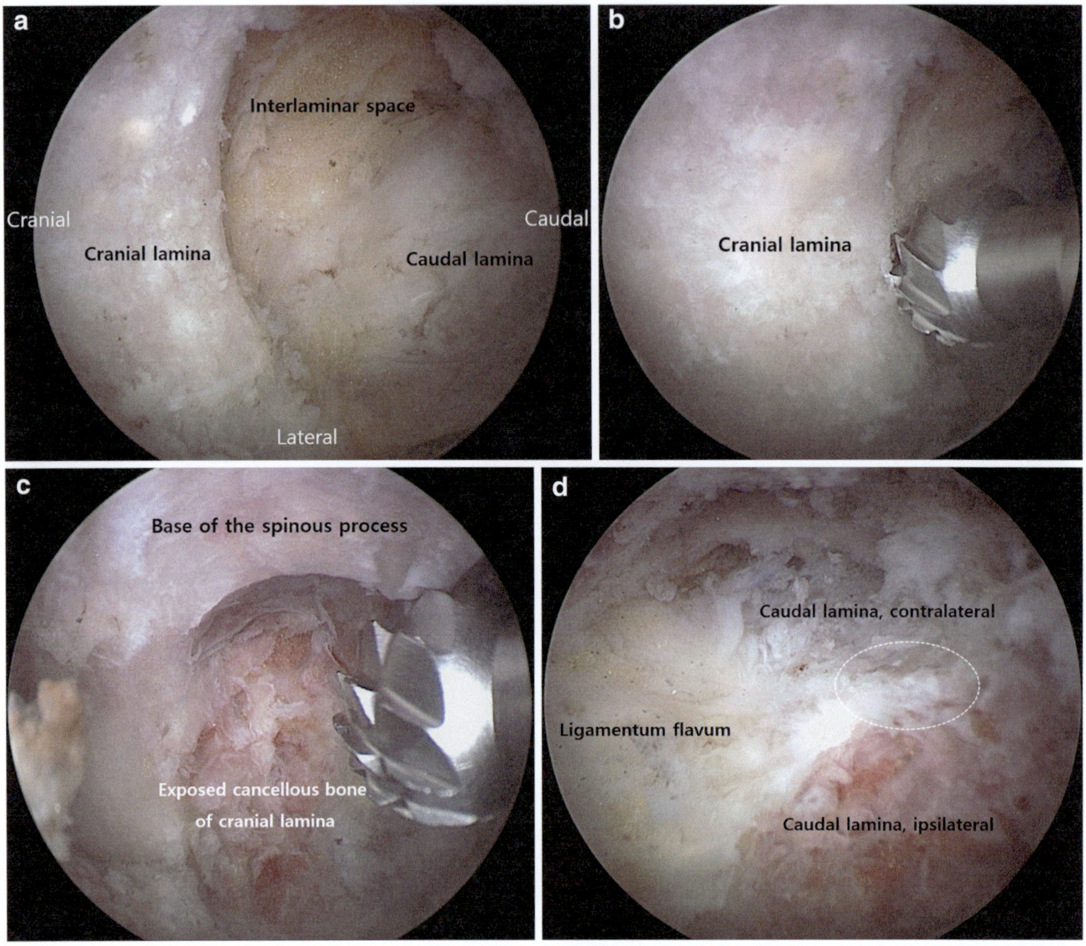


**Fig. 5** Serial sequence endoscopic images of the bone working. The surgical anatomy is first noted at the upper portion of the caudal lamina, the interlaminar space, and the inferior edge of the cranial lamina (**a**). The cranial lamina is removed starting at its inferior edge and then proceeding in a cranial direction (**b**). The base of the spinous process should be removed to provide better visualization and sufficient space for safe decompression at the contralateral side (**c**). Identification of the median crest of the upper part of the caudal lamina (white circle) and the contralateral side (**d**). Drilling of the median crest of the upper part of the caudal lamina (white circle) (e). Removed the median crest of the upper part of the caudal lamina (**f**). Identification of the cranial lamina at the contralateral side (**g**). Drilling of the cranial lamina at the contralateral side (**h**). Anatomical landmark for midline orientation. The white circle indicates the midline gap of the ligamentum flavum (**i**). Cranial bone working at the contralateral side using a diamond drill (**j**). Anatomical landmark for cranial bone working. The dotted line indicates the superior attachment of the ligamentum flavum (**k**). The upper portion of the caudal lamina and medial aspect of SAP are ground into a thin and translucent form using a diamond drill (**l**). Paper-thin, translucent form of the caudal lamina (**m**). Anatomical landmark for lateral bone working. The lateral end of bone working extends up to the medial edge of the SAP (white dotted curved line), which is located at the medial margin of the pedicle. Ipsilateral (**n**) and contralateral (**o**)

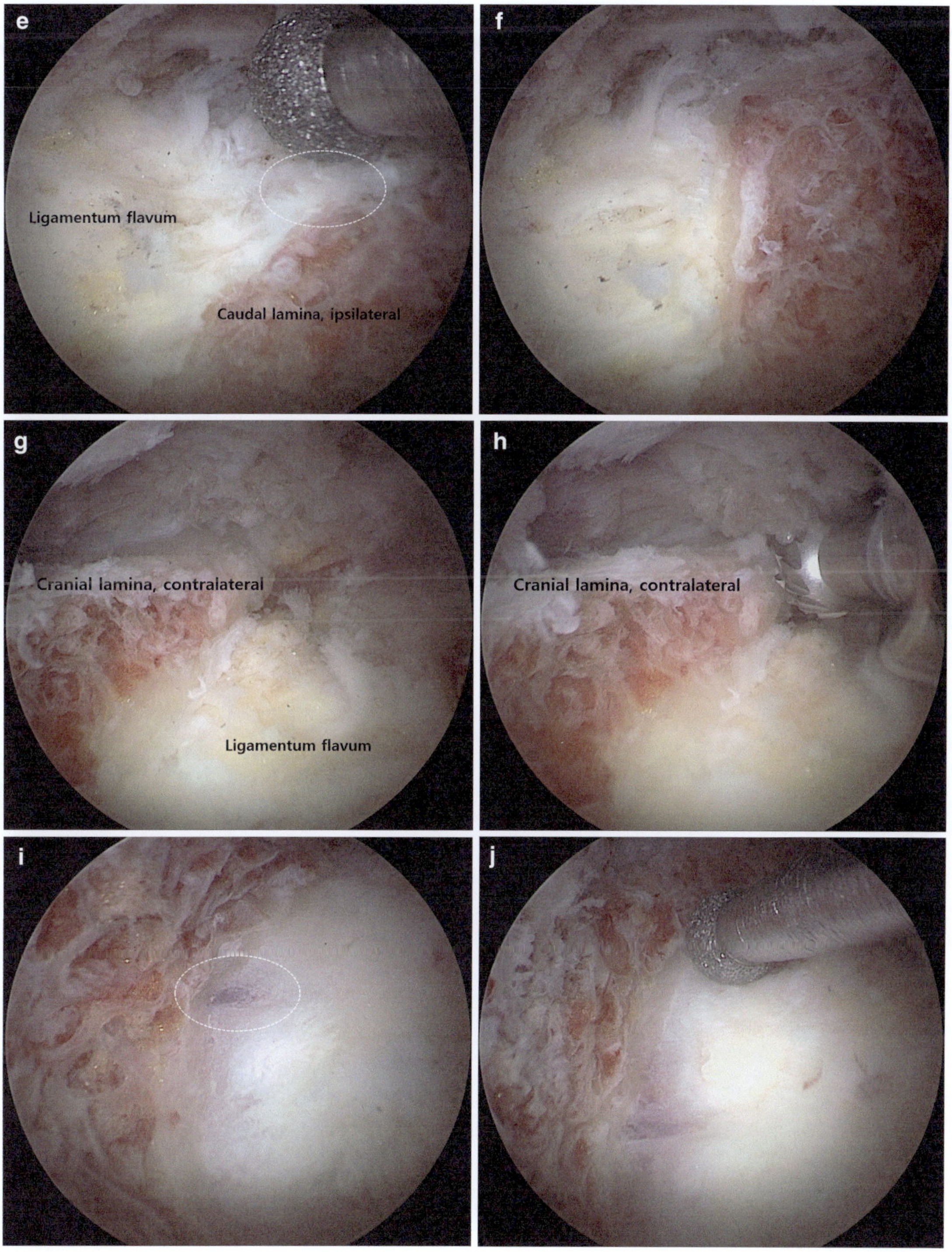


**Fig. 5** (continued)

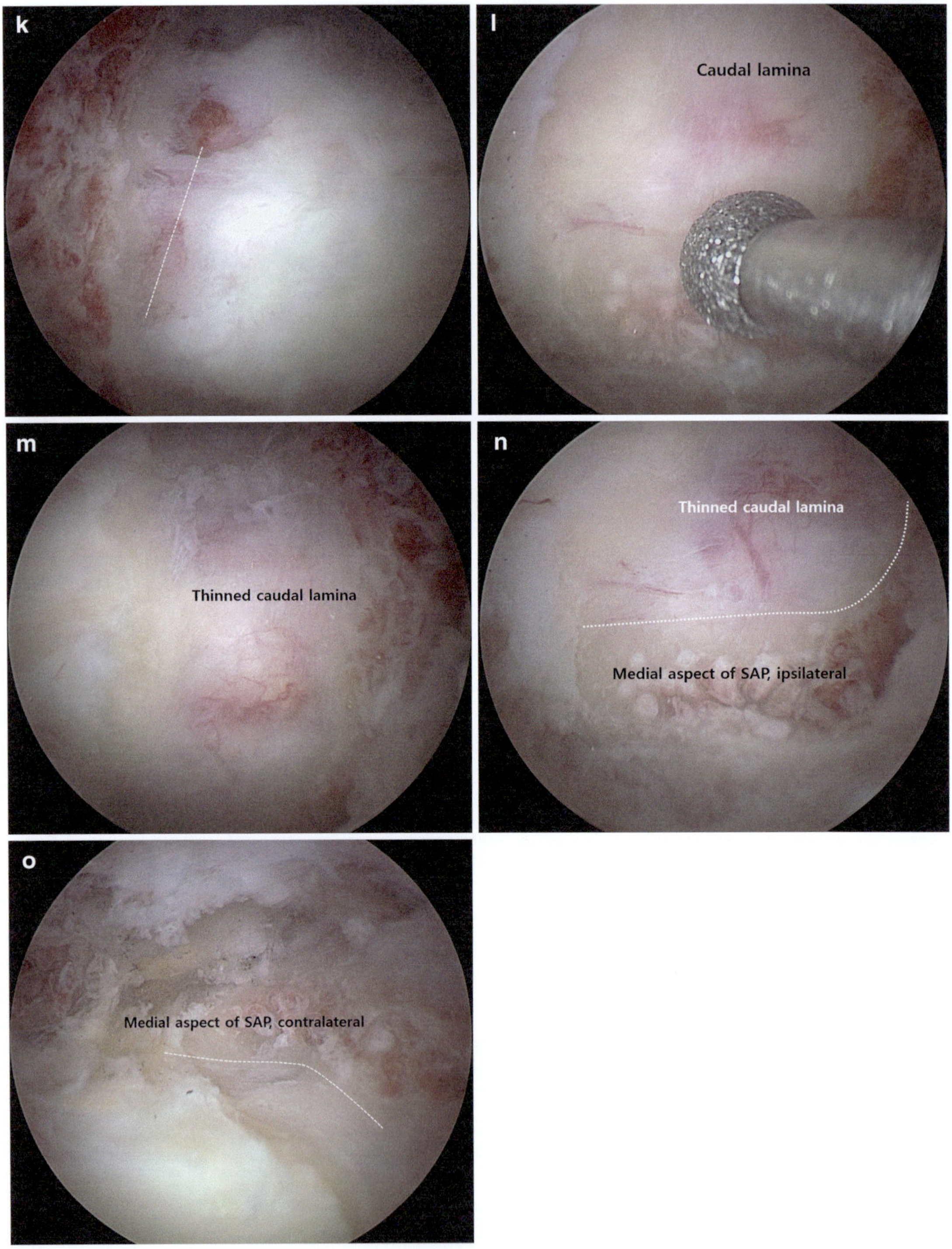


**Fig. 5** (continued)

the LF did not underlie beneath the upper portion of the caudal lamina. Hence, there was no soft tissue between the lamina and dural sac. The lateral end of bone working extended up to the medial edge of the SAP, which is located at the medial margin of the pedicle (Fig. 5n and o).

As suggested previously, no downward pressure should be exerted during any phase of bone working upon the underlying LF. Furthermore, as bone working is accomplished bilaterally, caution should be taken to preserve the LF, which is a safety protector, thereby covering the underlying spinal cord.

### 5.4 Removal of LF (Video 2)

After the completion of bone working, pituitary forceps are used to grasp and elevate the superficial layer of the LF without causing cord compression (Fig. 6a and b). Since the cervical spinal cord is sensitive to compression, the LF should be resected cautiously without causing spinal cord compression. Because cord compression is typically not severe around the superior attachment of the LF, it is gently detached with the hoot-type RF probe (Fig. 6c and d). The LF is cautiously detached using the 1-mm Kerrison rongeur or double-ended elevator that continues along the medial aspect of the SAP (Fig. 6e and f). Prior to the *en block* resection of the LF because of the abundance of the epidural blood vessels, coagulation with the RF probe could control bleeding (Fig. 6g). The LF is detached along its attachment to the lamina and is resected *en bloc* with pituitary forceps. The method for resecting the contralateral LF is the same as that mentioned above (Fig. 6h). When resecting the contralateral side of the LF, the surgeon should ensure that the spinal cord is not compressed by surgical instruments such as the Kerrison rongeur. Furthermore, it is important to thin out the caudal lamina and the medial aspect of the SAP sufficiently. The paper-thin residual lamina can be easily fractured, and the LF and residual lamina can be resected with the double-ended elevator. This technique can facilitate the *en block* resection of the deep layer of the LF without causing cord compression.

The lateral ends of decompression are the medial edge of the SAP and the lateral margin of the thecal sac, which are identified via endoscopic viewing (Fig. 6i). Finally, the free-floating dura mater is a sign of sufficient decompression under endoscopic guidance (Fig. 6j).

### 5.5 Foraminotomy

Additional foraminotomy could be performed if ipsilateral or contralateral foraminal stenosis is present. A detailed description of cervical foraminotomy by UBE is discussed in another chapter.

The diamond drill may be used to thin the medial aspect of the facet joint, and the 1-mm Kerrison rongeur or double-ended elevator could be used to perform foraminotomy (Fig. 7a–c). A higher degree of facet joint resection could be associated with instability and might predispose to kyphotic deformity. The association between the disc space and the nerve root in each segment is different, and surgeons should be knowledgeable about the anatomical relationship, achieve sufficient decompression, and prevent nerve root injury.

### 5.6 Two-Level Surgical Technique

For two-level decompression (e.g., C4–C5 and C5–C6), after docking on the C5 lamina, C5 bilateral total laminectomy with sparing of the tip of the spinous process is performed. Subsequently, partial laminectomy of the C4 level and partial laminectomy of the upper part of the C6 level, along with flavectomy are performed, and two-level decompression is completed.

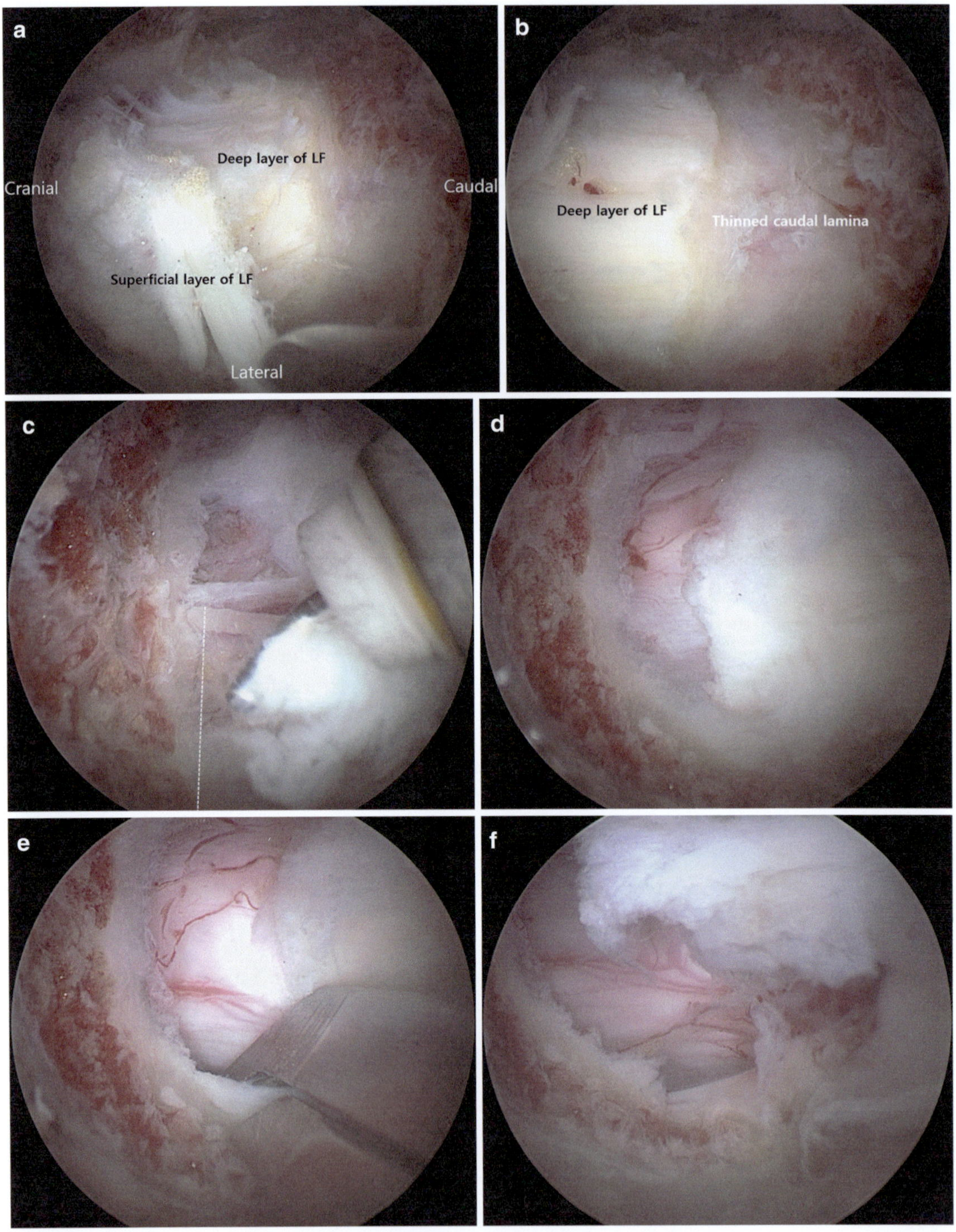


**Fig. 6** Endoscopic images showing the sequential steps of the removal of the ligamentum flavum. Detachment of the superficial layer of the ligamentum flavum (LF) (**a**). After removal of the superficial layer of the LF (**b**). The superior attachment of the LF (dotted line) is gently detached using a hoot-type RF probe (**c**). Detachment of the superior attachment of the LF (**d**). The LF is carefully detached using a 1 mm Kerrison rongeur that continues along the medial aspect of SAP (**e**). Detachment of the lateral attachment of the LF (**f**). Prior to *en bloc* removal of the LF, coagulation of the epidural vessel using the RF probe is helpful to control bleeding (**g**). After removal of the LF at the contralateral side (**h**). The lateral end of decompression is the medial edge of SAP, lateral margin of the thecal sac, and nerve root (white arrow), which are identified by endoscopic viewing (**i**). Free-floating dura mater is a sign of sufficient decompression under endoscopic guidance (**j**)

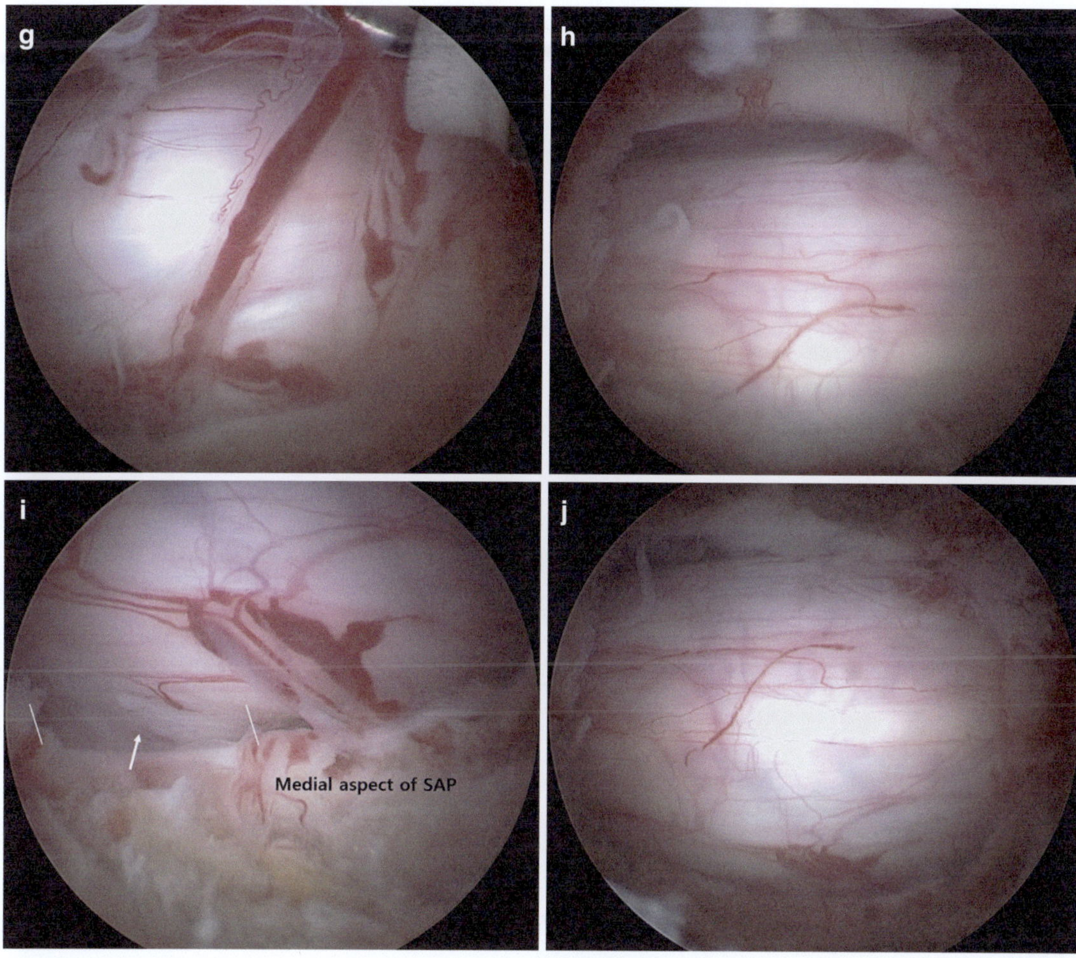


**Fig. 6** (continued)

## 5.7 Postoperative Drain

After completing the surgery, a Jackson–Pratt drain (100 cc) is inserted via the working portal to prevent hematoma. Caution should be taken to insert the Jackson–Pratt drain deeply as the tip of the drain could cause cord injury.

## 5.8 Postoperative Care

The patient could ambulate on the first day after surgery. Postoperative magnetic resonance imaging (MRI) should be performed within 2 days to assess for possible complications and decompression. Soft cervical neck collar must be used for 4 weeks.

## 5.9 Illustrated Cases

### 5.9.1 Case 1: Cervical Spondylosis on the C6–C7 Levels

A 66-year-old man presented with neurological symptoms in the bilateral upper extremities caused by compressive myelopathy because of cervical spinal stenosis at the C6–C7 levels for 6 months. He was treated conservatively for 3

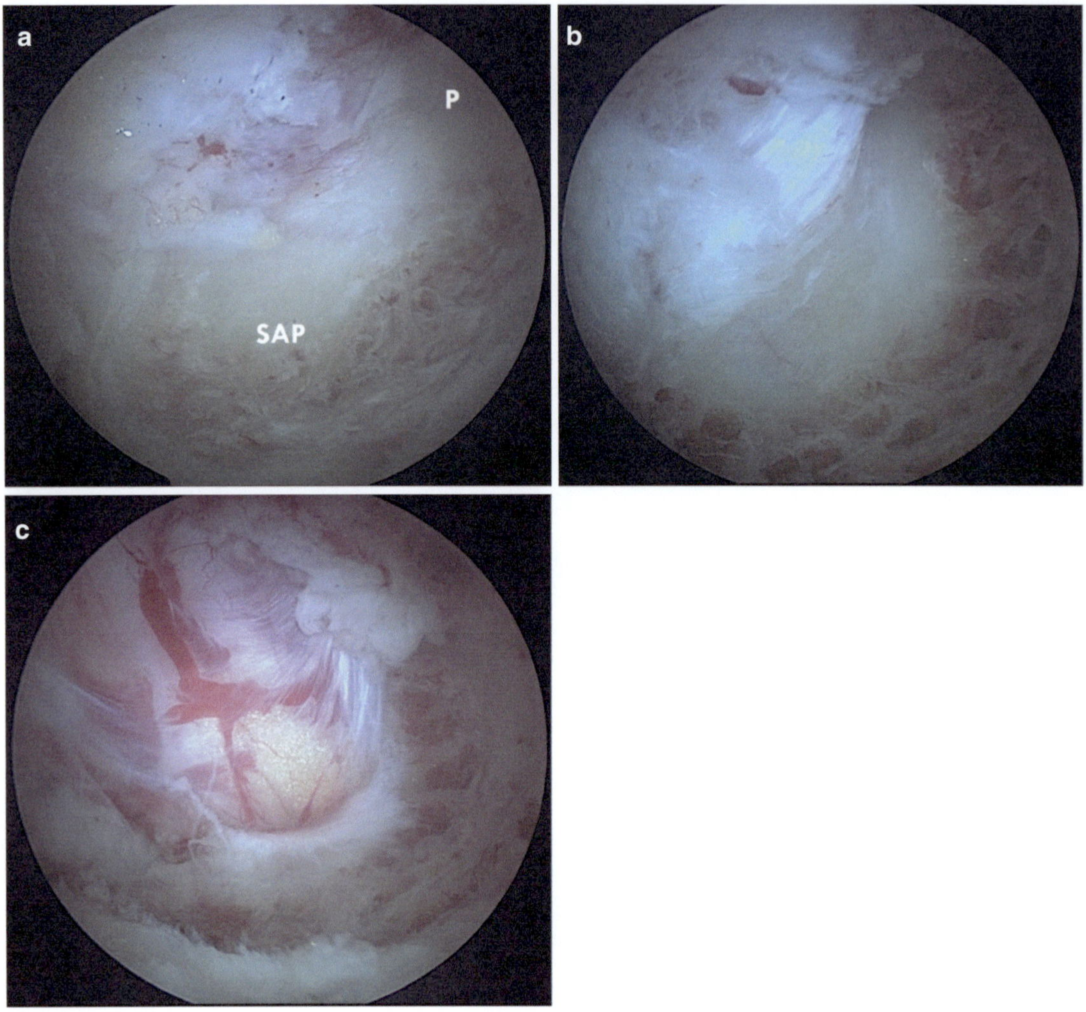


**Fig. 7** Endoscopic images showing the sequential steps of foraminotomy: identification of the medial aspect of the superior articular process (SAP) and pedicle (P) (**a**). Thinning out the medial aspect of the SAP (**b**). Confirmation of the nerve root (**c**)

months; however, his symptoms worsened. MRI revealed cervical spinal stenosis at the C6–C7 levels (Fig. 8a and b). Postoperative MRI revealed adequate decompression of the spinal cord at the C6–C7 levels (Fig. 8c and d). The symptoms improved significantly, and the patient did not present with symptoms of cervical myelopathy during follow-up.

### 5.9.2 Case 2: Cervical Spondylosis on the C4–C5, C5–C6, and C6–C7 Levels

A 70-year-old man presented with a 12-month history of CSM. On preoperative MRI (Fig. 9a–d), cervical spinal stenosis, which causes cord compression at the C4–C5, C5–C6, and C6–C7 levels, was identified. Cervical lam-

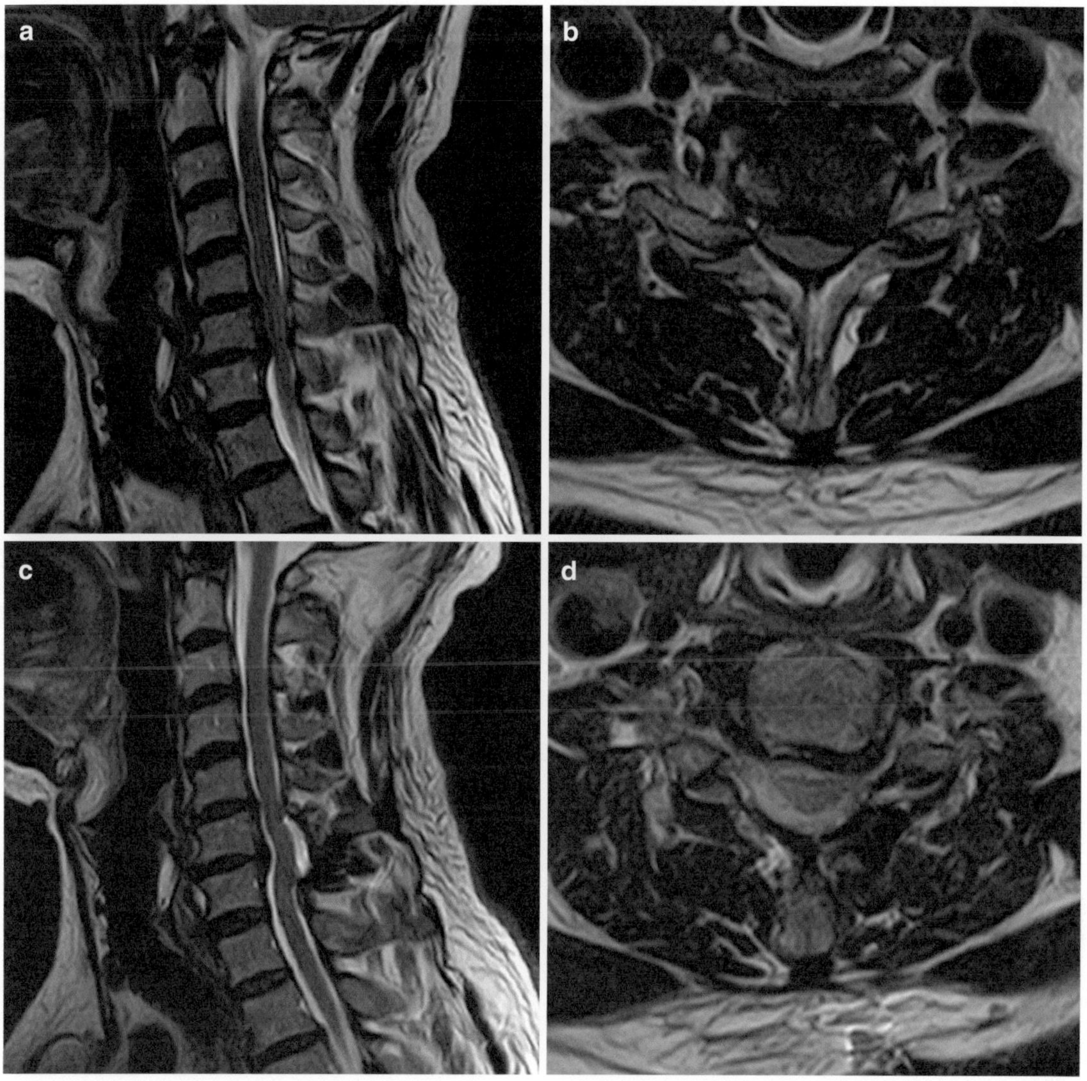

**Fig. 8** Images of a 66-year-old woman with cervical spinal stenosis at the C6–C7 level. Preoperative MRI shows cervical spinal stenosis at the C6–C7 level (sagittal: **a**, axial: **b**). Postoperative axial T2-weighted MRI shows sufficient decompression with minimal muscle injury (sagittal: **c**, axial: **d**).

inectomy by UBE at the C4–C5, C5–C6, and C6–C7 levels was performed from the left side. After surgery, the outcome was confirmed on postoperative MRI (Fig. 9e–h). During the 3-month follow-up, the patient's bilateral physical strength score returned to 5, and he could walk long distances.

### 5.9.3 Case 3: OPLL at the C4–C5 Levels

A 68-year-old man with CSM presented with bilateral arm numbness and spastic gait. Preoperative MRI and computed tomography (CT) scan showed spinal cord compression with OPLL at the C2-C5 levels with severe spinal cord

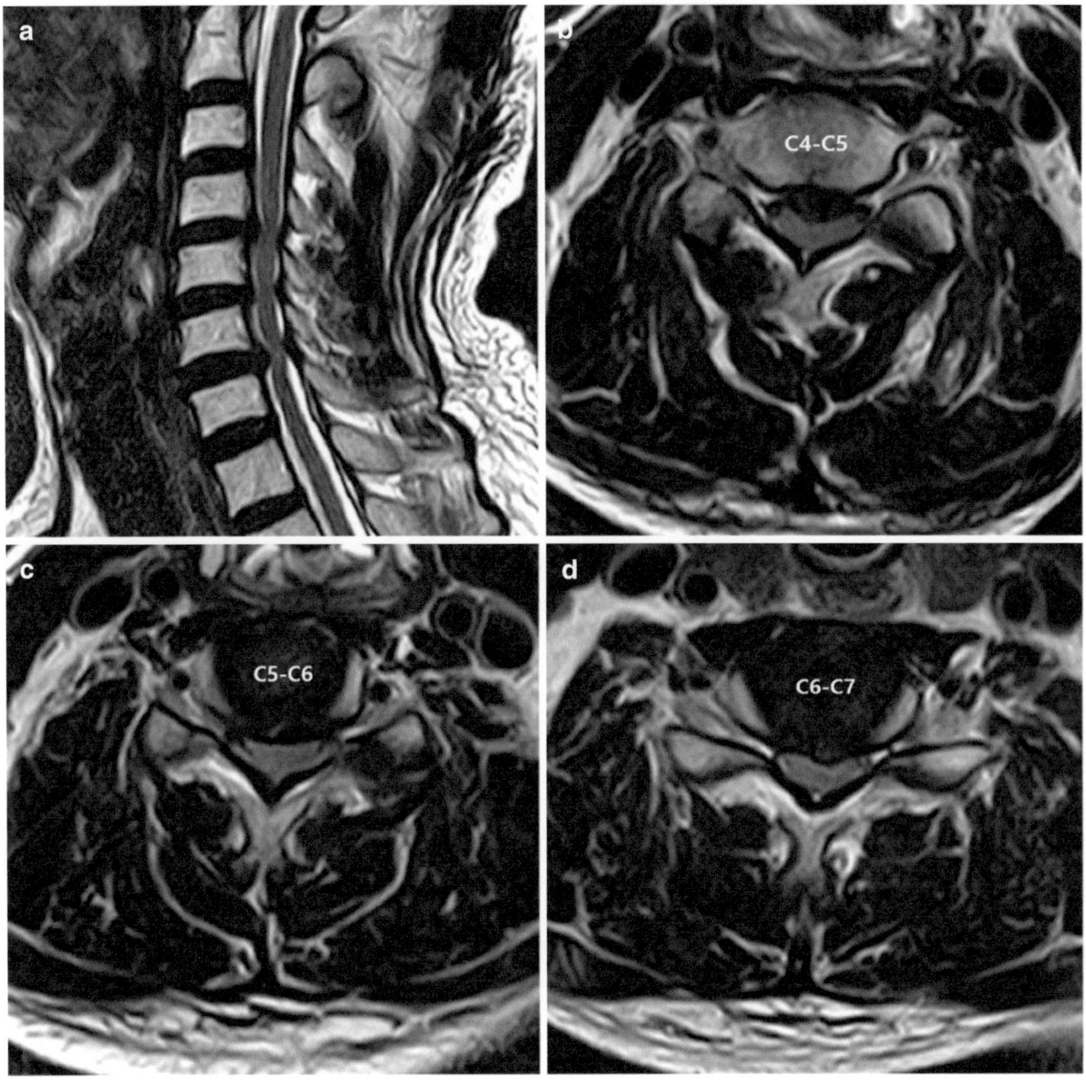


**Fig. 9** Images of a 70-year-old man with cervical spondylosis at the C4–C5, C5–C6, and C6–C7 levels. Preoperative MRI shows cervical spinal stenosis and compressing of the cord at the C4–C5, C5–C6, and C6–C7 levels. (MRI sagittal: **a**, axial: **b**, **c** and **d**). Postoperative axial T2-weighted MRI shows sufficient decompression of the cervical spondylosis (MRI sagittal: **e**, axial: **f**–**h**)

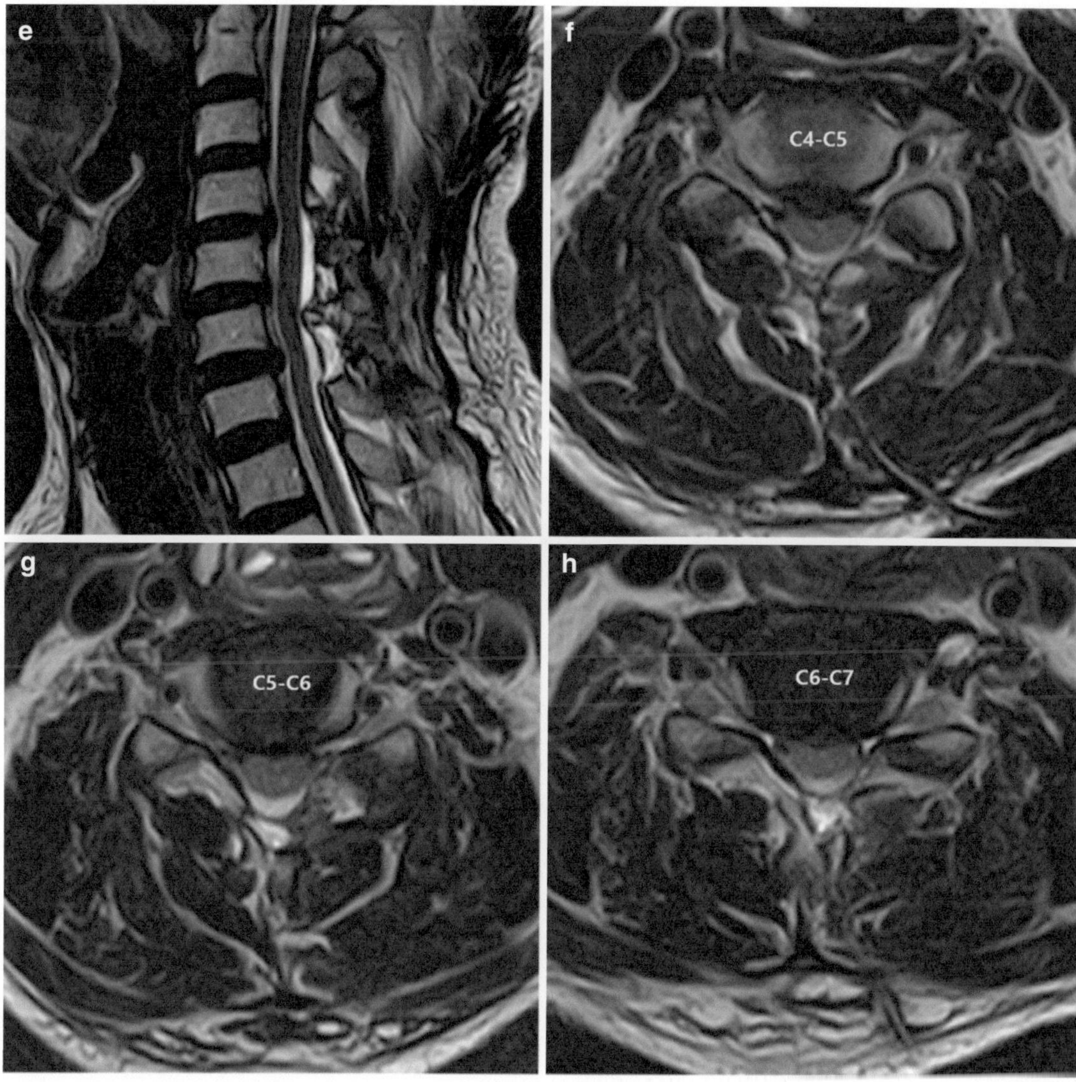


**Fig. 9** (continued)

compression at the C4–C5 levels (Fig. 10a and b). The patient underwent cervical laminectomy by UBE at the C4-C5 levels. Based on the postoperative MRI and radiography, spinal cord decompression was successfully managed (Fig. 10c and d). Postoperatively, the patient's symptoms disappeared, and recurrence was not observed during follow-up.

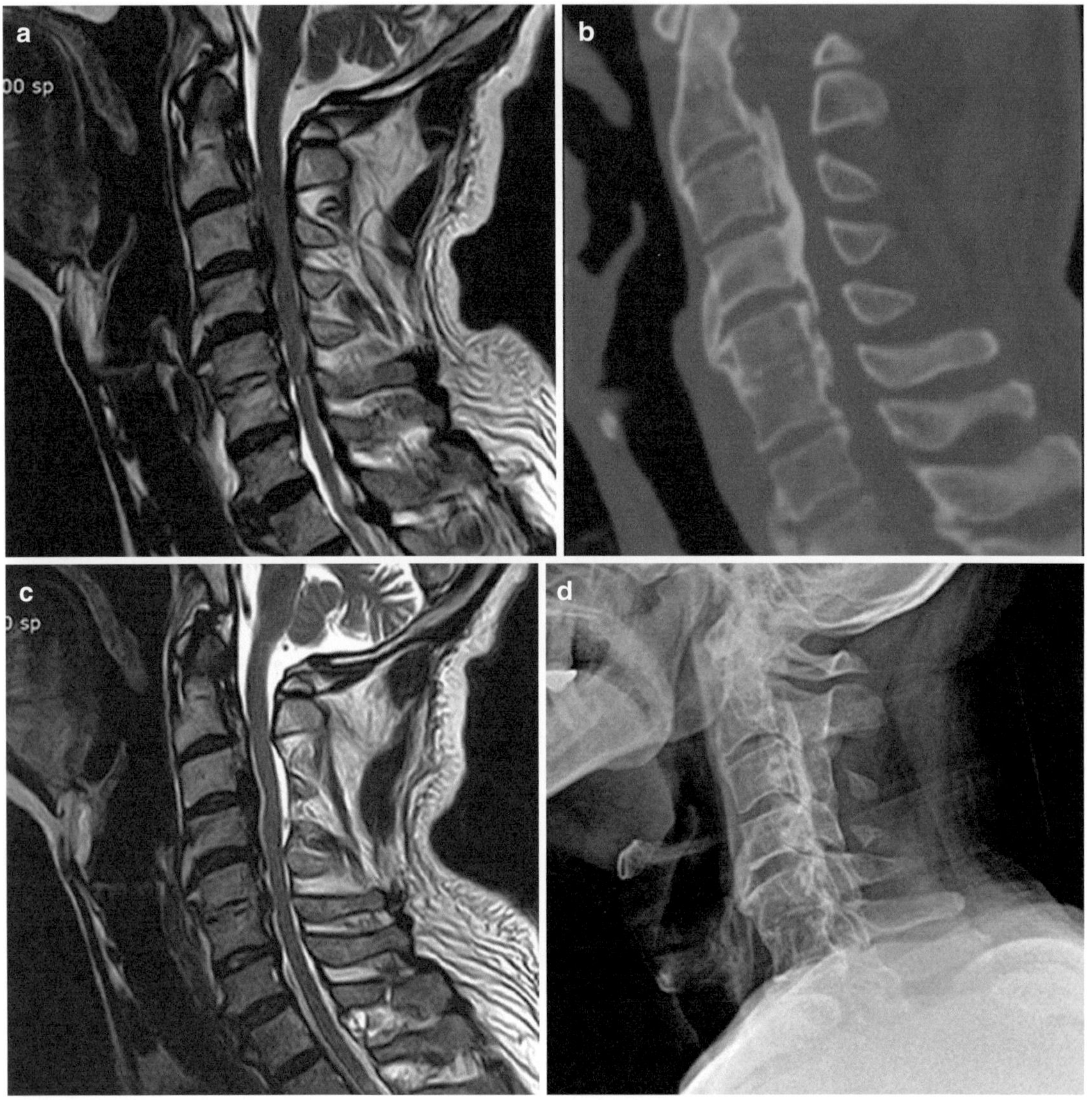

**Fig. 10** Images of a 68-year-old man with ossification of posterior longitudinal ligament (OPLL). Preoperative MRI and CT show OPLL and compressing of the cord at the C4–C5 level (MRI sagittal: **a**, CT sagittal. (**b**). Postoperative axial T2-weighted MRI shows decompression at the C4–C5 level (MRI sagittal: **c**, lateral radiography: **d**)

## 6 Prevention and Management of Complications

### 6.1 Cord Injury

Although retraction of the dura matter is occasionally required during lumbar surgery to decompress the contralateral side, this maneuver can be significantly dangerous when operating on the cervical spine and can lead to irreversible cord injury. When performing cervical laminectomy by UBE, strict adherence to a few principles is essential to prevent iatrogenic injury to the spinal cord. First, caution is taken to prevent exerting any pressure on the LF or spinal cord. Second, to prevent cord injury during bone working, the

LF is left as a protector until bone working is completed. Third, the base of the spinous process and median crest at the caudal lamina should be resected sufficiently. This provides enough working space particularly during contralateral decompression. Forth, the RF probe must be used with caution after LF resection. When using the RF probe around the spinal cord, surgeons should pay special attention to use it against the spinal cord with low voltage. Fifth, the placement of instruments into the stenotic spinal canal (e.g., the Kerrison rongeur) must be prevented due to the risk of cord injury. Therefore, it is safe to thin out the lamina with the diamond burr and then remove it with the doubled-ended elevator. Finally, caution should be taken while placing the semi-tubular retractor to ensure more fluid output at the cervical cord level, which is sensitive to pressure.

### 6.2 Dural Tear

A small dura tear can be managed with cautious packing with the fibrin collagen patch (TachoComb), bedrest for 5–7 days, and lumbar drain. If the dural defect is large and cannot be covered with the fibrin collagen patch, the dural defect should be repaired directly via dural suturing or conversion under microscopic surgery.

### 6.3 Postoperative Hematoma

Excessive intraoperative bleeding may lead to the overuse of the RF probe and subsequent cord injury. Therefore, caution must be taken to achieve meticulous hemostasis. Bony bleeding should be waxed immediately to reduce the risk of venous air embolism. Particular attention should be provided to epidural vessel bleeding during LF resection. The posterior epidural venous plexus is located in the anterior epidural fat of the LF. The posterior epidural venous plexus is irregular, and there are abundant lateral anastomoses. Based on the abovementioned anatomy, prior to LF resection, the judicious use of the RF probe and hemostatic agents (WoundClot or Gelfoam) are sufficient to control bleeding. To prevent postoperative hematoma, the Jackson–Pratt surgical drain (100 cc) must be placed through the working portal for 1 or 2 days.

## 7 Discussion (Surgical Tips and Pitfall)

Cervical laminectomy by UBE preserves the paraspinal muscle and ligament, which are resected during the conventional posterior approach, and it has advantages with regard to maintaining lordosis and decreasing axial neck pain. Although cervical laminectomy by UBE may not be the standard treatment for CSM, this technique should have broader applications in the future.

Although UBE has gained widespread popularity in recent years, cervical laminectomy by UBE is a technically demanding technique. However, if surgeons become comfortable with UBE and the use of this procedure increases, safety is also improved. Consequently, cervical laminectomy by UBE is only recommended if the surgeon has a sufficient experience in performing other procedures by UBE. Furthermore, surgeons should note the anatomical landmark and the following surgical tips of cervical laminectomy by UBE:

1. The docking point to the caudal lamina, rather than the cranial lamina, is not obstructed by the spinous process.
2. The resection of the base of the spinous process and median crest of the upper part of the caudal lamina can help achieve a sufficient space for contralateral decompression.
3. If the endoscope and instruments are hindered by the bifid or prominent tip of the spinous process, the tips of the spinous process are resected to establish a working space for decompression.
4. When performing contralateral decompression, subtotal laminectomy is conducted rather than sublaminar drilling to prevent LF compression.
5. The upper portion of the caudal lamina and medial aspect of the SAP are grounded into a

thin and translucent form to prevent the placement of instruments such as the Kerrison rongeur under the lamina.

6. During bone working, caution should be taken to preserve the LF, which is a safety protector, thereby covering the underlying spinal cord.
7. To prevent cord compression when resecting LF, it is important to thin out the caudal lamina and medial aspect of the SAP. Then, the LF should be resected with the pituitary forceps.
8. With consideration of technical difficulties, novice surgeons should not perform UBE on patients with severe CSM as they may exhibit major clinical characteristics and may have a poor prognosis.

## References

1. Li C, Tang X, Chen S, Meng Y, Zhang W. Clinical application of large channel endoscopic decompression in posterior cervical spine disorders. BMC Musculoskelet Disord. 2019;20(1):548.
2. Miyamoto H, Maeno K, Uno K, Kakutani K, Nishida K, Sumi M. Outcomes of surgical intervention for cervical spondylotic myelopathy accompanying local kyphosis (comparison between laminoplasty alone and posterior reconstruction surgery using the screw-rod system). Eur Spine J. 2014;23(2):341–6.
3. Hosono N, Yonenobu K, Ono K. Neck and shoulder pain after laminoplasty. A noticeable complication. Spine. 1996;21(17):1969–73.
4. Shiraishi T. Skip laminectomy—a new treatment for cervical spondylotic myelopathy, preserving bilateral muscular attachments to the spinous processes: a preliminary report. Spine J. 2002;2(2):108–15.
5. Zhang C, Li D, Wang C, Yan X. Cervical endoscopic laminoplasty for cervical myelopathy. Spine. 2016;41(Suppl 19):B44–51.
6. Park MK, Son SK, Park WW, Choi SH, Jung DY, Kim DH. Unilateral biportal endoscopy for decompression of extraforaminal stenosis at the lumbosacral junction: surgical techniques and clinical outcomes. Neurospine. 2021;18(4):871–9.
7. Park MK, Park SA, Son SK, Park WW, Choi SH. Clinical and radiological outcomes of unilateral biportal endoscopic lumbar interbody fusion (ULIF) compared with conventional posterior lumbar interbody fusion (PLIF): 1-year follow-up. Neurosurg Rev. 2019;42(3):753–61.
8. Heo DH, Lee DC, Park CK. Comparative analysis of three types of minimally invasive decompressive surgery for lumbar central stenosis: biportal endoscopy, uniportal endoscopy, and microsurgery. Neurosurg Focus. 2019;46(5):E9.
9. Heo DH, Hong YH, Lee DC, Chung HJ, Park CK. Technique of biportal endoscopic transforaminal lumbar interbody fusion. Neurospine. 2020;17(Suppl 1):S129–S37.
10. Ikuta K, Arima J, Tanaka T, Oga M, Nakano S, Sasaki K, et al. Short-term results of microendoscopic posterior decompression for lumbar spinal stenosis. Technical note. J Neurosurg Spine. 2005;2(5):624–33.

# Endoscopic Assistant Cervical Instrumentation

Man Kyu Choi, Jin Hwa Eum, and Dae-Hyun Kim

**Abstract**

Biportal endoscopic approaches may have expandability. Cervical posterior instrumentations usually need wide muscle dissection. Minimally invasive cervical approach can reduce iatrogenic muscle injury and postoperative wound pain. Minimally invasive cervical surgery can enhance recovery after surgery. Biportal endoscopic approaches may have expandability. We attempted the biportal endoscopy assistant cervical posterior instrumentations. We introduced and described the surgical technique for UBE-assisted posterior cervical instrumentation for lateral mass screw fixation in subaxial cervical spine and lag screw fixation for C2, different from the tubular retractor system.

**Supplementary Information** The online version contains supplementary material available at https://doi.org/10.1007/978-981-99-1133-2_11.

M. K. Choi
Department of Neurosurgery, Kyung Hee University College of Medicine, Seoul, South Korea

J. H. Eum
Department of Neurosurgery, Ain Al Khaleej Hospital, Abu Dhabi, UAE

D.-H. Kim (✉)
Department of Neurosurgery, Daegu Catholic University Medical Center, College of Medicine, Catholic University of Daegu, Daegu, South Korea
e-mail: daehkim@cu.ac.kr

**Keywords**

Biportal · Cervical · Endoscopy Instrumentation

## 1 Introduction

The primary goals of minimally invasive spine surgery are to reduce the iatrogenic muscle injury inherent to conventional open spine surgery, hopefully reducing postoperative pain and facilitating return to daily activities. Recently, one of the minimally invasive techniques, unilateral biportal endoscopic (UBE) surgery, has been adapted to the cervical, thoracic, and lumbar spine with good results [1–4]. UBE surgery was focused on decompressive technique for lumbar degenerative pathology in the early days, but gradually expanded to cervical and thoracic lesions, and has been widely adapted to lumbar fusion surgery [3, 5–7].

Minimally invasive access to the posterior cervical instrumentation was designed to exposure through a paramedian approach. Mikhael et al. described a surgical technique for cervical microforaminotomy and lateral mass screw fixation using a specialized tubular retractor system [8]. In cases of traumatic cervical injury, tubular retractor-assisted direct repair technique using lag screw for atypical hangman's fracture has also been shown to be a good outcome [9]. In what follows, the surgical technique for UBE-assisted posterior cervical instrumentation for lateral mass


H. S. Kim et al. (eds.), *Advanced Technique of Endoscopic Cervical and Thoracic Spine Surgery*,
https://doi.org/10.1007/978-981-99-1133-2_11

screw fixation in subaxial cervical spine and lag screw fixation for C2, different from the tubular retractor system, will be described in detail.

## 2 Surgical Anatomy (Fig. 1)

1. If the screw trajectory is too medial, cervical cord injury may occur, and if the screw trajectory is too lateral or medial angulation is insufficient, vertebral artery injury may occur (lag screw for C2).
2. Nerve root injury may occur if the lateral mass screw trajectory is incorrect, and if the screw penetration is too deep; vertebral artery injury is a rare complication that may occur if the trajectory is medial and the screw penetration is too deep (lateral mass screw for subaxial cervical spine).

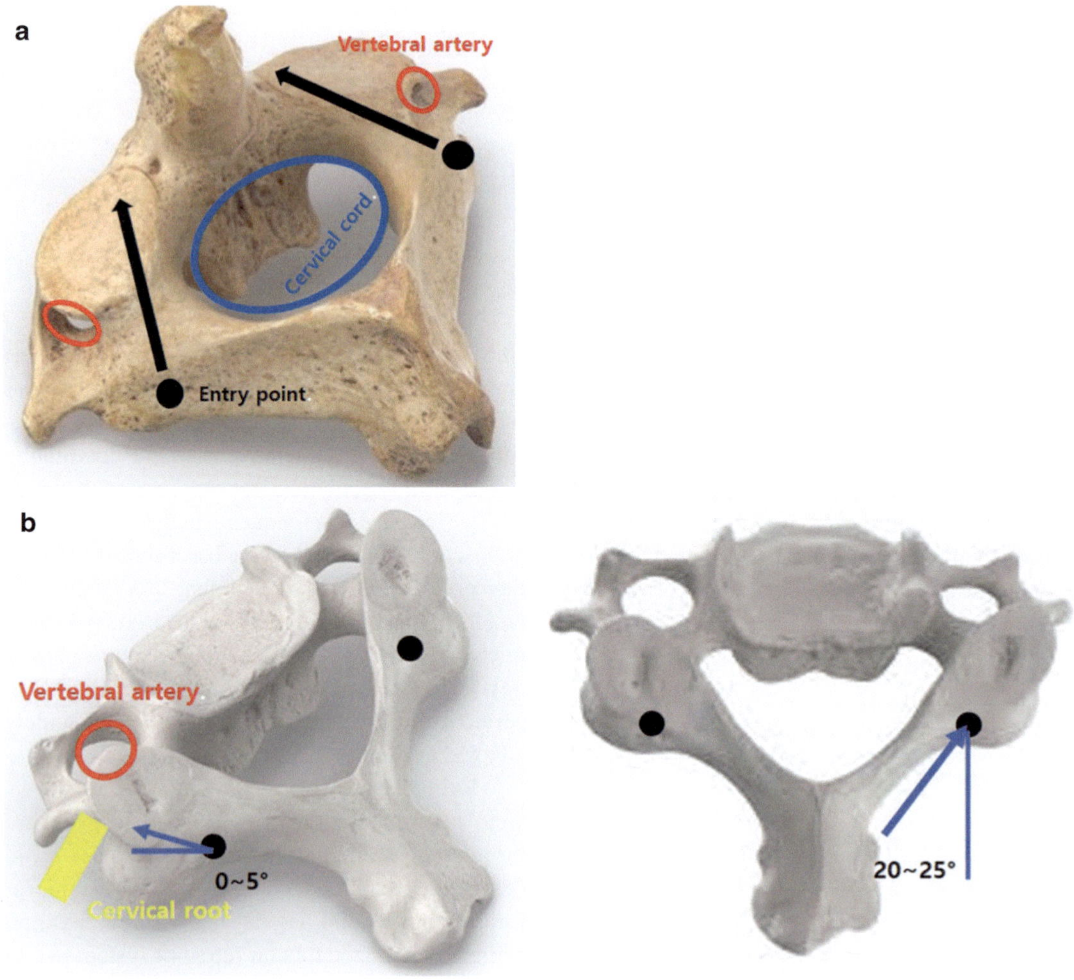


**Fig. 1** Schematic illustration of the C2 lag screw (**a**) and subaxial lateral mass screw (**b**)

## 3 Position (Fig. 2)

1. Mayfield tongs are applied; rigid fixation of the head to the table in the prone position.
2. The cervical spine should be slightly flexed and distracted.
3. The arms and elbows are placed adjacent to the torso and are well preserved to prevent mechanical pressure.
4. The shoulders are gently pulled caudad by taping.

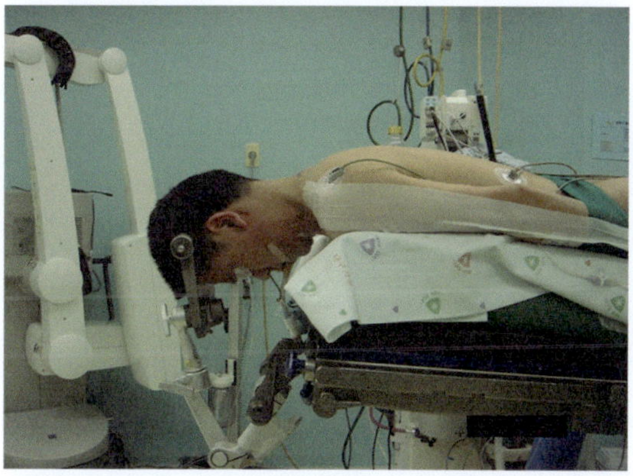

**Fig. 2** Mayfield tongs are applied, rigid fixation of the head to the table in the prone position. The neck should be slightly flexed, the arms and elbows are placed adjacent to the torso, and the shoulders are gently pulled caudad by taping

## 4 Surgical Instruments (Fig. 3)

During the procedure, 3.5-mm spherical bur and diamond drill, 0° 4-mm-diameter arthroscope, radiofrequency device, serial dilators, laminectomy instruments, and standard posterior screw instrument system, including drill sleeve, depth gauge, socket wrench, and sharp hook, were used.

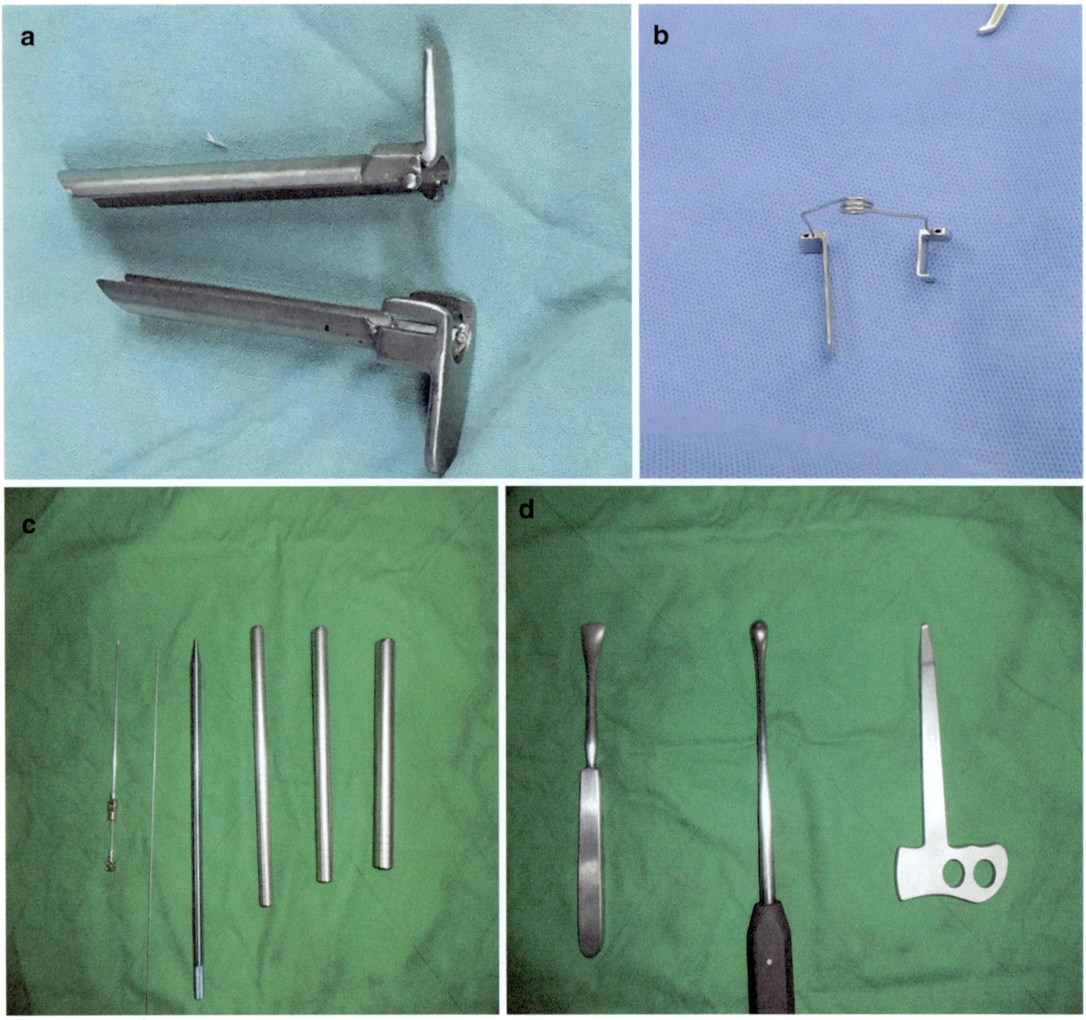


**Fig. 3** Various kinds of surgical instruments of biportal endoscopic cervical screw fixation. Working cannula (**a**), self-retracting working cannula (**b**), serial dilators (**c**), muscle detachers (**d**), 5-mm thoracoscopy port (**e**), and endoscopic retractor sheath and scope retractors (**f**)

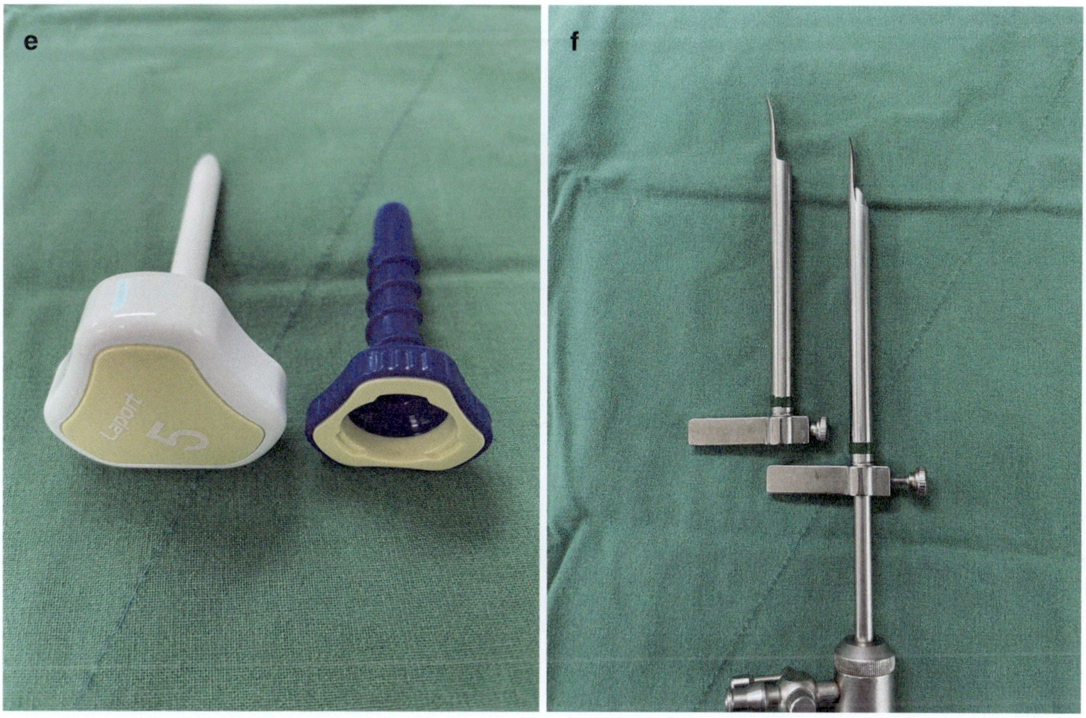


**Fig. 3** (continued)

## 5 Surgical Procedure

### 5.1 Step 1. Skin Mark, Incision, and Biportal Making (Fig. 4)

Under image intensification, intraoperative fluoroscopy is used to center the incision over the pathological level. The incision is typically 7–15 mm in length to accommodate the diameter of the scope and instruments. Two portals are made: one portal was used for endoscope and the other working portal was used for instruments. Portal entry point is determined according to the target level, cervical lordotic angle, and anatomical variation. Therefore, it is ideal to determine the skin entry point considering the cephalad and lateral angulation of the screws. Serial dilators were used to working portal and split the semispinalis cervicis and multifidus touching the spinous-lamina junction. Usually, dominant hand was used for working portal, and nondominant hand was used for endoscopic portals. Ipsilateral lamina and lateral mass were dissected and exposed using dissectors and radiofrequency (RF) probes. The lateral masses are fully exposed, extending to the lateral edges of the lateral mass and the facet joint at each fusion level.

### 5.2 Step 2. Determination of the Entry Point and Placing the Screw

1. C2 Lag Screw (Fig. 5, Video 1)

   Reduction of the fracture dislocation upon positioning was confirmed using intraoperative C-arm fluoroscopic images. After skin and fascia incision, the first dilator is advanced slowly through the musculature of the paraspinals under C-arm fluoroscopic guidance and docked at the screw entry point of the C2. The serial dilator is then toggled in the same direction of the screw insertion, and the field is cleared by an RF device. To avoid canal

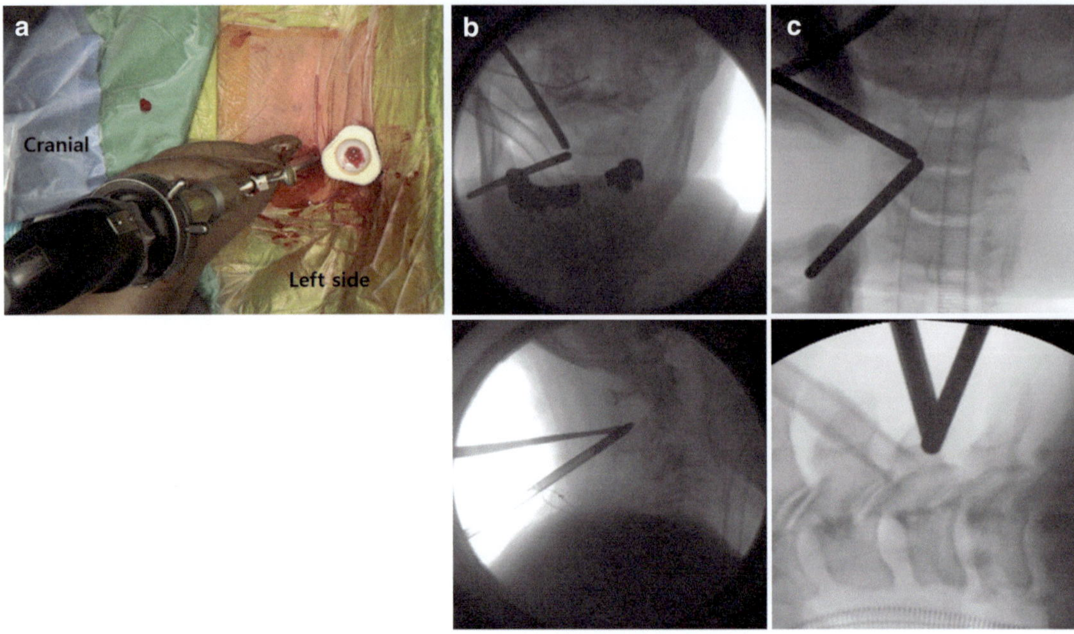


**Fig. 4** Overview of biportal endoscopic cervical fixation. Location of skin incision, biportal entry (**a**), and intraoperative fluoroscopic image (**b**) for C2 lag screw. (**c**) Subaxial lateral mass fixation

violation, the medial wall of the pedicle of C2 is confirmed using a freer double-ended elevator. After the trajectory is selected, a drill is inserted, and the pilot hole is made. A K-wire is carefully advanced under intraoperative fluoroscopic control to avoid cervical cord and vascular injuries. Subsequently, a 4-mm-diameter, self-tapped, cannulated screw is placed along a K-wire with/without washer.

2. Subaxial Lateral Mass Screw (Fig. 6)

   A high-speed drill is used to decorticate the bone at the entry point and create the starting hole. The hole should be made perpendicular to preserve the posterior cortex of the lateral mass. After entering into the lateral mass, tapping is then directed toward upward and lateral ventral corner toward the so-called "safe quadrant," with intraoperative fluoroscopic guidance. We used Kim's free-hand technique as a reference [10]. After a 3.5 mm tap is used, a probe is inserted before the screw to confirm that the lateral mass walls have not been violated. A depth gauge is inserted to measure the screw length, and an appropriately sized screw is inserted. In most cases, to preserve the normal anatomical landmarks, screw insertion is performed before posterior decompression procedures. Ipsilateral cervical laminectomy and bilateral decompression were performed. Rods of appropriate length were selected and bent to match the contour of the cervical spine, and secured to the screws by screw head nuts. Bone grafts from a dissected lower part of spinous processes and lamina were placed laterally on both sides of the joints. Additional two skin incisions were made contralaterally for contralateral lateral mass screw fixation with the same method. After bleeding control, a drainage catheter was inserted.

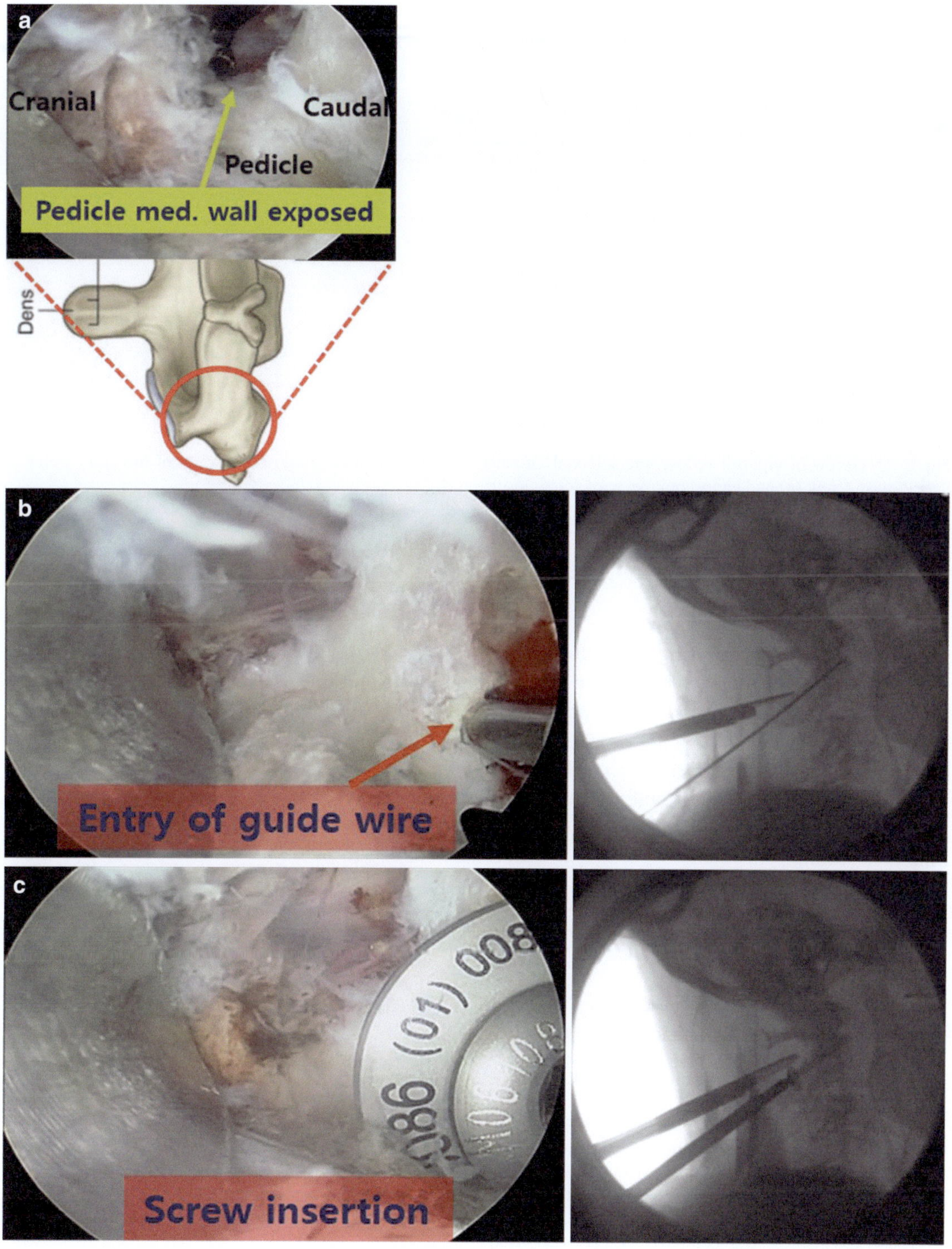


**Fig. 5** Overview of biportal endoscopic C2 lag screw fixation. Surgical anatomy of C2 (**a**), endoscopic view of the entry point of C2 lag screw and real-time intraoperative fluoroscopic image, (**b**) and endoscopic view of screw insertion and intraoperative fluoroscopic image (**c**)

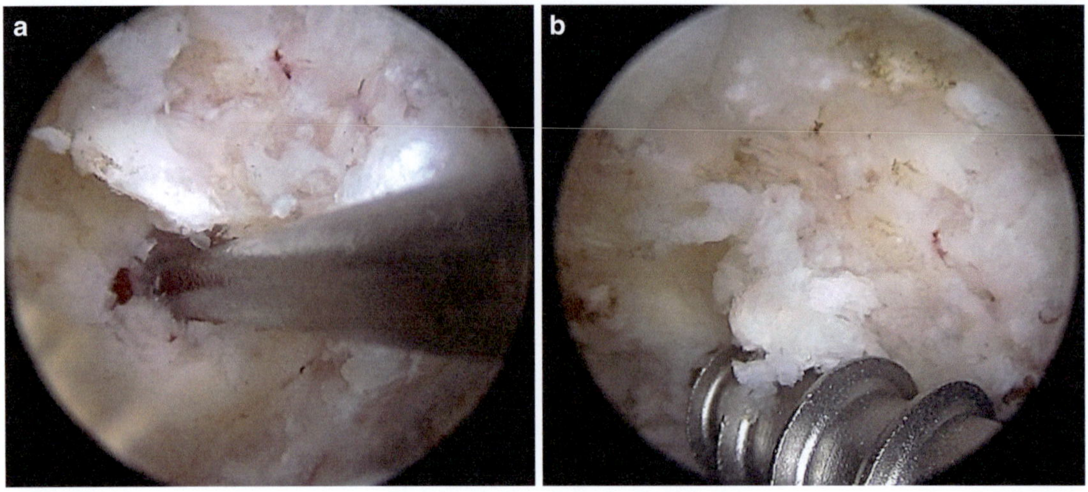

**Fig. 6** Overview of biportal endoscopic subaxial lateral mass screw fixation. Endoscopic view of the entry point of lateral mass screw (**a**) and endoscopic view of screw insertion (**b**)

## 6 Pitfall

Cervical instrumentation using a biportal endoscope can be performed under a clear surgical view using an optical lens and has the advantage of reducing damage to the paraspinal muscle compared to conventional open surgery. However, unlike the cervical procedure centered on decompression, it is technically demanding and time-consuming.

## References


1. Kim J, Heo DH, Lee DC, Chung HT. Biportal endoscopic unilateral laminotomy with bilateral decompression for the treatment of cervical spondylotic myelopathy. Acta Neurochir. 2021;163(9):2537–43.
2. Heo DH, Lee N, Park CW, Kim HS, Chung HJ. Endoscopic unilateral laminotomy with bilateral discectomy using biportal endoscopic approach: technical report and preliminary clinical results. World Neurosurg. 2020;137:31–7.
3. Lin GX, Huang P, Kotheeranurak V, Park CW, Heo DH, Park CK, Park JY, Kim JS. A systematic review of unilateral biportal endoscopic spinal surgery: preliminary clinical results and complications. World Neurosurg. 2019;125:425–32.
4. Heo DH, Son SK, Eum JH, Park CK. Endoscopic IUB: fully endoscopic lumbar interbody fusion using a percutaneous unilateral biportal endoscopic technique: technical note and preliminary clinical results. Neurosurg Focus. 2017;43(2):E8.
5. Kim N, Jung SB. Percutaneous unilateral biportal endoscopic spine surgery using a 30-degree arthroscope in patients with severe lumbar spinal stenosis: a technical note. Clin Spine Surg. 2019;32(8):324–9.
6. Park MK, Park SA, Son SK, Park WW, Choi SH. Clinical and radiological outcomes of unilateral biportal endoscopic lumbar interbody fusion (ULIF) compared with conventional posterior lumbar interbody fusion (PLIF): 1-year follow-up. Neurosurg Rev. 2019;42(3):753–61.
7. Heo DH, Sharma S, Park CK. Endoscopic treatment of extraforaminal entrapment of L5 nerve root (far out syndrome) by unilateral biportal endoscopic approach: technical report and preliminary clinical results. Neurospine. 2019;16(1):130–7.
8. Mikhael MM, Celestre PC, Wolf CF, Mroz TE, Wang JC. Minimally invasive cervical spine foraminotomy and lateral mass screw placement. Spine. 2012;37(5):E318–22.
9. Man Kyu C, Youngseok K, Ki Hong K, Dae-Hyun K. Direct trans-pedicular screw fixation for atypical hangman's fracture: a minimally invasive technique using the tubular retractor system. J Clin Neurosci. 2019;70:146–50.
10. Kim SH, Seo WD, Kim KH, Yeo HT, Choi GH, Kim DH. Clinical outcome of modified cervical lateral mass screw fixation technique. J Korean Neurosurg Soc. 2012;52(2):114–9.

# Part IV

# Thoracic - Introduction

# Anatomical Considerations for Thoracic Endoscopic Spine Surgery

Junseok Bae and Dong Hwa Heo

**Abstract**

The surgical approach to the thoracic spine has a high incidence of approach-related complications. Due to the complexity of the thoracic spine, there are several conventional open surgical techniques, but the advantage of direct visualization is often related to a potential risk of pulmonary complications, extensive bone resection, and a wide range of instrumentations. Endoscopic surgery can minimize the incidence of complications by preserving bone and joint tissue. Understanding the surgical anatomy is important for minimally invasive surgery, especially endoscopic surgery. It is also very important to understand the preoperative radiological anatomy for successful endoscopic thoracic spine surgery. We introduce the surgical anatomy and radiological anatomy of the posterior and transforaminal endoscopic approaches in the thoracic spine.

J. Bae
Endoscopic Spine Surgery Center, Neurosurgery, Champodonamu Spine Hospital, Seoul, South Korea

D. H. Heo (✉)
Neurosurgery, Wooridul Spine Hospital, Gangnam, South Korea

**Keywords**

Thoracic endoscopic approach · Thoracic spine · Anatomy · Transforaminal approach Surgical anatomy

## 1 Transforaminal Approach

### 1.1 Identifying the Surgical Level

Accurate localization of index level during the surgery is very important and often mistaken in the thoracic spine. Double-check the surgical level during the surgery. Since rib count is often misleading, authors recommend counting the pedicle to confirm the vertebra level in the AP fluoroscopic view for the upper and mid-thoracic spine (Fig. 1a). The lower thoracic spine can be counted up from the sacrum in the lateral fluoroscopic view (Fig. 1b). If the patient has an instrumented vertebra, it may be more helpful to check the level, so it should be checked before surgery. T12 ribs are an important landmark of level marking (Fig. 1c).

In preoperative MRI and CT scans, it may be also difficult to confirm the level only with the image of the thoracic spine. Therefore, it is necessary to add a sagittal scan of a wide field of view, including the cervical spine to confirm the correct level (Fig. 2).


H. S. Kim et al. (eds.), *Advanced Technique of Endoscopic Cervical and Thoracic Spine Surgery*,
https://doi.org/10.1007/978-981-99-1133-2_12

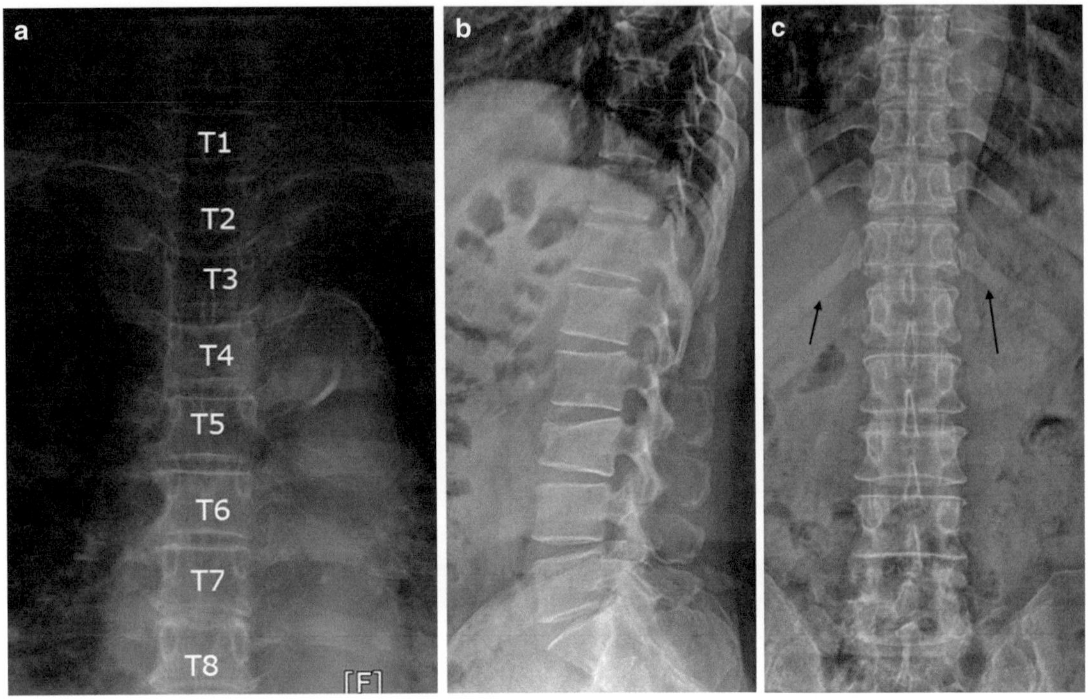


**Fig. 1** Accurate localization of index level during the surgery is important in the thoracic spine. Counting the pedicle number to confirm the vertebra level in the AP fluoroscopic view for the upper and mid thoracic spine. (**a**) The lower thoracic spine can be counted up from the sacrum in the lateral fluoroscopic view. (**b**). T12 ribs are a good landmark of level confirmation in AP vie (**c**, arrows)

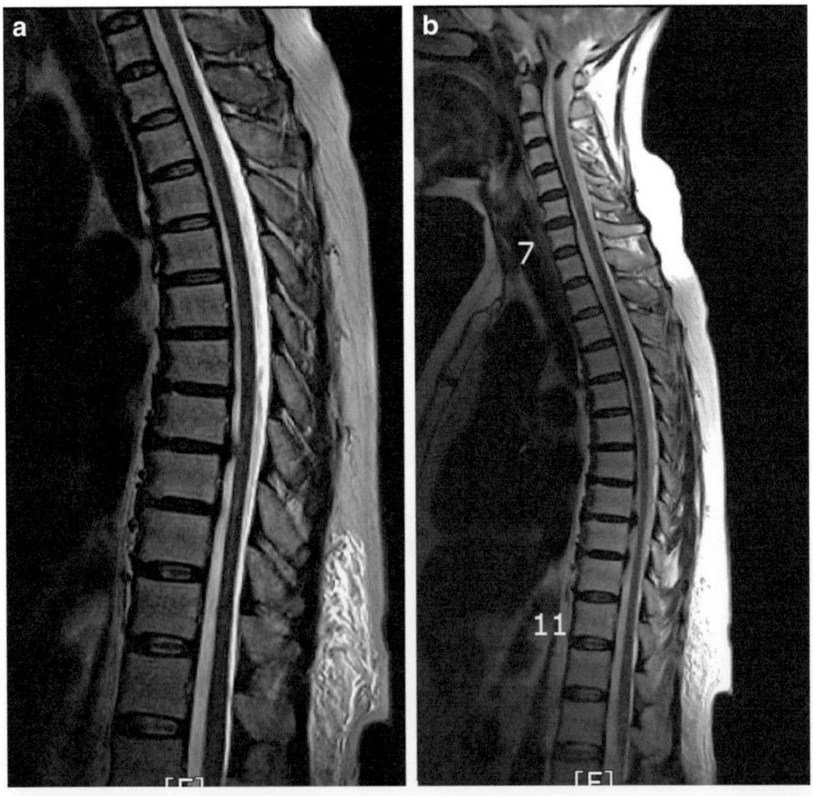


**Fig. 2** In preoperative MRI, it may be also difficult to confirm the level only with the image of the thoracic spine (**a**). It is necessary to check a sagittal scan of a wide field of view, including the cervical spine to confirm the correct level (**b**)

### 1.2 Intervertebral Neural Foramen

The neural foramen in the thoracic spine is different from the lumbar spine. The height of the neural foramen is smaller, the extraforaminal space becomes narrower by the costovertebral joint, and the width of the foramen becomes wider because of the coronal-oriented facet joint [1]. From T1 to T10, the intervertebral foramen in the thoracic spine is characterized by the head of the closet rib, superior articular process, and ventral aspect of facet joint, pedicle, ligamentous and capsular attachment, and the intervertebral disc. Neural foramen in the T10–11 and T11–12 levels is similar to the upper lumbar spine because the 11th and 12th ribs do not play a role in the structure [2, 3] (Fig. 3).

The upper 1/3 of the neural foramen is occupied by the corresponding exiting nerve root. There is little safe room for the transforaminal approach. For these anatomical limitations, extensive foraminoplasty is the key step for the transforaminal approach. Entering posterolaterally, a foraminotomy is performed to enlarge cannula access to the inner foraminal zone. The articular facet is undercut and the rib head is trimmed with an endoscopic reamer or high-speed burr [4].

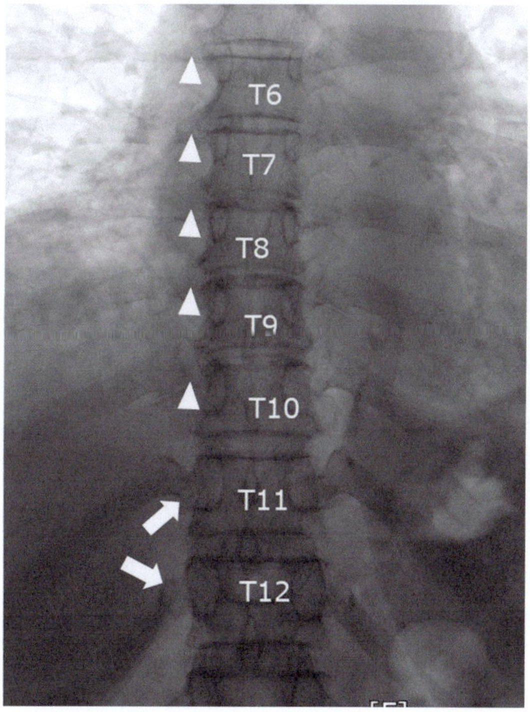


**Fig. 3** The neural foramen in the thoracic spine is bordered by the rib head (arrowhead) laterally above the T9–10 level. Neural foramen in the T10–11 and T11–12 level is similar to the upper lumbar spine because the 11th and 12th rib head (arrow) is attached to the lateral vertebral body

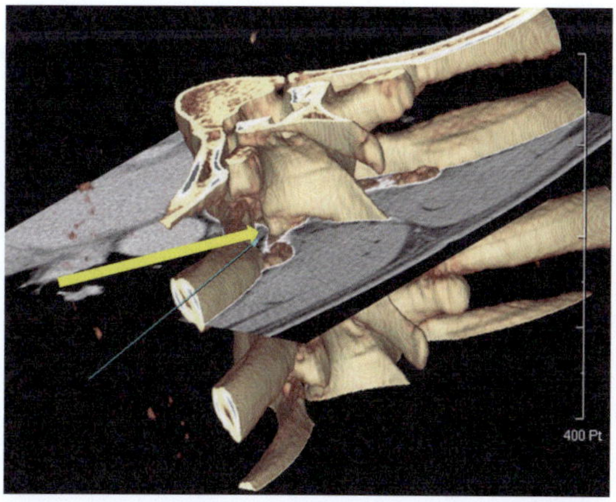


**Fig. 4** Approaching the endplate parallel to the endplate (green arrow) interferes with the transverse process, so it should be approached at an oblique angle (yellow arrow)

The transverse process of the thoracic spine is relatively long and protruded posterolateral from the pedicle and laminar junction. Approaching the endplate parallel to the endplate interferes with the transverse process, so it should be approached at an oblique angle (Fig. 4).

### 1.3 Spinal Canal

Surgical access to the thoracic spinal canal is limited by the anatomical constraints of the rib attachments. The spinal cord at the thoracic level is particularly vulnerable to surgical intervention. The natural thoracic kyphosis flattens the dural sheath against the disc's posterior margin, and the spinal cord's mobility is limited within the canal by the denticulate ligaments. In addition, the ratio of cord diameter to that of the canal leaves little space around the cord and, at some levels, the medullary vascularization is limited. Therefore, the outside-in technique should be considered in very limited cases to avoid spinal cord retraction. The inside-out technique is safe not only for para-median disc herniation but for central disc herniation [5]. The thoracic intervertebral disc appears heart-shaped in its axial plane view, which allows direct endoscopic visualization of the central disc space (Fig. 5).

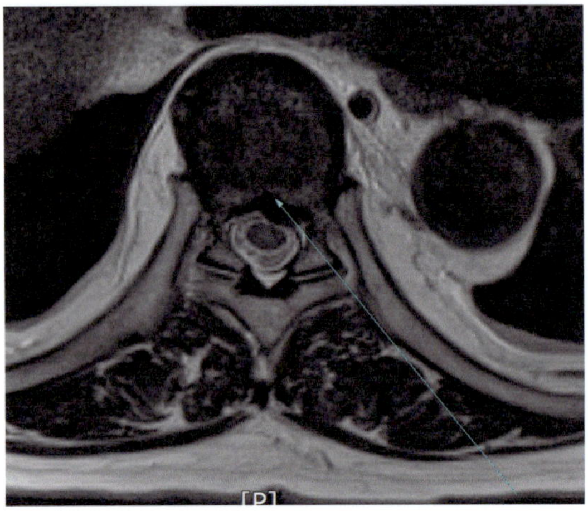

**Fig. 5** The thoracic intervertebral disc appears heart-shaped in its axial plane view, which allows direct endoscopic visualization of the central disc space (arrow)

## 1.4 Endoscopic Anatomy of Transforaminal Approach

Endoscopic surgical anatomy is similar to that of the lumbar transforaminal approach. The inside-out approach allows clear neural anatomy to be visualized after full decompression. After internal decompression, the posterior longitudinal ligament (PLL) and herniated fragment are seen (Fig. 6a). Partial resection of the PLL layer and posterior annulus is exposing the ventral epidural space. PLL resection is mandatory in case of trans-ligamentous herniation. Epidural-free pulsation or inspection of ventral dura is a sign of full decompression (Fig. 6b). Surgery can be finished at this stage.

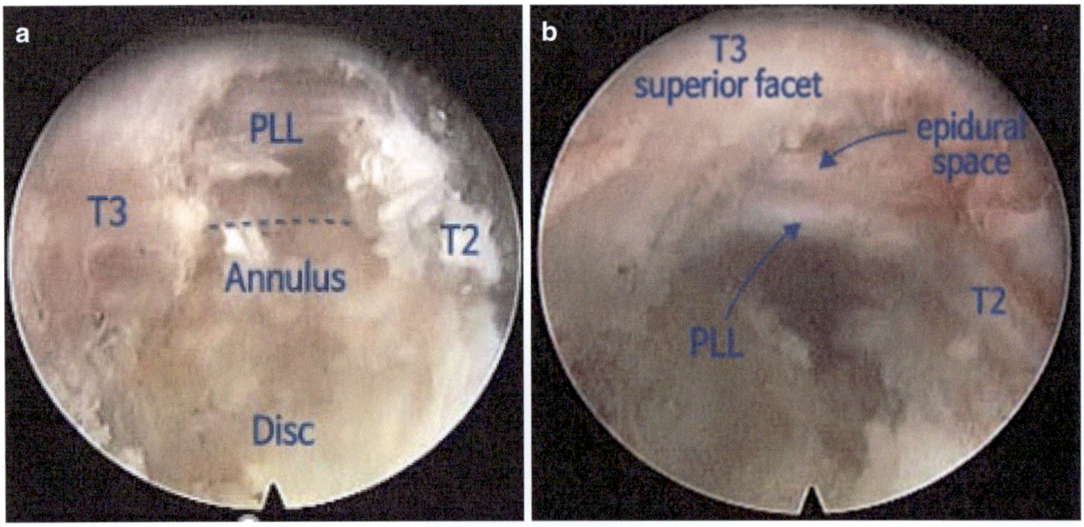


**Fig. 6** (**a**) After internal decompression, the posterior longitudinal ligament (PLL) and herniated fragment are seen. (**b**) Epidural-free pulsation or inspection of ventral dura is a sign of full decompression

## 2 Posterior Approach

### 2.1 Radiological Anatomy

In posterior endoscopic approaches using biportal or uniportal endoscopic systems, decompressive thoracic laminectomy or thoracic discectomy was usually performed [6, 7]. Preoperative CT images were important for preoperative surgical planning of posterior thoracic endoscopic surgery. Interlaminar space was usually lower than intervertebral disc space (Fig. 7a). Therefore, we should do superior-wide laminotomy over the disc space for complete decompression. Pedicles were an important landmark for an endpoint of thoracic endoscopic laminectomy. In a posterior endoscopic laminectomy, we tried to do complete decompression from pedicle to pedicle (Fig. 7b).

Axial CT images were also important for the decision-making of surgical treatment (Fig. 8a and b). In patients having dural calcifications with ossification of ligamentum flavum, microscopic surgery may be better than endoscopic decompression. Dural calcification related to ossification of ligamentum flavum may have a high possibility of dural injury and incomplete decompression (Fig. 8a). Thoracic CT images can reveal the presence of calcification of herniated thoracic disc (Fig. 8b).

### 2.2 Endoscopic Anatomy of Posterior Thoracic Approaches

Unilateral thoracic laminotomy with bilateral decompression was usually attempted for thoracic stenosis or thoracic ossification of ligamentum flavum (Fig. 9a). Midline laminotomy of spinous process base is important in a thoracic endoscopic laminectomy. After ipsilateral laminotomy, ipsilateral and contralateral ligamentum flavum should be seen (Fig. 9a). Ossification of ligamentum flavum is usually located under the normal ligamentum flavum (Fig. 9b). Ossification of ligamentum flavum was attached to lower lam-

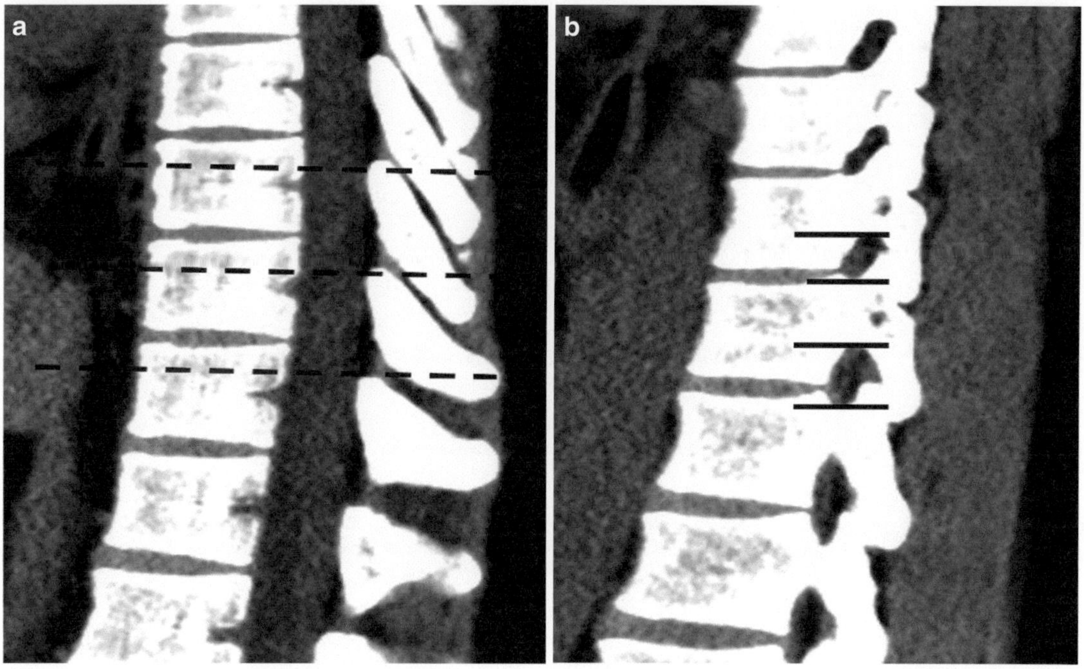


**Fig. 7** Sagittal CT images of the thoracic spine. Interlaminar space is lower than the disc space (**a**). The pedicle margin is an important landmark of endoscopic posterior thoracic decompression. Laminotomy should be performed from pedicle to pedicle (**b**)

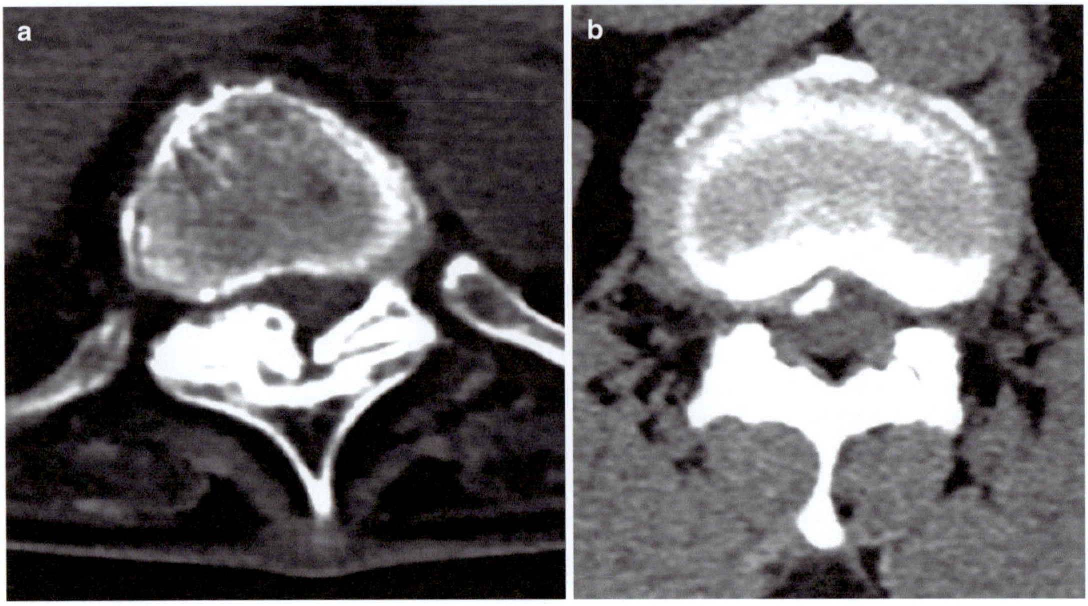

**Fig. 8** CT axial images of the thoracic spine. Ossification of ligamentum flavum was detected in the thoracic area (**a**). There was a high possibility of dural calcification and dura adhesion (**a**). CT images reveal the calcification of herniated thoracic disc (**b**)

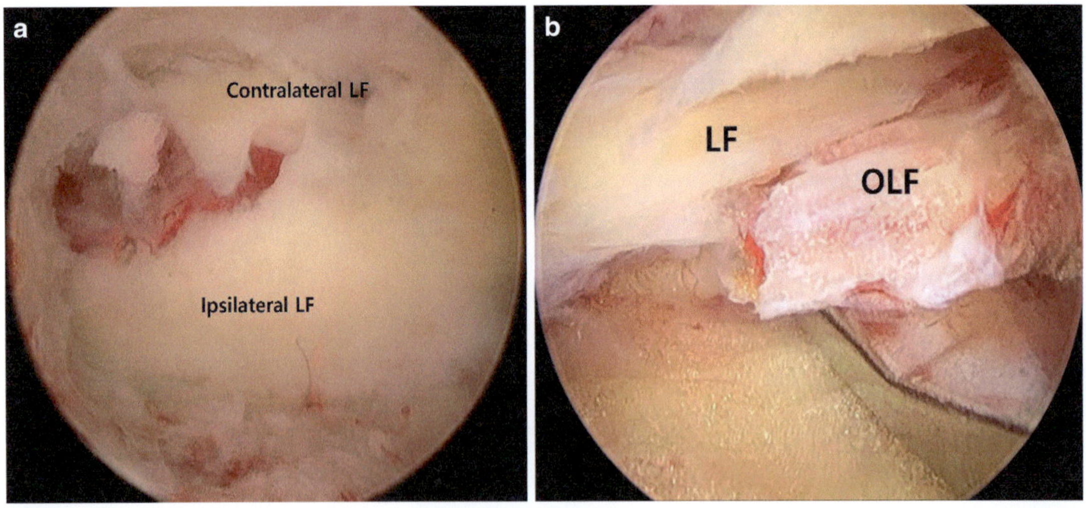


**Fig. 9** Intraoperative endoscopic images of posterior thoracic approach. The endoscopic images of unilateral thoracic laminotomy with bilateral decompression show ipsilateral and contralateral ligamentum flavum (**a**). The ossification part of ligamentum flavum was usually located under normal soft ligamentum flavum (**b**)

inae and superior articular process (Fig. 10). Before removal of ossified ligamentum flavum, laminar superior articular process should be exposed after thoracic laminotomy.

After laminotomy and removal of ligamentum flavum, the medial border of the pedicle was palpated for confirmation of complete decompression of the thoracic central canal (Fig. 11).

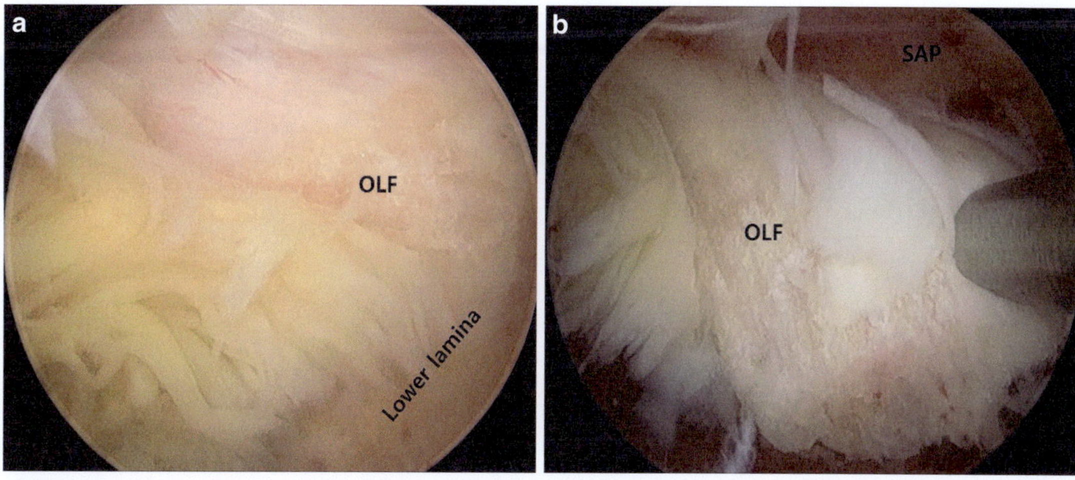


**Fig. 10** Intraoperative endoscopic images of ossification of ligamentum flavum in the thoracic spine. Ossified ligamentum flavum was attached to the lower laminae (**a**). The lateral part of the ossification of ligamentum flavum was attached to the superior articular process (**b**)

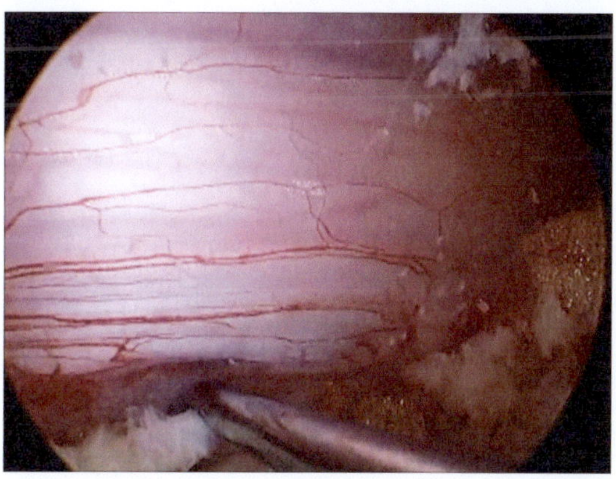

**Fig. 11** Fully decompression status of the thoracic central canal. The medial border of the pedicle should be checked using a dissector or a probe

## References


1. Bae J, Chachan S, Shin SH, Lee SH. Percutaneous endoscopic thoracic discectomy in the upper and midthoracic spine: a technical note. Neurospine. 2019;16(1):148–53.
2. Choi G, Munoz-Suarez D. Transforaminal endoscopic thoracic discectomy: technical review to prevent complications. Neurospine. 2020;17(Suppl 1):S58–65.
3. Wagner R, Telfeian AE, Iprenburg M, Krzok G, Gokaslan Z, Choi DB, et al. Transforaminal endoscopic foraminoplasty and discectomy for the treatment of a thoracic disc herniation. World Neurosurg. 2016;90:194–8.
4. Choi KY, Eun SS, Lee SH, Lee HY. Percutaneous endoscopic thoracic discectomy; transforaminal approach. Minim Invasive Neurosurg. 2010;53(1):25–8.
5. Bae J, Lee SH, Wagner R, Shen J, Telfeian AE. Full endoscopic surgery for thoracic pathology: next step after mastering lumbar and cervical endoscopic spine surgery? Biomed Res Int. 2022;2022:8345736.
6. Kang MS, Chung HJ, You KH, Park HJ. How I do it: biportal endoscopic thoracic decompression for ossification of the ligamentum flavum. Acta Neurochir (Wien). 2022;164(1):43–7.
7. Kim HS, Wu PH, Kim JY, Lee YJ, Kim DH, Lee JH, et al. Comparative clinical and radiographic cohort study: uniportal thoracic endoscopic laminotomy with bilateral decompression by using the 1-block resection technique and thoracic open laminotomy with bilateral decompression for thoracic ossified ligamentum flavum. Oper Neurosurg (Hagerstown). 2022;22:391.

# Part V

# Thoracic - Uniportal

# Transformational Thoracic Discectomy

Junseok Bae, Jin-Sung Kim, and Gun Choi

**Abstract**

Thoracic disc herniation is a relatively rare and various symptom making it difficult to diagnose. Due to the complexity of neural and vascular structure, surgical treatment of thoracic disc herniation is challenging. Transforaminal access offers a safe surgical corridor into the thoracic spinal canal. Under local anesthesia, direct discectomy with endoscopic visualization through a transforaminal approach is an effective treatment method for the selected groups of patients with thoracic disc herniation.

**Keywords**

Endoscopic thoracic discectomy
Transforaminal approach · Foraminoplasty
Thoracic disc herniation · Awakened surgery

**Supplementary Information** The online version contains supplementary material available at https://doi.org/10.1007/978-981-99-1133-2_13.

J. Bae (✉)
Department of Neurosurgery, Wooridul Spine Hospital, Seoul, South Korea

J.-S. Kim
Department of Neurosurgery, Seoul St. Mary's Hospital, Seoul, South Korea

G. Choi
Department of Neurosurgery, Pohang Woori Spine Hospital, Pohang, South Korea

## 1 Introduction

Thoracic disc herniation is rare compared with lumbar disc or cervical disc herniation, accounting for 0.25–0.5% of disc disease [1–3]. However, the diagnosis of thoracic disc herniation is increasing with the development of diagnostic methods such as magnetic resonance imaging (MRI). In patients with symptomatic thoracic disc herniation, clinical manifestations can be dynamic and progressive. Progressive myelopathy or voiding difficulty, lower limb motor weakness, and patients with radiculopathy not responding to conservative therapy are candidates for decompression surgery [4–6].

Kambin introduced the concept of posterior-lateral disc decompression in 1983. Endoscopic discectomies were developed into effective treatment methods for many herniated disc patients. However, compared to open surgery, endoscopic decompression is difficult to apply for all forms of disc herniation due to its small operating field, limited equipment availability, and limited working mobility. Therefore, it is very important to establish an appropriate indication.

Transforaminal endoscopic thoracic discectomy (TETD) can minimize the incidence of postoperative spinal instability by minimizing



H. S. Kim et al. (eds.), *Advanced Technique of Endoscopic Cervical and Thoracic Spine Surgery*,
https://doi.org/10.1007/978-981-99-1133-2_13

the resection of bone and joint tissue. It can be performed under local anesthesia and has a faster recovery than open surgery. In addition, there is little traction on the nerve, which can reduce nerve edema, and it does not cause excessive nerve tissue exposure, thus minimizing postoperative neural adhesion. Indications for endoscopic discectomy are becoming increasingly widespread due to patient needs and the development of endoscopic devices [1–3, 7, 8].

## 2 Indications

- Symptomatic soft disc herniation of paramedian, foraminal, or central disc space.
- Condition that failed to improve symptoms after intensive conservative treatment, including transforaminal epidural block and physical therapy.
- Calcified disc herniations, concomitant ossification of the posterior longitudinal ligament (OPLL) or ossification of the ligamentum flavum (OLF), significant myelopathy causing prominent neurological deterioration, history of trauma, and worker's compensation claim were excluded.

## 3 Anesthesia and Position

The patient is positioned face down on a radiolucent operating table and on a Wilson frame, with the side to be operated on facing the surgeon. The arms are supported on arm boards over the head. As only mild sedation and local anesthesia are used, the extremities, buttocks, and shoulders can be prevented from jerking with tape if necessary. The marking of the level to be operated and the point of entry into the skin are made with the aid of C-arm images in the visualization and axial profile, corroborating the preoperative planning previously measured by computed tomography or magnetic resonance. Using the axial image of the level to be operated on, draw a line from the center of the protrusion through the edge of the facet joint and extend to the skin, joining another line drawn from that point to the midline. After the patient's position, the surgeon faces the side to be operated on, and the assistant nurse stands on the surgeon's right side and next to her the table with the instruments. Video tower, C-arm, and laser generator are on the other side of the patient, facing the surgeon (Fig. 1). All procedures were performed under local anesthesia with conscious sedation.

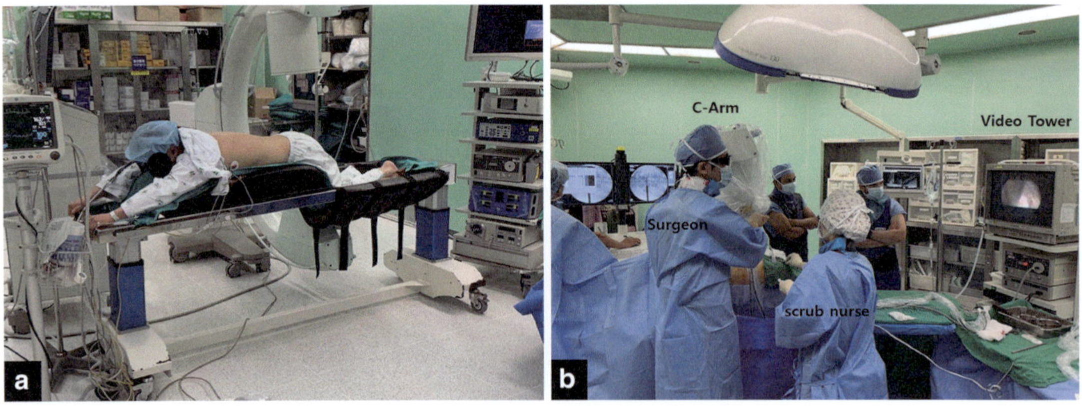


**Fig. 1** Patient's position (**a**) and positions of medical staffs (**b**) during TETD

## 4 Special Instrument

Although the basic mechanics of instruments for the thoracic transforaminal endoscopy system is very similar to the lumbar endoscopy system, the subtle variations in angles, diameters, and length of instruments hold the key to the successful execution of thoracic endoscopic surgery.

1. Thoracic endoscopes differ from other spinal endoscopes in the following ways [2]:
   - They are angled at 45°. This allows us to work with a steeper access route and much shorter in length as the thoracic spine does not have much soft-tissue cover dorsally.
   - They are smaller in diameter to accommodate space restriction in the thoracic spine.
2. Endo-reamers/endo drills are available in various sizes and angles. They are used for undercutting the superior facet or removal of a part of the vertebral body. They can also be used to make a hole in the annulus and allow easy passage of the dilator. They can also be used for the removal of small osteophytes or calcified disk material.
3. Instruments for discectomy are endoscopic forceps and dissecting instruments. There are rigid or articulating forceps either up-biting or down-biting figures. The jaws can be serrated or nonserrated. Radiofrequency probes can be used as a dissector and coagulator of soft tissue.

## 5 Procedures

An appropriate skin entry point was determined by drawing a line from the posterior annulus at the mid-pedicular level to the lateral margin of facet join on axial computed tomography (CT) scan cuts (Fig. 2). The skin entry point was commonly located at 5–6 cm from the midline. Although the scapular does move laterally with lifting arms, there is a limitation of the lateral access point. Extensive foraminotomy is thus required. The outline of foraminoplasty may be similar to other thoracic levels. However, a steeper approach requires more aggressive tech-

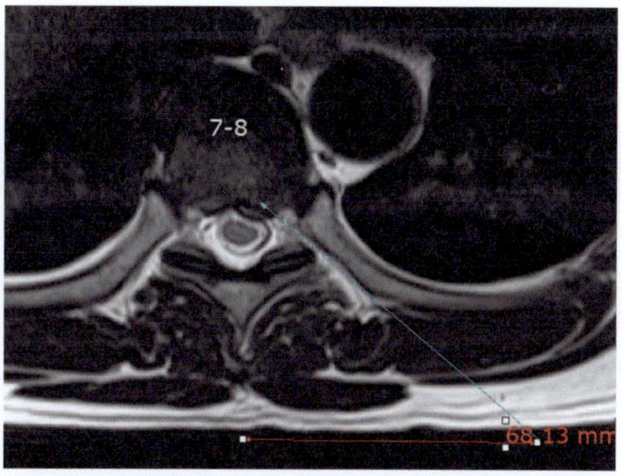


**Fig. 2** The skin entry point was determined by drawing a line from the posterior annulus at the midpedicular level to the lateral margin of the facet joint on axial computed tomography scan or magnetic resonance imaging, usually located approximately 6–7 cm from the midline

niques using reamers. On lateral fluoroscopic view, approach angle was measured by drawing an oblique line from the posterior endplate of the lower vertebra passing the tip of the superior articular process along with its inclination. This is to avoid a thick transverse process obstructing the working trajectory.

After infiltration of local anesthetics, an 18-gauge needle is advanced along the planned trajectory under lateral fluoroscopic view to the lateral aspect of the superior facet. A guidewire was inserted through the needle. Epidurography was performed, followed by an epidural block. Discography was performed by injecting a mixture of radiopaque dye (Telebrix; Guerbet, France), indigo carmine (Carmine; Korea United Pharmaceutical, Yoenki, Korea), and normal saline in a 2:1:2 ratio. Indio carmine stains the degenerated acidic nucleus blue and helps in identifying the herniated disc fragment.

Foraminoplasty was performed using a serial dilating side-cutting drill, reamer, or high-speed drill (Fig. 3). A beveled 5.8-mm outer diameter working cannula was then placed on the posterior disc space (Fig. 4). Then, the 3.1-mm endoscope (TESSYS thx, Joimax GmbH, Germany) was introduced. Under the direct visualization, a blue-stained annular surface and herniated disc fragment could be identified. By removing the annulus of the outer layer and the internal layer of the posterior longitu-

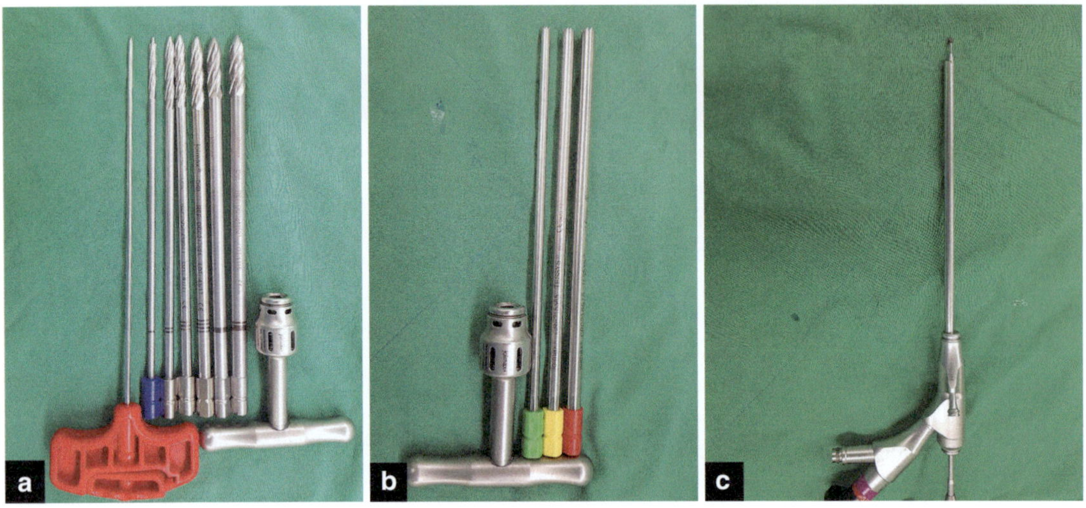


**Fig. 3** Special surgical instrument used for foraminoplasty: (**a**) manual bone drill, (**b**) manual bone reamer, and (**c**) endoscopic high-speed burr

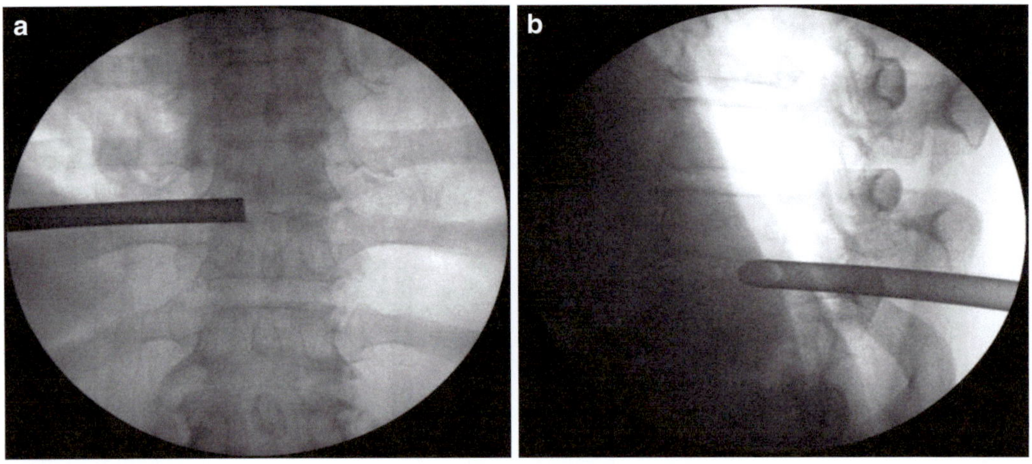


**Fig. 4** Fluoroscopic view of transforaminal working channel placement. Note that it is located on the medial pedicle line on the AP view (**a**) and the posterior vertebral line on the lateral view (**b**)

dinal ligament (PLL) with a side-firing laser, the blue-stained herniated fragment was released from anchoring. Then the fragment was removed using microforceps (Video 1). Since thoracic disc herniation is mostly chronic and contained herniation with or without partial calcification, resection of PLL is not always necessary, and soft herniation decompression is the goal of surgery. After adequate decompression, ventral epidural space and thecal sac were visible. Epidural pulsation can be observed even when the PLL remains.

The skin was closed with a single subcuticular suture and a sterile dressing was applied.

## 6 Illustrated Cases

### 6.1 Case 1

A 30-year-old male presented with mid-thoracic back pain of 3 years duration. MRI thoracic spine showed left paramedian TDH at the T8–9 level. He underwent PETD under local anesthesia. Postoperatively patients showed significant improvements in both VAS and ODI scores. Using modified Macnab's criteria, the clinical outcome was categorized as good and it was maintained during 12 months of postop follow-up (Fig. 5).

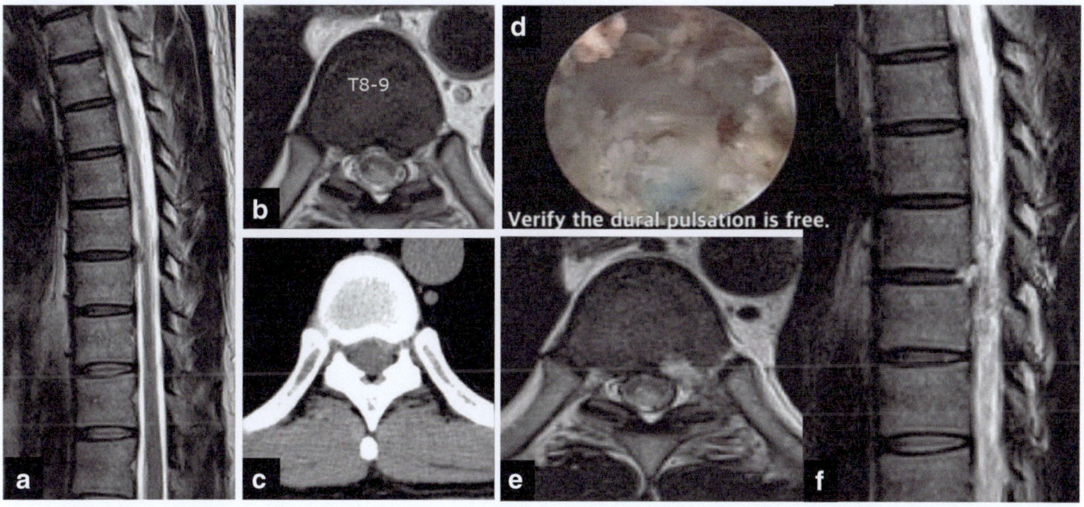


**Fig. 5** Case presentation of a 30-year-old male, presented with mid-thoracic back pain of 3 years duration. Preoperative sagittal (**a**) and axial (**b**) magnetic resonance image (MRI) and CT scan (**c**) showed paramedian soft disc herniation at the T8–9 level. Transforaminal endoscopic discectomy was done (**d**). Postoperative axial (**e**) and sagittal (**f**) MRI showed full decompression, and the patient's pain improved

## 6.2 Case 2

A 46-year-old male patient suffering from thoracic back pain and chest discomfort for 1 year was diagnosed as paramedian TDH at the T2–3 level. TETD was performed under local anesthesia. After surgery, the patient's pain decreased (VAS 7 to 1) (Fig. 6).

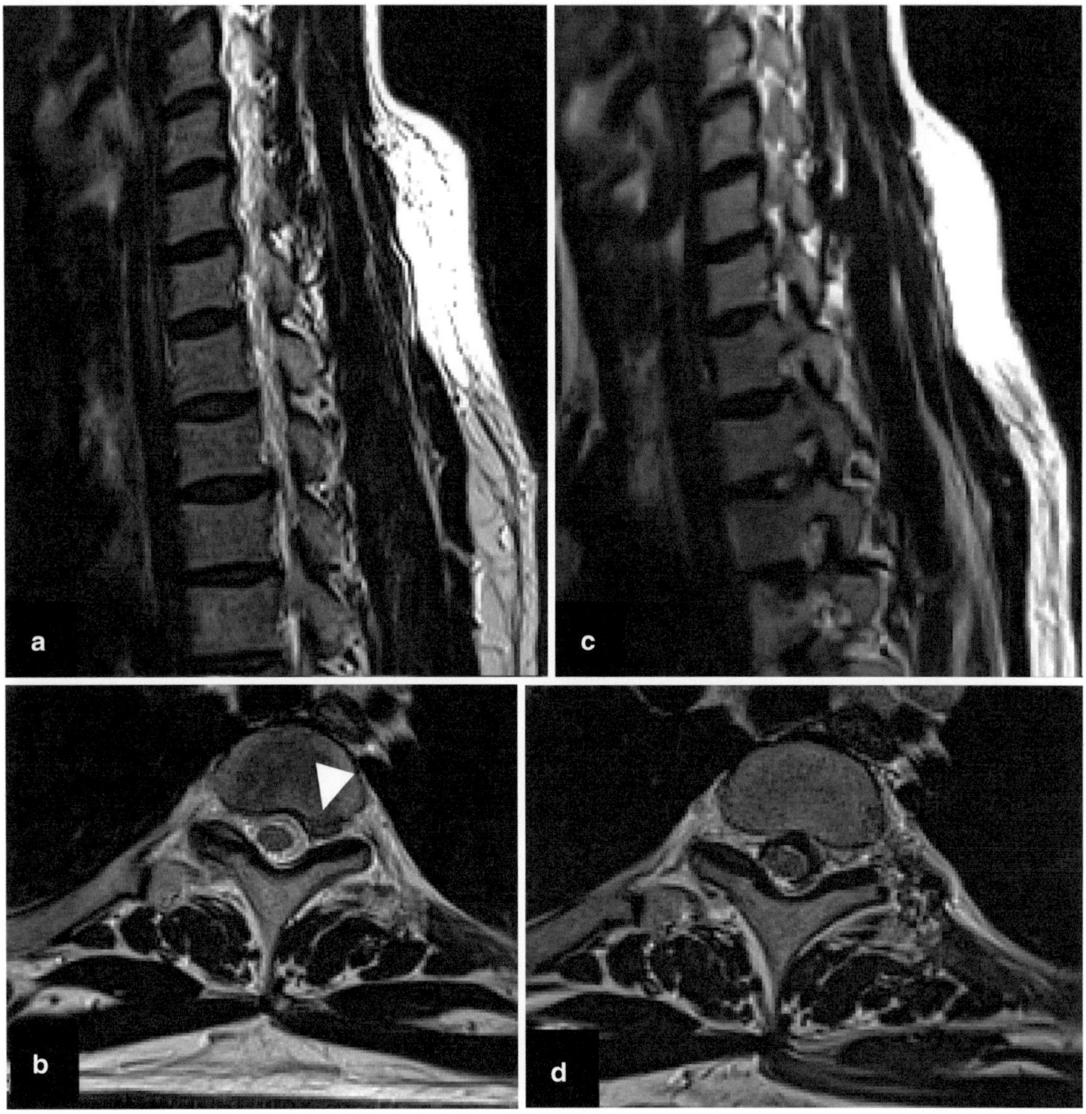


**Fig. 6** Case presentation of a 46-year-old male patient suffering from thoracic back pain and chest discomfort. Preoperative sagittal (**a**) and axial (**b**) MRI showed foraminal soft disc herniation at the T2–3 level. TETD was performed under the local anesthesia. Postoperative MRI showed full decompression (**c**, **d**). After surgery, the patient's pain decreased

## 7 Prevention and Management of Complications

The proximity of major vascular, visceral, and neurological structures during TETD is a real concern. Understanding of three-dimensional anatomy, sufficient experience with spinal endoscopy techniques, and expert patient selection to get optimum results are necessary. To achieve a safe surgical trajectory into the spinal canal, foraminoplasty is an essential step [1–3, 6, 8]. A safe corridor is mapped on the preoperative MRI to avoid the lung and the ribs. Another special consideration is given to the dural sac to spinal canal ratio. The needle trajectory for transforaminal aims to allow access as close as possible to the ventral surface of the dural sac avoiding injury of the dura mater. Reamer and bone drills allow removal of the ventrolateral portion of the superior facet to unveil the ventral pathology. Recurrent disc herniation is not uncommon but repeated TETD can be a surgical option. As in the case of recurrent disc herniation after transforaminal endoscopic lumbar discectomy, there is little epidural adhesion after TETD, and repeated TETD is a safe procedure.

## 8 Discussion

Transforaminal endoscopic thoracic discectomy (TETD) can minimize the incidence of postoperative spinal instability by minimizing the resection of bone and joint tissue. It can be performed under local anesthesia and has a faster recovery than open surgery.

The distance from the midline to the skin entry point can be calculated in the axial image of the MRI, usually 5–7 cm. An access angle of about 45–60° is recommended for the removal of the disc in the subarticular zone.

The neural foramen in the lower thoracic spine is similar to the upper lumbar spine. Rib head attached on index vertebra. The superior articular process is relatively small. The transforaminal approach can be performed without foraminoplasty.

In the upper and middle thoracic spine, anatomical barriers are more complex with the widened transverse process, cranial attachment of the rib head at the disc level, and coronal-directed facet joint complex resulting in narrow neural foramen [9]. Extensive foraminoplasty is mandatory for the TETD. Thoracic vertebral bodies appear heart-shaped when viewed from above. The left–right width increases from T4 to T12 with a trapezoid in shape. In central extruded disc or broad-based disc herniation, paracentral intra-annular placement of working cannular can permit good endoscopic visualization. Surgical planning of TETD is different from TELD in this respect of anatomical characteristics.

The presence of calcification is important in decision-making. Hard disc or calcified disc causes severe epidural adhesion, making it difficult in dissecting or complete decompression. Moreover, accompanied dural ossification or ventral dural erosion is a risk factor of the intra-operative dural leak. Intradural disc herniation is very rare but can be observed in a chronic lesion with calcifications. A preoperative CT scan should be performed to exclude these cases.

## References

1. Choi G, Munoz-Suarez D. Transforaminal endoscopic thoracic discectomy: technical review to prevent complications. Neurospine. 2020;17(Suppl 1):S58–65.
2. Bae J, Chachan S, Shin SH, Lee SH. Transforaminal endoscopic thoracic discectomy with foraminoplasty for the treatment of thoracic disc herniation. J Spine Surg. 2020;6(2):397–404.
3. Wagner R, Telfeian AE, Iprenburg M, Krzok G, Gokaslan Z, Choi DB, et al. Transforaminal endoscopic foraminoplasty and discectomy for the treatment of a thoracic disc herniation. World Neurosurg. 2016;90:194–8.
4. Shen J, Shaaya E, Bae J, Telfeian AE. Endoscopic spine surgery of the cervicothoracic spine: a review of current applications. Int J Spine Surg. 2021;15(suppl 3):S93–S103.
5. Gibson RDS, Wagner R, Gibson JNA. Full endoscopic surgery for thoracic pathology: an assessment of supportive evidence. EFORT Open Rev. 2021;6(1):50–60.
6. Cho JY, Lee SH, Jang SH, Lee HY. Oblique paraspinal approach for thoracic disc herniations using tubu-

lar retractor with robotic holder: a technical note. Eur Spine J. 2012;21(12):2620–5.
7. Bouthors C, Benzakour A, Court C. Surgical treatment of thoracic disc herniation: an overview. Int Orthop. 2019;43(4):807–16.
8. Choi KY, Eun SS, Lee SH, Lee HY. Percutaneous endoscopic thoracic discectomy; transforaminal approach. Minim Invasive Neurosurg. 2010;53(1):25–8.
9. Bae J, Chachan S, Shin SH, Lee SH. Percutaneous endoscopic thoracic discectomy in the upper and midthoracic spine: a technical note. Neurospine. 2019;16(1):148–53.

# Thoracic Full Endoscopic Unilateral Laminotomy with Bilateral Decompression (TE ULBD)

Pang Hung Wu, Hyeun Sung Kim, and Il-Tae Jang

**Abstract**

Thoracic spinal decompression surgery for degenerative spinal disease and, in particular, thoracic-ossified ligamentum flavum faced several challenges: (1) presence of lung, pleura, and major vessels in proximity; (2) thoracic level has higher risk of wrong-level surgery; (3) density of neural element in thoracic cord with high risk of paralysis in cord compression/retraction; and (4) dura adhesion from the thoracic-ossified ligamentum flavum. There are several advantages of thoracic endoscopic spine surgery to optimize the surgical performance of the thoracic-ossified ligamentum flavum decompression: (1) high magnification provides clarity in visualization; (2) presence of working channel within the endoscope allows efficient precise placement of instruments to the region for decompression; and (3) less soft-tissue damages in exposure of region for decompression due to small diameter endoscope. These inherent advantages of spinal endoscopy allowed a systematic decompression of the thoracic-ossified ligamentum flavum as a single block off the dura of thoracic spinal cord. This chapter describes the nuances, tips, and tricks to perform full endoscopic unilateral laminotomy with bilateral decompression one-block resection technique for the thoracic-ossified ligamentum flavum.

**Keywords**

Ossified ligamentum flavum · Thoracic spinal decompression · Thoracic endoscopic unilateral laminotomy with bilateral decompression · Thoracic spinal endoscopy

**Supplementary Information** The online version contains supplementary material available at https://doi.org/10.1007/978-981-99-1133-2_14.

P. H. Wu
Nanoori Gangnam Hospital, Spine Surgery, Seoul, South Korea

National University Health System, JurongHealth Campus, Orthopaedic Surgery, Singapore, Singapore

H. S. Kim (✉) · I.-T. Jang
Nanoori Gangnam Hospital, Spine Surgery, Seoul, South Korea

## 1 Introduction

Thoracic myelopathy is an important cause of myelopathy. It is an important differential diagnosis to cervical myelopathy in patients presenting with unsteady gait. The common causes of thoracic myelopathy include facet hypertrophy and arthropathy, thoracic disc herniation, ossification of the posterior longitudinal ligament, and ossified ligamentum flavum (OLF) [1, 2]. Surgical decompression is recommended for these symptomatic thoracic myelopathy patients who had progressive deterioration and refractory



H. S. Kim et al. (eds.), *Advanced Technique of Endoscopic Cervical and Thoracic Spine Surgery*, https://doi.org/10.1007/978-981-99-1133-2_14

to conservative management [3]. Traditionally, open or minimally invasive thoracic laminectomy or unilateral laminotomy with bilateral decompression using a microscope with or without tubular retractor were options of surgical treatment in this group of patients. Perioperative complications in these surgeries are commonly described in the literature, with dural tears and CSF leaks being more commonly described. Less commonly described but catastrophic complication of neurological deterioration can happen during thoracic decompression [3]. As open decompression in thoracic spine might require significant bony removal and posterior spinal element disruption during decompression, instrumented stabilization and fusion procedure is common after thoracic decompression [2]. After surgical decompression in thoracic myelopathy, most literature suggests that there is some improvement in the Japanese Orthopaedic Association (JOA) score; however, the postoperative functional status remains fair [4].

Endoscopic spine surgery (ESS) had evolved from transforaminal endoscopic lumbar discectomy to a wide spectrum of surgical techniques as technological and technical improvements were made in endoscope lens optics, instruments, and handling. Current indications had broadened ESS indications to include degenerative spinal conditions of the cervical, thoracic, and lumbar regions [5, 6]. In thoracic spine, in order to decompress the spinal cord, uniportal full endoscopic thoracic approach is divided into two main approaches: anterior and posterior procedures. Transforaminal endoscopic thoracic discectomy (TETD) is the workhorse of anterior endoscopic approach to decompress soft thoracic disc. Extended indications of TETD include thoracic spinal stenosis from the degenerated disc or calcified disc [5, 6]. While TETD is perhaps the least invasive approach to thoracic spine, there is an inherent catastrophic danger of lung and segmental vessels and large vessel injuries as these vital structures are very close to the docking point in the TETD technique. In addition, TETD has limited efficacy in decompression of the thoracic spinal canal as it has limited access to posterior elements of the spinal segment, and its efficacy to decompress facet hypertrophy and ossified ligamentum flavum is very limited. Posterior endoscopic approach: thoracic endoscopic unilateral laminotomy with bilateral decompression (TE-ULBD) docks at laminofacet (V point) with serial dilation and retractor working tube. This minimizes soft-tissue damages as muscle dissection is minimal. The endoscope's optical lens, in-flow and out-flow irrigation channel, as well as working channel are all encased within the 10-mm-outer diameter endoscope. The 15–30 degrees angular lens allows wide-view angle to visualize under magnification while decompression is performed. Direct delivery of instruments through the endoscope's working channel under magnified endoscopic vision is possible through uniportal endoscope; hence, there is potential in improving safety and minimizing soft-tissue damages during the decompressive procedure.

The authors had previously described the technique of lumbar endoscopic unilateral laminotomy with decompression in 12 steps [7]. Adaptation of this technique can be applied for thoracic endoscopic decompression. The technical details are highlighted in this chapter.

## 1.1 Advantages

- Direct docking of working retractor cannula minimizes soft-tissue damages.
- Magnified visualization provides clarity of neural elements and in experienced hands can reduce rate of dura tear during separation of ossified yellow ligament and adhesions from compressive soft and bony tissues.
- Constant saline irrigation decreases infection rate and washout debris to provide improved visualization.
- Decrease postoperative morbidity: blood loss, perioperative pain and opioids requirement, wound care, and length of stay are shown to be beneficial [8].
- Endoscopic decompression has the potential to decompress sufficiently without causing instability with preservation of posterior spinal elements.

### 1.2 Disadvantages

- Steep learning curve in using endoscopic equipment in cord-level surgery.
- Duration of surgery is directly proportional to the number of levels of surgery; hence, <3 level surgeries are recommended.
- Limited capacity for instrumentation if needed at the thoracic level.
- Not recommended for patients with a significant neurological deficit with motor weakness.

## 2 Clinical Indications

- Symptomatic thoracic myelopathy
- Thoracic radiculopathy with failed conservative treatment

## 3 Radiographic Indications

- Sato types: lateral, extended, enlarged, and fused types of OLF [9]
- Facet arthropathy and facet cyst leading to spinal cord compressive myelopathy
- Central large/calcified disc
- Ossified posterior longitudinal ligament (OPLL)

## 4 Radiographic Relative Contraindications

- Tuberous type of OLF.
- Multiple (>3) levels of contiguous compression.
- Dural ossification with tram track and comma sign may have higher rate of dural tear [10].

## 5 Contraindications

- Tumor, infection, or traumatic injury leading to spinal cord compression
- Patients with a significant neurological deficit with motor and/or sensory deficit
- Spinal instability

## 6 Anatomical Considerations

There are significant anatomical variations in thoracic spinal anatomy compared to the lumbar spine that should be carefully analyzed before planning for thoracic endoscopic decompression. Thoracic vertebrae canal and foramen diameter and area generally increase in a cephalad to the caudal direction. The superior articular facet is facing dorsally and upward as well as flat and oval when it arises out from the pediculo-laminar junction. The corresponding inferior articular facet is facing medially and downward in order to articulate as the thoracic facet joint. The medial portion of the facet joint forming the junction with the upper region of the caudal thoracic lamina is an important landmark for docking of the working retractor cannula for TE-ULBD. The thoracic spinal cord has the narrowest space compared to its cervical and lumbar counterparts. Thoracic spine is kyphotic compared to lordotic cervical and lumbar spinal regions. This explains why thoracic cord is particularly sensitive to compression from disc and/or ligamentum flavum or facet hypertrophy. Within the intradural compartment, there is a higher proportion of nerve, that is, rootlets and cord to cerebral spinal fluid than other spinal regions, which explains why the thoracic region is particularly sensitive to heat injury, vibration, and retraction from surgery due to the lack of CSF buffer. Thoracic ribs attachment and thoracic cage's rigidity are advantageous for thoracic spine that helps limit the amount of movement compared to the cervical and lumbar spine. Ligamentum flava in thoracic spine are paired ligaments running from cephalad lamina to caudal lamina. Ligamentum flavum is the thinnest in cervical spine with increasing thickness toward the thoracic and the thickest in the lumbar spine. Each ligamentum flavum passes ventral and inferior to the cephalad lamina and the dorsal superior aspect of caudal lamina. The lateral extension of the thoracic ligamentum flavum is less lateral compared to the lumbar ligamentum flavum (Fig. 1). Hence, there is

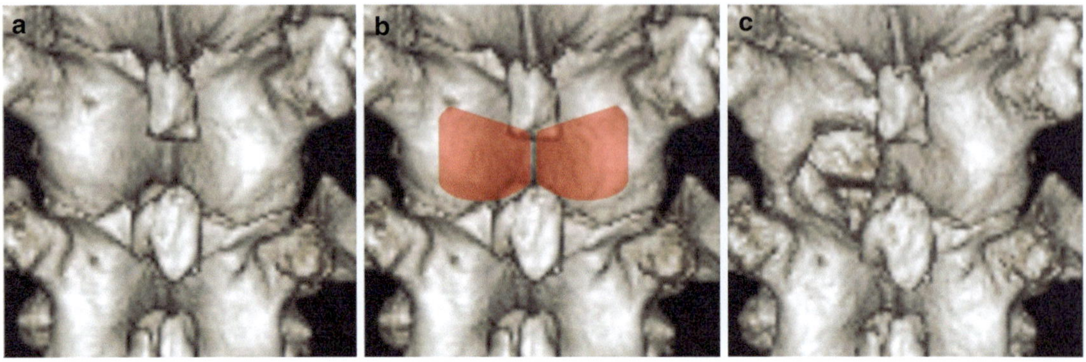


**Fig. 1** (**a**) Preoperative 3D image of thoracic vertebra. (**b**) The extent of the ligamentum flavum to be removed in thoracic endoscopic unilateral laminotomy with bilateral decompression for the thoracic ossified ligamentum flavum. (**c**) Postoperative 3D image of left thoracic endoscopic unilateral laminotomy with bilateral decompression and ipsilateral laminotomy performed with over-the-top decompression of the contralateral side preserving posterior spinal structures

lower incidence of thoracic disk herniation compared to the lumbar and cervical spine [11]. Thoracic compression from OLF and OPLL is more common due to genetic and biosocial factors in the Asian population compared to the Western population [11, 12].

## 7 Preoperative Surgical Planning

The patients are evaluated with the modified JOA score for thoracic myelopathy. They present with lower limb myelopathy symptoms, such as unsteady gait, motor, and lower limbs' sensory impairment. Red flag and late presentation includes urinary and bowel incontinence [13]. Preoperative anteroposterior, lateral, flexion, and extension plain radiographs (XR), computer tomography (CT), and magnetic resonance imaging (MRI) of the thoracolumbar spine were performed. A plain radiograph is necessary to count the levels and assess any lumbosacral junctional transitional changes and abnormal ribs configurations. Sato et al. classified OLF into five types using CT scan axial cut images. (A) Lateral type, which means ossification of only the capsular portion of the ligamentum flavum. (B) Extended type, which means extended ossification of the interlaminar portion. (C) Enlarged type, which means anteromedial thickening and enlargement of ossification. (D) Fused type, which means fusion of the bilateral ossified masses at the midline. (E) Tuberous type, which means anterior growth of the fused mass of ossification [14]. CT also predicts whether there is any dural ossification such as comma sign and tram track sign [10]. OPLL and calcified disc are well visualized with CT scan. The MRI evaluation of the whole spine helps in discovering multiple OLFs, thoracic disc and facet hypertrophies, and double crush syndrome. It also helps in assessing signal changes in the spinal cord. This is important information required prior to surgery. CT and MRI also help in planning which side of the spine compression is more significant. The operating surgeon would stand and perform the surgery on the side with more significant compression.

## 8 Anesthesia and Positioning

Patients undergo general anesthesia, intravenous antibiotics, intravenous tranexamic acid, and calf pumps if no contraindications to their usage. The patient is positioned prone on Wilson frame on top of the radiolucent operating table with thorax and abdomen free of external pressure. The patient's arms are tucked longitudinally and padded next to the patient for upper thoracic spine, while for lower thoracic spine, upper limbs can be supported on the side with side extension table with elbow padding. The hips and knees are flexed slightly with padding.

## 9 Thoracic Endoscopic Equipment

- Uniportal Stenosis Decompression Endoscope: 15° lens, 125-mm length, 6-mm inner working channel diameter, 10-mm-outer endoscope diameter (approximate: varies according to the design and trademark of endoscopic companies)
- Endoscopic drill
  - Diamond burr size 3–4.5 mm for stenosis decompression
- Fluid pump for continuous irrigation
- Radiofrequency ablator
- Video endoscopic tower
- Working cannula (retractor cannula)
- Endoscopic guide needle
- Obturator (for sequential dilation)
- Endoscopic Kerrison rongeur
- Endoscopic pituitary forceps
  - Upward
    Fine forceps for soft tissue
    Large forceps for disc and ligament
  - Forward
  - Flexible
- Penfield dissector

## 10 Surgical Steps

### 10.1 Step 1: Entry Point Marking

#### 10.1.1 Identification of the Surgical Level and Safe Docking of the Endoscope

The surgeon stands on the side with a greater degree of stenosis on the CT and MRI scans (Fig. 2). The skin is marked to the correct level of thoracic spine under the fluoroscopic guidance of anteroposterior (AP) and lateral views. The intersection of medial pedicle line and mid disc line on the AP view and on the lateral view of the mid disc of the correct surgical level is known as the "V" point. It is named V point as the confluence of cephalad and caudal laminar facet junction has a V-shaped intraoperative endoscopic view (Fig. 3) [15].

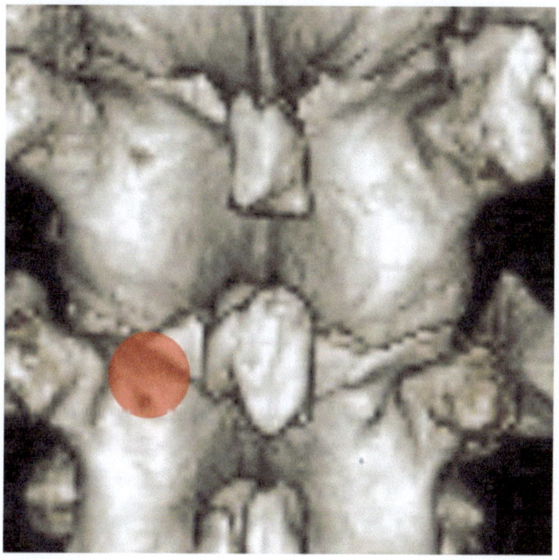

**Fig. 2** Docking point is on the symptomatic side over the V point

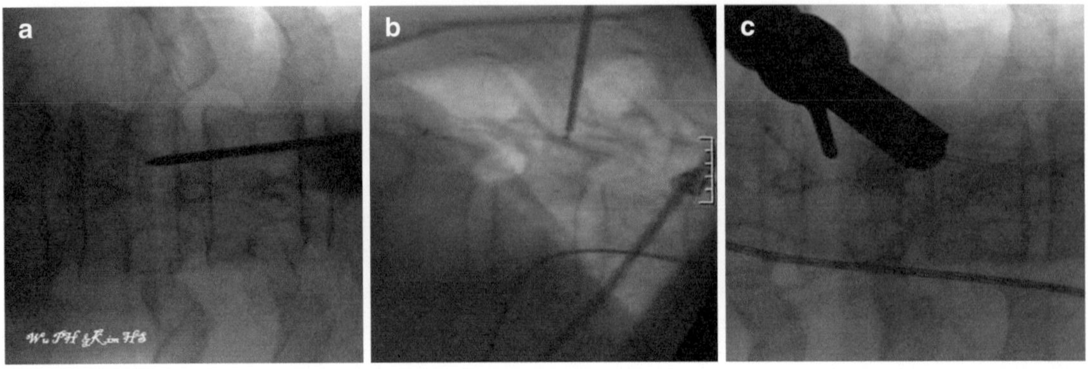

**Fig. 3** Intraoperative fluoroscopic picture of the docking point. (**a**) Docking on the junction of the medial aspect of the left facet joint, caudal lamina, and cephalad lamina with guidewire placed through skin and fascia incision on the AP view and "V" point. (**b**) Lateral view. (**c**) Serial dilation followed by docking of and docked on the isthmus. Serial dilators were employed with obturators followed by the insertion of a 13.7-mm outer diameter beveled tip working cannula on the "V" point

## 10.2 Step 2: Approach and Docking

A 1-cm skin and 3-cm fascia were incised, followed by serial dilation and an endoscopic working retractor cannula slide through the dilators to allow smooth insertion of an endoscope. We used a working cannula of 13.7-mm outer diameter and 10.2-mm inner diameter with a 10.0-mm endoscope with a 6-mm working channel. The procedure was performed under continuous irrigation with normal saline at hydraulic pressures not exceeding 25–30 mm Hg.

## 10.3 Step 3: Soft-Tissue Dissection

Once docking on the V point was performed, we used endoscopic radiofrequency ablation device to dissect the interlaminar rotatores muscle and expose the capsule of the facet joint, and cranial and caudal lateral parts of the bony lamina to expose the endoscopic bony "V" point. We assessed the facet joint's midpoint under endoscopic vision to prevent over-resection of the facet joint. We preserve the pars interarticularis to maintain segmental stability of the thoracic level of decompression.

## 10.4 Step 4: Bony Decompression

Endoscopic drilling was performed from medial to lateral and cephalad direction. One needs to be careful to preserve half of the inferior articular facet. Endoscopic drilling subsequently focuses on the cephalad lamina and the base of the spinous process. Endoscopic drilling was performed till the edge of the flavum was left with a paper-thin membrane of the ligamentum flavum covering the epidural space is seen. Endoscopic drilling was performed with over-the-top decompression to the contralateral-side cephalad lamina and contralateral ventral portion of IAP and medial edge of SAP to the contralateral lateral edge of the ligamentum flavum. This is followed by endoscopic drilling on the ipsilateral followed by contralateral caudal lamina till the contralateral edge of the ligamentum flavum was paper thin (Fig. 4).

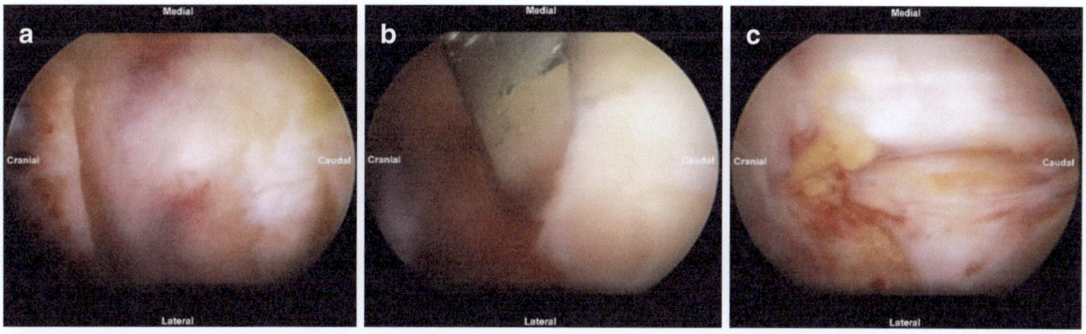


**Fig. 4** Intraoperative endoscopic pictures showing steps of decompression. (**a**) Final cephalad drilling point: boundary of cranial tip of the calcified ligamentum flavum and upper laminae. (**b**) The calcified ligamentum flavum from cranial attachment. (**c**) Final check on the free epidural space

### 10.5 Step 5: Ligamentum Flavum Decompression

After drilling of all edges of the ligamentum flavum, the thinned-out edges of flavum are gently lifted off from the underlying dura by a blunt endoscopic penfield or forceps. We can retrieve ligamentum flavum as an entire block with forceps or Kerrison rongeurs (Fig. 4).

### 10.6 Step 6: Final Assessment of Adequacy of Decompression and Status of Neural Elements Prior to Skin Closure

Neural elements and dura are checked for any defects, and there should be good thoracic cord pulsation under the irrigation fluid. Both lateral edges of the dura should be clearly defined. Unlike lumbar spine, we should not retract the cord at any point in time during the assessment. A drain was inserted under the direct endoscopic vision and anchored, and typically it will be removed on postoperative day 1. The skin was closed in layers.

## 11 Complications

The possible complications are wrong-level surgery, excessive facet resection leading to instability, exiting nerve root injury (dysesthesia, motor, and sensory deficit), spinal cord injury leading to neurological deficit, incomplete decompression, recurrence of stenosis, and the progression of degeneration. Dura tear is common in open surgery, but the authors find in their endoscopic practice with careful endoscopic drilling and gentle lifting off the ligamentum flavum from dura, and there is less incidence of dura tear.

## 12 Postoperative Care

The patient can be prescribed with a brace for comfort and soft-tissue recovery. They mobilized on the same day and can be discharged from the hospital when the drain is removed. The drain is typically removed on postoperative day 1. We found that there is significant remodeling of the bony elements of thoracic spine after decompression with gradual increment in the size of the facet joint (Figs. 5, 6, and 7).

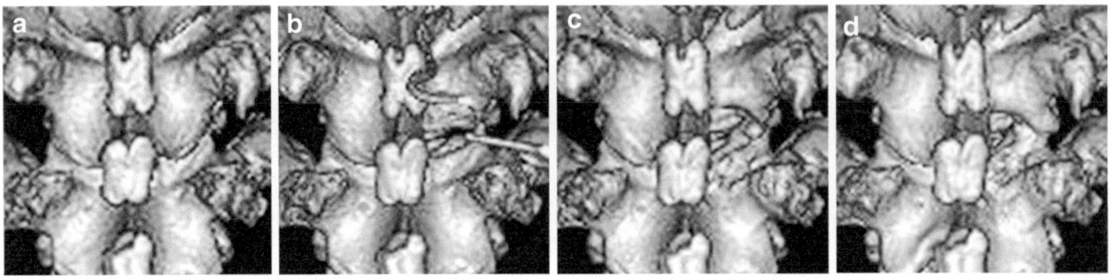


**Fig. 5** Remodeling pattern of thoracic laminectomy. Preoperative (**a**), postoperative day (**b**) 6 months follow-up (**c**), and 18 months follow-up CT images (**d**). 18 months follow-up CT showed further remodeling and increment of the resected facet joint (**d**)

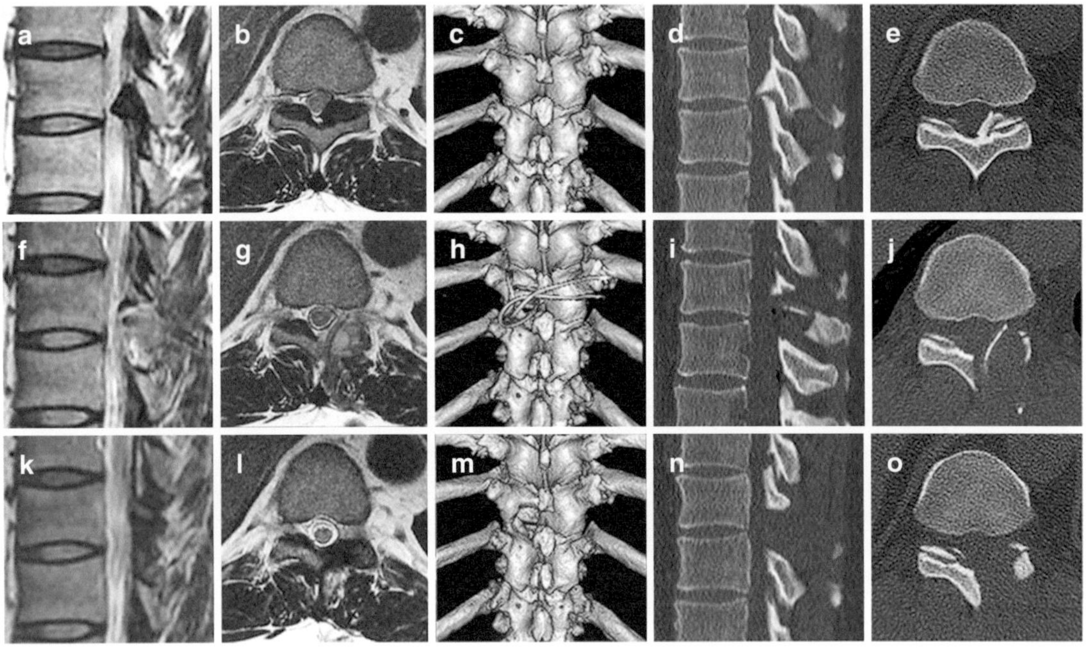


**Fig. 6** A 50-year-old male with severe thoracic back pain and myelopathy symptoms. Sagittal and axial MRI cut of the affected T9/T10 segment with left-sided thoracic OLF causing cord compression (**a** and **b**). Preoperative CT scan 3D reconstruction revealed thoracic OLF with thoracic cord compression (**c**, **d**, and **e**). Postoperative radiological images show marked improvement with complete removal of the ossified ligamentum flavum completely (**f**, **g**, **h**, **i**, and **j**). There seems to be over-resection of the facet joint of the left thoracic T9/10, but the patient is asymptomatic. Postoperative 6 months follow-up radiological images show remodeling of the facet joint with increment in size of facet over 6 months (**k**, **l**, **m**, **n**, and **o**)

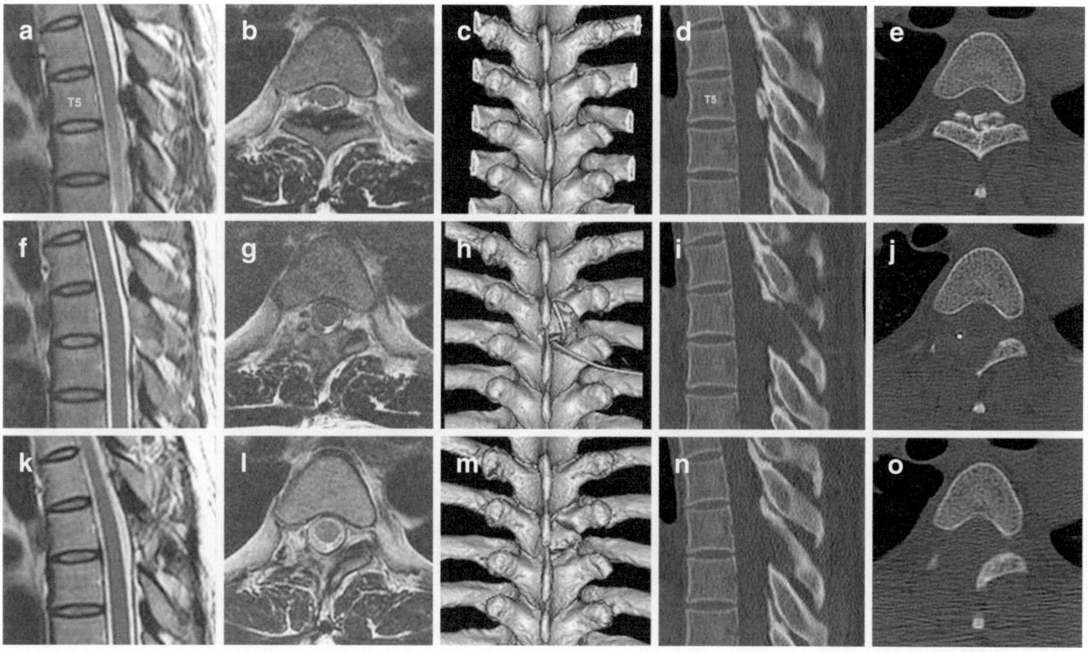

**Fig. 7** A 31-year-old male with severe thoracic back pain. (**a**) and (**b**) show preoperative sagittal and axial MRI cut of the affected T5/6 segment with right-sided thoracic OLF causing cord compression. Preoperative CT scan 3D reconstruction, and sagittal and axial cut of the same segment show that there is bilateral ossified ligamentum flava in this patient (**c**, **d**, and **e**). Postoperative 1-week radiological images reveal the completely removed ossified ligamentum flavum (**f**, **g**, **h**, **i** and **j**). At 6 months follow-up, CT images show remodeling of the facet joint with increment in size of the facet over 6 months and adequate decompression was maintained (**k**, **l**, **m**, **n**, and **o**)

## 13 Discussion: Surgical Tips and Pitfalls

Open decompression of thoracic spine has a long history of success and produced good overall clinical results but a significant perioperative complication rate. Some of the common and dreaded complications are dura tear and neurological deficits [3]. These complications can lead to poor surgical outcomes. The surgeon should carefully evaluate the possibility of dura adhesion preoperatively by evaluating the CT and MRI images. CT scan findings such as (1) the "tram track sign," where there was a hyperdense bony excrescence with a hypodense center, and (2) the "comma sign," where there was evidence of ossification of one-half of the circumference of the dura mater, are radiological signs of possible dense dura adhesion [10]. In such cases, surgeons should consider leaving a thin layer of OLF by a floating technique [16].

Endoscopic spine surgery has advantage over open traditional surgery due to the optimal optical view with the endoscopic lens with magnified and clear visualization of the structures that endoscopic drilling was performed upon. With such strong magnification and clarity of vision by irrigation, we can drill the lamina and ossified ligamentum flavum layer by layer carefully till only a thin membrane of OLF is above the epidural space and subsequently decompress the flavum by gently lifting the OLF off the dura. It is known that a steep learning curve is associated with endoscopic spine surgery [17]. Surgeons who would like to perform TE-ULBD technique should first be familiar with the technique of LE-ULBD of lumbar spinal stenosis [7].

## 14 Conclusions

Uniportal thoracic endoscopic laminotomy and bilateral decompression is a safe and effective technique for thoracic decompression in surgeons who have experience in spinal endoscopy.

## References


1. Tang CYK, Cheung JPY, Samartzis D, et al. Predictive factors for neurological deterioration after surgical decompression for thoracic ossified yellow ligament. Eur Spine J. 2017;26(10):2598–605. https://doi.org/10.1007/s00586-017-5078-7.
2. Yamazaki M, Mochizuki M, Ikeda Y, et al. Clinical results of surgery for thoracic myelopathy caused by ossification of the posterior longitudinal ligament: operative indication of posterior decompression with instrumented fusion. Spine (Phila Pa 1976). 2006;31(13):1452–60. https://doi.org/10.1097/01.brs.0000220834.22131.fb.
3. Osman NS, Cheung ZB, Hussain AK, et al. Outcomes and complications following laminectomy alone for thoracic myelopathy due to ossified ligamentum flavum: a systematic review and meta-analysis. Spine (Phila Pa 1976). 2018;43(14):E842–e8. https://doi.org/10.1097/brs.0000000000002563.
4. Kim J-K, Ryu H-S, Moon BJ, et al. Clinical outcomes and prognostic factors in patients with myelopathy caused by thoracic ossification of the ligamentum flavum. Neurospine. 2018;15(3):269–76. https://doi.org/10.14245/ns.1836128.064.
5. Wu PH, Kim HS, Raorane HD, et al. Safe extraforaminal docking and floating technique in transforaminal endoscopic discectomy for thoracolumbar junction for calcified disc herniation: a case report and technical review junction for calcified disc herniation. J Minim Invasive Spine Surg Tech. 2020;5(1):26–30. https://doi.org/10.21182/jmisst.2019.00066.
6. Xiaobing Z, Xingchen L, Honggang Z, et al. "U" route transforaminal percutaneous endoscopic thoracic discectomy as a new treatment for thoracic spinal stenosis. Int Orthop. 2019;43(4):825–32. https://doi.org/10.1007/s00264-018-4145-y.
7. Kim H-S, Wu PH, Jang I-T. Lumbar endoscopic unilateral laminotomy for bilateral decompression outside-in approach: a proctorship guideline with 12 steps of effectiveness and safety. Neurospine. 2020;17(Suppl 1):S99–S109. https://doi.org/10.14245/ns.2040078.039.
8. Kim HS, Wu PH, Jang I-T. Development of endoscopic spine surgery for healthy life: to provide spine care for better, for worse, for richer, for poorer, in sickness and in health. Neurospine. 2020;17(Suppl 1):S3–8. https://doi.org/10.14245/ns.2040188.094.
9. Sato T, Kokubun S, Tanaka Y, et al. Thoracic myelopathy in the japanese: epidemiological and clinical observations on the cases in miyagi prefecture. Tohoku J Exp Med. 1998;184(1):1–11. https://doi.org/10.1620/tjem.184.1.
10. Muthukumar N. Dural ossification in ossification of the ligamentum flavum: a preliminary report. Spine (Phila Pa 1976). 2009;34(24):2654–61. https://doi.org/10.1097/BRS.0b013e3181b541c9.
11. Han S, Jang IT. Prevalence and distribution of incidental thoracic disc herniation, and thoracic hypertrophied ligamentum flavum in patients with back or leg pain: a magnetic resonance imaging-based cross-sectional study. World Neurosurg. 2018;120:e517–e24. https://doi.org/10.1016/j.wneu.2018.08.118.
12. Kyung-Chung K, Chong-Suh L, Seung-Kee S, et al. Ossification of the ligamentum flavum of the thoracic spine in the Korean population. J Neurosurgery Spine. 2011;14(4):513–9. https://doi.org/10.3171/2010.11.SPINE10405.
13. Zhang J, Wang L, Li J, et al. Predictors of surgical outcome in thoracic ossification of the ligamentum flavum: focusing on the quantitative signal intensity. Sci Rep. 2016;6(1):23019. https://doi.org/10.1038/srep23019.
14. Sato T. Surgical treatment for ossification of ligamentum flavum in the thoracic spine and its complications. Spine Spinal Cord. 1998;11:505–10.
15. Quillo-Olvera J, Lin G-X, Kim J-S. Percutaneous endoscopic cervical discectomy: a technical review. Ann Transl Med. 2018;6(6):100. https://doi.org/10.21037/atm.2018.02.09.
16. Li Z, Ren D, Zhao Y, et al. Clinical characteristics and surgical outcome of thoracic myelopathy caused by ossification of the ligamentum flavum: a retrospective analysis of 85 cases. Spinal Cord. 2016;54(3):188–96. https://doi.org/10.1038/sc.2015.139.
17. Lee C-W, Yoon K-J, Kim S-W. Percutaneous endoscopic decompression in lumbar canal and lateral recess stenosis - the surgical learning curve. Neurospine. 2019;16(1):63–71. https://doi.org/10.14245/ns.1938048.024.

# Part VI

# Thoracic - Biportal

# Thoracic Decompressive Laminectomy by Unilateral Biportal Endoscopy

Ji Yeon Kim, Cheol Woong Park, Dong Chan Lee, and Choon Keun Park

**Abstract**

Biportal endoscopic surgery carries the benefits of less intraoperative bleeding, fast postoperative recovery, and preservation of motion segments. With the development of instruments and techniques, the biportal endoscopic system can access the contralateral side through unilateral thoracic laminotomy. The unrestricted use of the two hands through two independent portals facilitates intimate drilling of the lamina, thoracic ossification of the ligamentum flavum (OLF), and epidural dissection in every corner of the spinal canal. Thoracic myelopathy caused by OLF was successfully treated using the posterior biportal endoscopic approach.

**Keywords**

Endoscopy · Biportal · Stenosis
Laminectomy · Thoracic · Ossification

## 1 Advantages of the Biportal Endoscopic Approach for Thoracic Decompressive Laminectomy

Decompression surgery is typically required in patients with neurological symptoms of thoracic myelopathy due to canal stenosis with ossification of the ligamentum flavum (OLF). Open microscopic posterior laminectomy with or without fusion is usually performed to treat thoracic OLF; however, it carries the risk of severe paraspinal soft-tissue damage and excessive bleeding and may cause iatrogenic spinal instability [1].

Biportal endoscopic surgery carries the benefits of preserving normal structures, less intraoperative bleeding, fast postoperative recovery, and preservation of motion segments [2]. With the development of instruments and techniques, the biportal endoscopic system can access the contralateral side through unilateral cervical laminotomy. Accordingly, biportal endoscopic unilateral laminotomy with bilateral decompres-

**Supplementary Information** The online version contains supplementary material available at https://doi.org/10.1007/978-981-99-1133-2_15.

J. Y. Kim
Department of Neurosurgery, Spine Center, Seran Hospital, Anyang, South Korea

C. W. Park (✉)
Department of Neurosurgery, Spine Center, Daejeon Woori Hospital, Daejeon, South Korea

D. C. Lee
Department of Neurosurgery, Spine Center, Seran Hospital, Anyang, South Korea

Department of Neurosurgery, Spine Center, Wiltse Memorial Hospital, Suwon, South Korea

C. K. Park
Department of Neurosurgery, Spine Center, Wiltse Memorial Hospital, Suwon, South Korea



H. S. Kim et al. (eds.), *Advanced Technique of Endoscopic Cervical and Thoracic Spine Surgery*,
https://doi.org/10.1007/978-981-99-1133-2_15

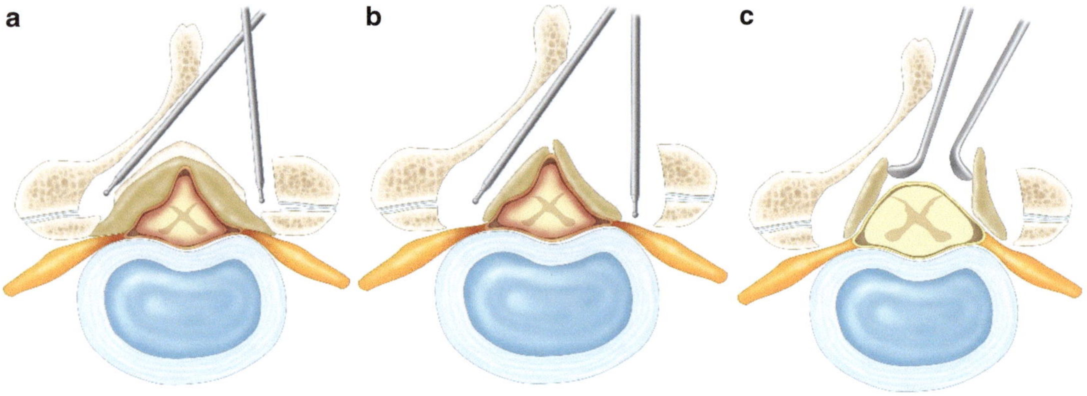


**Fig. 1** Surgical steps of biportal endoscopic unilateral laminotomy with bilateral decompression to treat thoracic myelopathy due to bilateral OLF. (**a**) Bilateral laminar thinning and marginal cutting are performed using an endoscopic diamond drill. (**b**) After removal of the thinned lamina, the bulky OLF is also thinned using layer-by-layer drilling. The thinned OLF is then floated by marginal drilling and cutting. (**c**) The floating OLF is elevated by fine dissectors and removed in an en bloc pattern

sion (ULBD) has been successfully performed to treat cervical spondylotic myelopathy [3].

Biportal endoscopic surgery could also be attempted for the treatment of thoracic myelopathy using two portals for the free movement of an endoscope and optimized instruments [3]. The unrestricted use of the two hands facilitates intimate drilling of the lamina, thoracic OLF, and epidural dissection in every corner of the spinal canal.

Biportal endoscopic ULBD was successfully performed to remove thoracic OLF in patients with myelopathy. The lamina and OLF were first thinned by drilling and then removed using an en bloc pattern (Fig. 1) different from the full endoscopic removal of OLF in a piecemeal removal pattern [2].

## 2 Indications and Contraindications

Preoperative computed tomography (CT) is critical to determine the location and morphology of the thoracic OLF, the degree of invasion of the spinal canal, and the extent of dural ossification.

The biportal endoscopic approach can be used in selective patients with one or two levels of thoracic stenosis.

### 2.1 Indication

1. Thoracic stenosis due to OLF and hypertrophied ligamentum flavum with or without myelopathy.
2. Unilateral or bilateral thoracic OLF without dural ossification signs, such as tram track sign, comma sign, and bridge sign, on preoperative CT images [4].
3. Thoracic stenosis with ossification of ligamentum flavum (OPLL) involves less than 50% of the spinal canal.

### 2.2 Relative Contraindications

1. Multiple-level thoracic stenosis involves more than three levels in the continuous and intermittent types.
2. Thoracic stenosis with disc herniation

### 2.3 Contraindications

1. Thoracic stenosis with segmental instability
2. Thoracic stenosis with OPLL or herniated disc involving more than 50% of the spinal canal

3. Thoracic OLF with definite signs of dural ossification on preoperative CT images [4]
4. Thoracic OLF with tuberous type of Sato classification on preoperative CT images [5]

In cases of contraindications, open microscopic surgery can be considered instead of biportal endoscopic surgery. In particular, open surgery with wide laminectomy should be performed in patients with definite signs of dural ossification [4] and tuberous type of Sato classification [5] on preoperative CT images.

## 3 Anesthesia and Position

Biportal endoscopic surgery was performed under general endotracheal anesthesia in the prone position, and the back was slightly flexed with a radiolucent Wilson frame. A compression-free sponge device was placed under the patient's face. The thoracic spine has a long prominent curve and different spatial orientation between the upper and lower thoracic vertebrae. Therefore, adjusting the operation level to a flat position is essential to decrease the fatigue of the shoulder and wrist of the surgeon.

## 4 Special Instruments

Several optimized surgical instruments are essential for a safe and successful neural decompression at the thoracic spinal level while avoiding spinal cord injury.

1. A 3.5-mm and 3.0-mm endoscopic diamond drill for thinning the thoracic lamina and bulky OLF.
2. Working cannula to maintain proper outflow of saline and prevent increased water pressure into the spinal cord.
3. Scope self-retractor to protect surrounding structures during drilling.
4. Arthroscopic meniscus scissors to remove fragments of the lamina and OLF, which are attached to the dura and ligamentum flavum.

## 5 Surgical Steps of the Biportal Endoscopic Posterior Approach for Bilateral OLF

### 5.1 Making of Two Portals

Two 1-cm skin incisions were made; subsequently, serial dilators were inserted to create an endoscopic and working portal. The surgeon stood on the left side of the patient. The endoscopic and working portals were made on the medial border of the upper and lower thoracic level pedicles in the anteroposterior view (Fig. 2a). If the portals are created closer to the midline, more violations of the midline structures, such as the spinous process and interspinous ligament, are necessary to access the contralateral side using the endoscope and instruments. Otherwise, more laterally created portals can induce more ipsilateral facet joint violation and increase the risk of spinal cord injury by passing instruments over the thecal sac with a shallow approach angle (Fig. 2b). We used biportal endoscopic systems (4-mm, 0° endoscope), a tool-kit set, and a radiofrequency (RF) system [3, 6, 7].

### 5.2 Bilateral Cortical Bone Drilling Overlying the OLF (Videos 1 and 2)

First, we exposed the entire ipsilateral lamina, facet joint, and interlaminar window using dissectors and an RF probe (Fig. 3a). The ipsilateral and midline parts of the outer cortical bone were removed by endoscopic drilling, and a contralateral sublaminar drilling was performed while retaining the spinous process and contours of the outer cortical bone (Fig. 3b). Initial laminar drill-

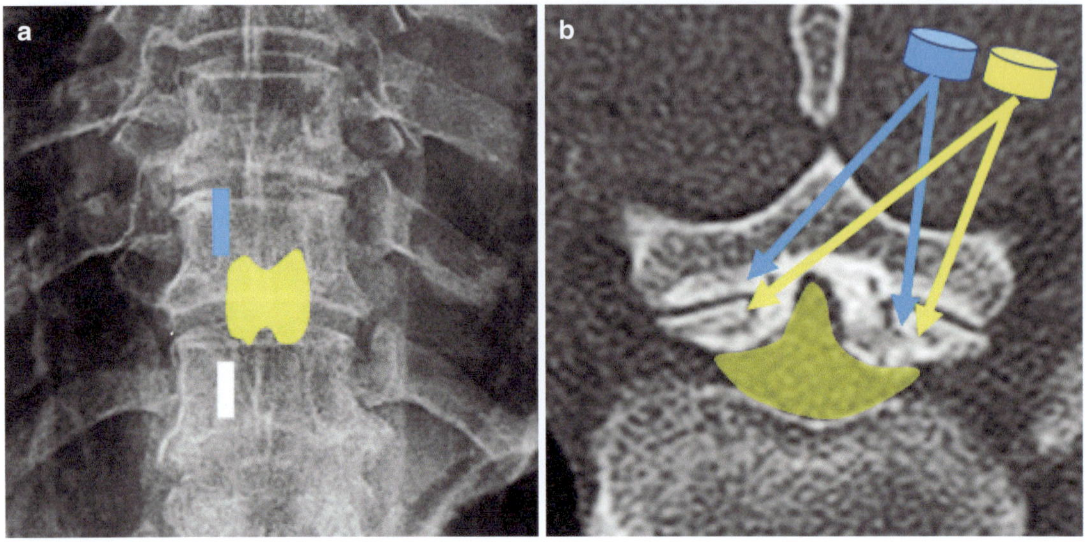


**Fig. 2** (**a**) Skin incision points of two portals with a left-sided approach for bilateral thoracic OLF removal at the T10–T1 level (blue line, endoscopic portal; white line, working portal). The estimated boundary of the OLF is represented with a yellow butterfly-like figure. (**b**) The ideal position of the portal and surgical trajectory on the bilateral lateral border of the OLF (blue-colored illustrations). More laterally created portals could induce more facet joint violation and spinal cord injury by passing instruments over the thecal sac with a shallow approach angle (yellow-colored illustration)

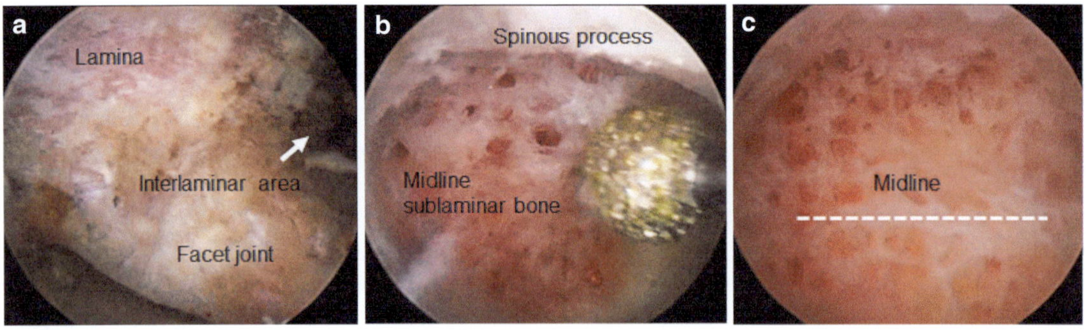


**Fig. 3** (**a**) The ipsilateral lamina, facet joint, and interlaminar window were exposed using dissectors and a radiofrequency (RF) probe. (**b**) Contralateral sublaminar drilling was performed while retaining the spinous process and contours of the outer cortical bone. (**c**) Initial laminar drilling was performed widely over the estimated boundary of the OLF (white dotted line: midline)

ing was performed widely over the estimated boundary of the OLF, laterally with the bilateral medial border of the facet joints and superiorly with the lower edge of the upper-level pedicle (Fig. 3c). We can confirm the boundary of the initial drilling area with an intraoperative X-ray if surgeons are not sure about the drilling margin with endoscopic vision.

## 5.3 Layer-by-Layer Thinning and Cutting of the Bilateral Lamina (Videos 3 and 4)

We performed lamina thinning using the over-the-top technique (Videos 3 and 4), drilling the bilateral exposed cancellous bone remaining in the inner cortical bone (Fig. 4a and b).

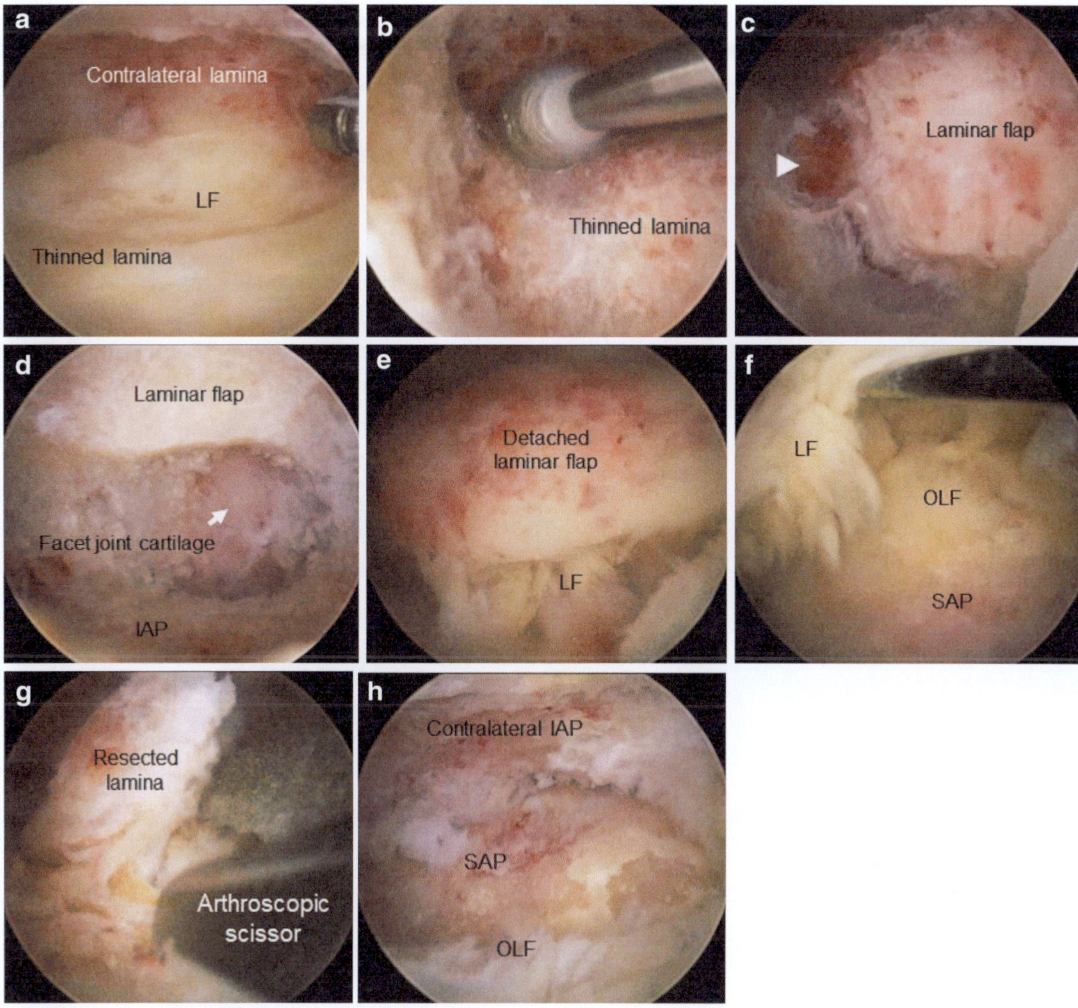


**Fig. 4** Intraoperative endoscopic photos of the laminar thinning and cutting steps. (**a**) After laminar thinning, the remaining inner cortical bone and LF are exposed. (**b**) Marginal drilling of the inner cortical bone is performed until it becomes paper thin. (**c**) Further drilling of the thin paper-like marginal tract caused the breakage, and the epidural space is exposed through the breakage parts (white arrowhead). (**d**) Ipsilateral facet joint cartilage was exposed after laminar marginal drilling through the medial part of the facet joint. (**e**, **f**) The laminar flap was elevated using dissectors to detach from the OLF and LF. (**g**) If the laminar flap adhered severely to the dura, we could cut the adhesion tissues using arthroscopic scissors. (**h**) The outer contour of the OLF and bilateral SAP are confirmed after removal of the lamina. OLF, ossification of the ligamentum flavum; LF, ligamentum flavum; SAP, superior articular process; IAP, inferior articular process

Subsequently, the inner cortical bone was drilled along the medial part of the bilateral facet joints and the proximal end of the ligamentum flavum, similar to thin paper (Fig. 4c). Lateral marginal drilling should be performed, including the medial part of the facet joint, even with facet joint violation. We could access the lateral edge of the OLF and cut the OLF safely through the tract created by drilling the medial facet joint (Fig. 4d). The drilled margin was cut using a fine dissector, and a flap of the bilateral inner cortical bone was created (Fig. 4e). We then elevated the secured laminar flap with dissectors and removed the flap with forceps and endoscopic scissors (Fig. 4f and g). We confirmed the outer contour of the OLF and bilateral superior articular process (SAP) after removing the lamina (Fig. 4h).

### 5.4 Floating and Removal of the OLF (Video 5)

The OLF was fused with the bilateral medial part of the SAP; thus, we exposed the connection site between the OLF and SAP to cut the OLF along the bilateral lateral edge (Fig. 5a–c). We estimated the boundary of the OLF with the lateral border of the cranially exposed thecal sac. We decreased the size of the bulky OLF by endoscopic drilling in a layer-by-layer pattern and obtained a clear endoscopic view of the contralateral corners. Subsequently, the bilateral lateral border of the OLF was drilled until it became paper thin and was cut using fine dissectors and a 1-mm Kerrison punch (Fig. 5a–d). The flap of the bilateral OLF with the ligamentum flavum was detached from the bony margin and floated dorsally into the free space created by laminec-

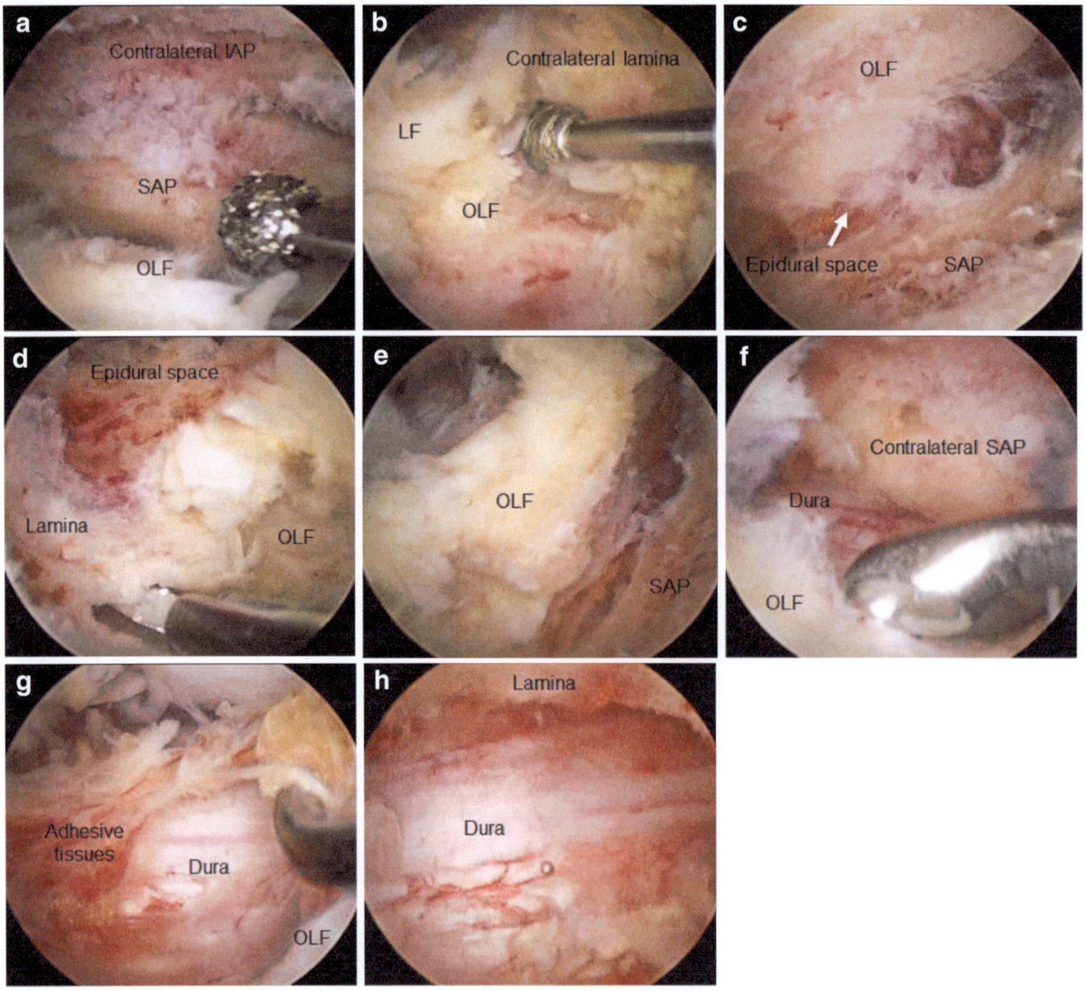


**Fig. 5** Intraoperative endoscopic photo of the thoracic OLF removal steps. (**a**, **b**) Contralateral OLF is cut with the drilling of the OLF lateral border. (**c**) Ipsilateral OLF is also cut with marginal drilling from the SAP. (**d**) The LF is detached from the lamina using fine punches. (**e**) The detached OLF flap is floated, and neural compression is partially relieved. (**f**) Contralateral OLF is removed first. (**g**) Subsequently, the ipsilateral OLF is removed after meticulous epidural dissection. (**h**) The entirely decompressed thecal sac is found

tomy (Fig. 5e). At this time, spinal cord compression was partially relieved, which could decrease the risk of spinal cord injury while manipulating and removing the OLF. Subsequently, a bilateral OLF flap was removed after careful epidural dissection using the fine dissector under direct endoscopic vision (Fig. 5f and g). The OLF of the contralateral side was usually removed first, retaining the ipsilateral OLF to avoid accidental spinal cord injury by passing the instrument over the thecal sac (Fig. 5f). A sufficiently decompressed thecal sac with free dural pulsation was found after clear removal of the OLF and hypertrophied ligamentum flavum (Fig. 5h). A drainage catheter was inserted to prevent epidural hematoma and complete the operation.

## 6 Surgical Steps of the Biportal Endoscopic Posterior Approach for Unilateral OLF (Video 6)

The surgical steps of making portals and working space were the same for unilateral and bilateral types of OLF. Initial laminar drilling was performed widely over the estimated boundary of the OLF medially by crossing the midline and laterally to the medial border of the ipsilateral facet joints. Sufficient drilling of the spinolaminar part was essential to create space for the unrestricted use of an endoscopic drill and instrument during the procedures in the midline part (Fig. 6a and b). The exposed cancellous bone was removed using an endoscopic drill, and marginal inner cortical bone drilling was performed along the midline and proximal end of the ligamentum flavum and the medial part of the ipsilateral facet joint (Fig. 6c and d). The drilled bony margin was cut using a fine dissector, and a flap of the ipsilateral thinned lamina was created (Fig. 6e). We then removed the detached laminar flap and attached the ligamentum flavum with dissectors and forceps (Fig. 6f). We confirmed the outer contour of the OLF fused with SAP (Fig. 6g). If the OLF was bulky on the preoperative CT image, the OLF was thinned using a layer-by-layer drilling pattern. Subsequently, the ipsilateral lateral border of the OLF was drilled until it became paper thin and cut using fine dissectors and a 1-mm Kerrison punch (Fig. 6h and i). The detached OLF was elevated after careful epidural dissection and removed using fine dissectors and forceps (Fig. 6j). Successful removal of OLF and neural decompression was performed (Fig. 6k).

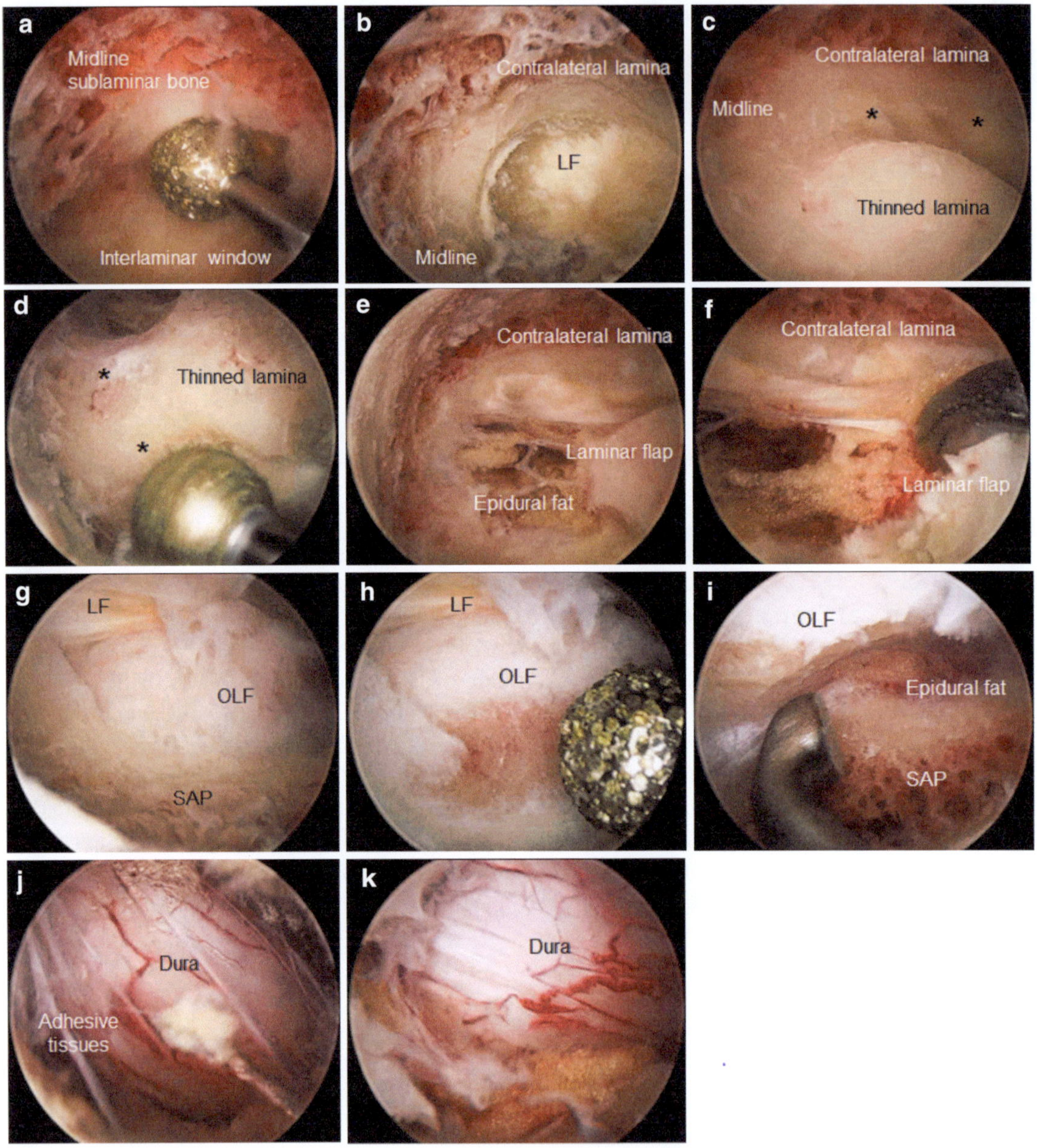


**Fig. 6** Intraoperative endoscopic photos of biportal endoscopic unilateral OLF removal. (**a**) Drilling the midline part of the spinolaminar junction. (**b**) Contralateral sublaminar drilling to expose the midline part of the ligamentum flavum. (**c**) Laminar thinning and contralateral marginal drilling along the medial border of the OLF (*, a tract of marginal drilling). (**d**) Marginal drilling along the cranial and lateral border of the OLF (*, a tract of marginal drilling). (**e**) The laminar flap is detached from the drilled bony margin, and the epidural space is exposed. (**f**) The laminar flap is removed using dissectors and forceps. (**g**) After the laminar flap is removed, the outer surface of the OLF and a connection site to the SAP. (**h, i**) The lateral border of the OLF is drilled and cut using dissectors and punches. (**j**) The OLF and ligamentum flavum are removed after epidural dissection. (**k**) A sufficient neural decompression is found

## 7 Illustrated Cases

**Case 1** A 75-year-old male presented with insidious-onset motor weakness and gradual progression of the lower extremities. Preoperative magnetic resonance (MR) images revealed central thoracic stenosis at the T10–T11 level, which compressed the secondary ligament flavum hypertrophy of the spinal cord. Preoperative CT images showed bilateral fused OLF without signs of dural ossification (Fig. 7). We performed a biportal endoscopic unilateral T10 laminotomy with bilateral decompression at the T10–T11 level using a left-sided approach. Postoperative MR images showed a fully decompressed dural sac after removing the OLF and bilaterally preserved facet joints (Fig. 7). We found the contour of the laminotomy area on postoperative radiography. Myelopathic symptoms gradually improved after surgery.

**Case 2** A 73-year-old female presented with a gradual progression of motor weakness in the lower extremities. The patient complained of radicular pain in the left lower extremity. Preoperative MR images revealed central thoracic stenosis at the T9–T10 level, which compressed the spinal cord secondary ligament flavum hypertrophy. Preoperative CT images showed bilateral nonfused OLF without signs of dural ossification (Fig. 8). We performed a biportal endoscopic unilateral T9 laminotomy with bilateral decompression at the T9–T10 level using a left-sided approach. Postoperative MR images showed a sufficiently decompressed dural sac. Furthermore, more than half of the bilateral facet joints were preserved after removal of the OLF (Fig. 8). Postoperatively, the symptoms of neurological deficits and radicular pain improved significantly.

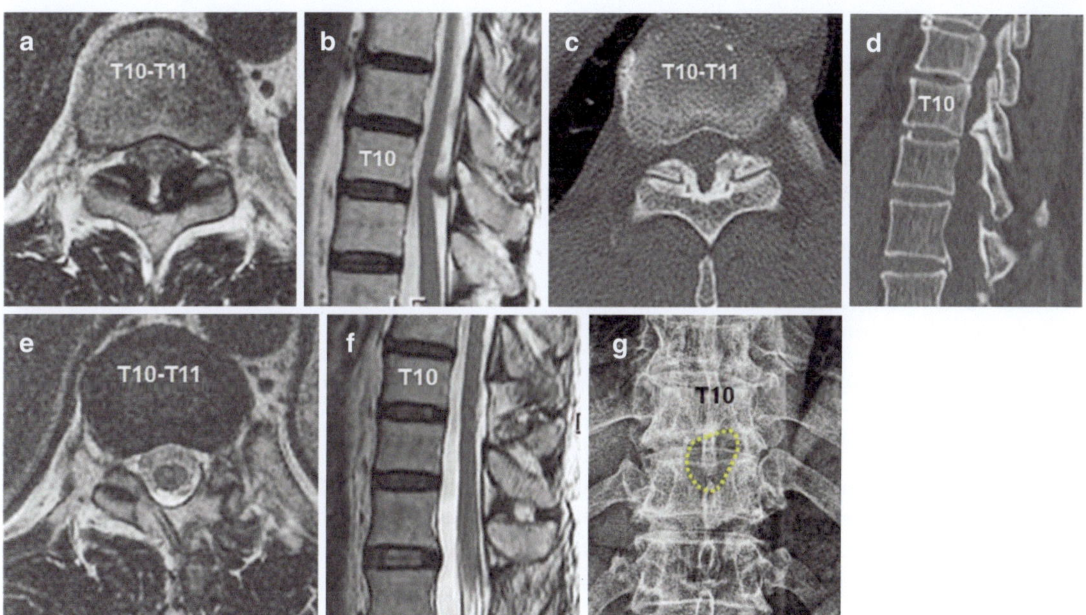


**Fig. 7** Left-sided biportal endoscopic approach for the treatment of thoracic canal stenosis by OLF at the T10–T11 level. (**a**, **b**) Preoperative T2-weighted MR images show thoracic canal stenosis. (**c**, **d**) Preoperative CT images reveal a bilaterally fused thoracic OLF. (**e**, **f**) Postoperative MRI show a fully expanded dural sac without remained OLF. (**g**) Postoperative X-ray image reveals the contour of the bilateral laminotomy area

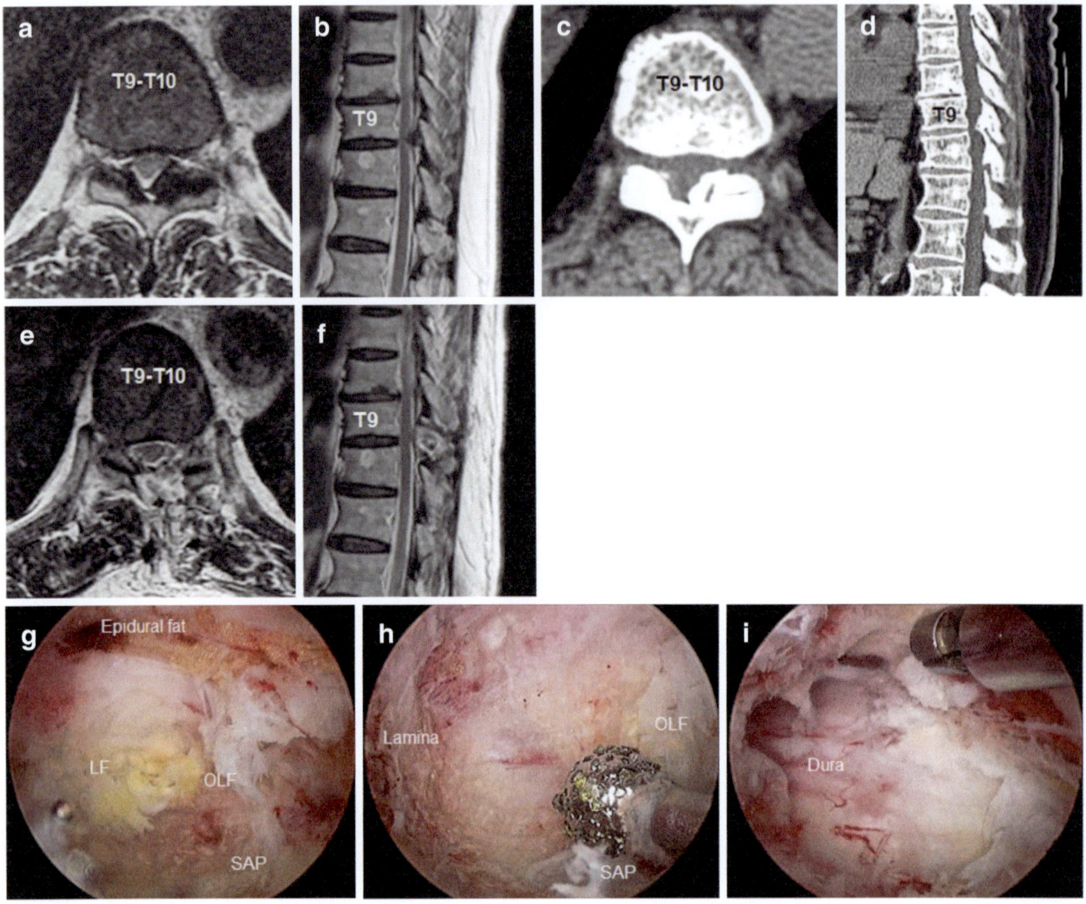


**Fig. 8** Left-sided biportal endoscopic approach for the treatment of thoracic canal stenosis and OLF at the T9–T10 level. (**a**, **b**) Preoperative T2-weighted MR images show thoracic canal stenosis. (**c**, **d**) Preoperative CT images reveal bilaterally nonfused thoracic OLF. (**e**, **f**) Postoperative MRI shows a sufficiently expanded dural sac with well-preserved bilateral facet joints. (**g**) After removing the lamina, the OLF and hypertrophied ligamentum flavum are exposed. (**h**) Marginal drilling is performed along the lateral and cranial borders of the OLF. (**i**) A fully decompressed dural sac is found after OLF removal

**Case 3** A 43-year-old female presented with mid-back and left chest wall pain with gradual progression for 3 years of conservative treatment. Preoperative MR images revealed left dominant thoracic canal stenosis at the T8–T9 and T9–T10 levels (Fig. 9). We performed biportal endoscopic unilateral laminotomy and OLF removal using a left-sided approach. Postoperative MR images showed a sufficiently decompressed dural sac while preserving the facet joints (Fig. 9). Postoperatively, the symptoms of back and chest wall pain improved significantly.

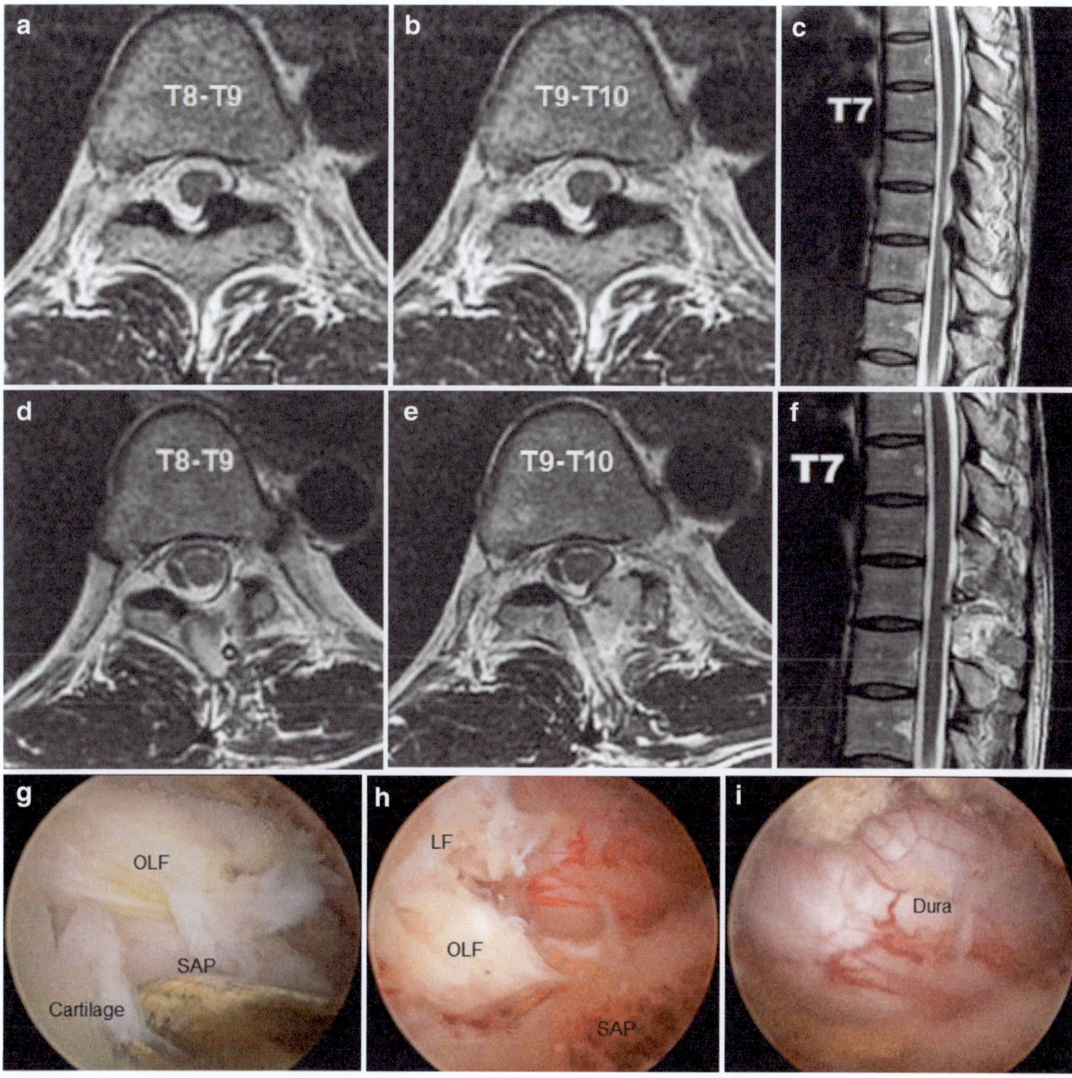


**Fig. 9** Left-sided biportal endoscopic approach for treating thoracic canal stenosis and OLF to the left of the T8–T9 and T9-T10 levels. Preoperative T2-weighted MR images show the thoracic canal stenosis on the left side (**a**–**c**). Postoperative MRI shows a sufficiently expanded dural sac with well-preserved bilateral facet joints (**d**–**f**). After removal of the lamina, the OLF, hypertrophied ligamentum flavum, and facet joint cartilage are exposed (**g**). After cutting the OLF using the endoscopic drill, the detached OLF is removed (**h**). A fully decompressed dural sac is found after the removal of OLF (**i**)

## 8 Prevention and Management of Complications

The best way to avoid serious complications is to maintain surgical steps and appropriate indications.

Wide bilateral laminectomy, including the medial part of the facet joints, is essential to obtain the space for drilling and cutting the lateral edge of the OLF, while the dura is covered by the OLF and ligamentum flavum.

Narrow laminectomy and early dural exposure induce repetitive dural manipulation, while OLF severely compresses the spinal cord (Video 7). Instrument insertion between the dura and the OLF for epidural dissection or laminar punching causes spinal cord compression (Video 8). Additional pressure on the compressed spinal cord by the instruments can cause irreversible neural injury in the neurologically impaired state. Furthermore, if contralateral laminar drilling was performed while the dura was exposed through the narrow laminectomy area, the risk of dural tear and direct spinal cord injury might be increased even during the careful drilling procedure (Video 9). Therefore, it would be better to use over-the-top decompression with an en bloc removal pattern to treat the thoracic OLF safely in the neurologically impaired state [3]. The inside-out approach used in lumbar decompression surgery [8] should not be applied to thoracic spinal decompression surgery (Video 3).

Drilling of the OLF after floating can cause direct spinal cord injury. If thinning of the bulky OLF is necessary, the OLF should be carefully drilled in a side-to-side pattern before marginal cutting.

If incidental durotomy occurs during biportal endoscopic surgery, the hole should be repaired using a fibrin sealant patch or suture-less clip. However, if the endoscopic repair fails, open microscopic surgery should be performed for complete dural repair [9].

Continuous saline infusion pressure to the spinal cord may increase epidural pressure and induce spinal cord injury [10]. We should carefully monitor the good patency of the saline outflow and recommend saline infusion pressures below 30 mmHg.

Massive use of RF in epidural vessels may induce spinal cord injury, and we recommend a foamy hemostatic agent for diffuse and multifocal epidural bleeding.

A drainage catheter was inserted to prevent postoperative epidural hematoma, and the drainage bag was kept under negative pressure for approximately two days after surgery.

Intraoperative electrophysiological monitoring may prevent iatrogenic spinal cord injury.

## 9 Discussion (Surgical Tips and Pitfalls)

We recommend informing the patient about the benefits of surgery and the potential risks of this technique. This procedure has the advantages of minimal invasiveness in treating thoracic OLF through a biportal endoscopic approach, while minimizing facet joint violation and preserving paraspinal soft tissues, and additional posterior instrumentation can be avoided. We preoperatively informed the patients about the possibility of conversion to open microscopic surgery if insufficient decompression or incidental durotomy is expected due to dural adhesions.

Sufficient bony decompression should be prioritized over preservation of the facet joints in thoracic spinal decompression surgery. Laminectomy was usually extended to the medial part of the bilateral facet joints to expose the lateral border of the thoracic OLF and detach the OLF from the SAP by marginal drilling (Fig. 10a). If the facet joint space and joint cartilage were not exposed after laminar drilling, it might be insufficient bone drilling within the OLF boundary. Furthermore, early dural exposure and piecemeal OLF removal are inevitable (Fig. 10b). However, violation of the medial part of the facet joints may not induce stability problems due to minimal invasiveness in preserving the paraspinal muscular ligamentous structures and more than half of the bilateral facet joints.

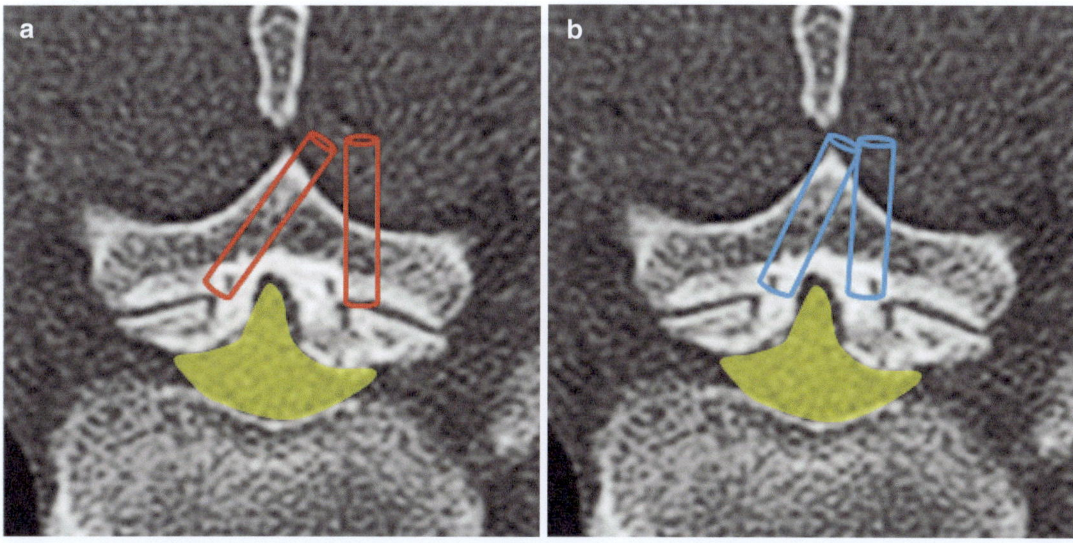


**Fig. 10** (**a**) The laminar drilling should be extended until the medial part of the facet joint space is exposed to create the surgical tract to the lateral border of the bilateral OLF. (**b**) Narrow laminar drilling along the medial border of the facet joints could induce early dural exposure before OLF removal and insufficient neural decompression. Yellow-colored figure: compressed spinal cord

We recommend exposing the entire contour of the ipsilateral lamina, facet joint, spinous process, and interlaminar window before starting bone drilling. Clear anatomical identification aids in determining the extent of bony removal of the lamina and facet joints for successful neural decompression with minimized dural manipulation.

If the OLF has signs of dural ossification and shows the bilateral tuberous type of Sato classification on preoperative CT images, open microscopic surgery with wide laminectomy should be considered instead of biportal endoscopic surgery.

**Conflicts of Interest** None.

**Disclosure of Funding** None.

## References

1. Osman NS, Cheung ZB, Hussain AK, Phan K, Arvind V, Vig KS, et al. Outcomes and complications following laminectomy alone for thoracic myelopathy due to ossified ligamentum flavum: a systematic review and meta-analysis. Spine (Phila Pa 1976). 2018;43(14):E842–e8.
2. Lin YP, Lin R, Chen S, Rao SY, Zhao S, Wen T, et al. Thoracic full-endoscopic unilateral laminotomy with bilateral decompression for treating ossification of the ligamentum flavum with myelopathy. Ann Transl Med. 2021;9(12):977.
3. Kim J, Heo DH, Lee DC, Chung HT. Biportal endoscopic unilateral laminotomy with bilateral decompression for the treatment of cervical spondylotic myelopathy. Acta Neurochir (Wien). 2021;163(9):2537–43.
4. Muthukumar N. Dural ossification in ossification of the ligamentum flavum: a preliminary report. Spine (Phila Pa 1976). 2009;34(24):2654–61.
5. Sato T, Kokubun S, Tanaka Y, Ishii Y. Thoracic myelopathy in the Japanese: epidemiological and clinical observations on the cases in Miyagi Prefecture. Tohoku J Exp Med. 1998;184(1):1–11.
6. Heo DH, Hong YH, Lee DC, Chung HJ, Park CK. Technique of biportal endoscopic transforaminal lumbar interbody fusion. Neurospine. 2020;17(Suppl 1):S129–s37.
7. Park JH, Jang JW, Park WM, Park CW. Contralateral keyhole biportal endoscopic surgery for ruptured lumbar herniated disc: a technical feasibility and early clinical outcomes. Neurospine. 2020;17(Suppl 1):S110–s9.
8. Lim KT, Meceda EJA, Park CK. Inside-out approach of lumbar endoscopic unilateral laminotomy for bilateral decompression: a detailed technical description,

rationale and outcomes. Neurospine. 2020;17(Suppl 1):S88–s98.

9. Heo DH, Ha JS, Lee DC, Kim HS, Chung HJ. Repair of incidental durotomy using sutureless nonpenetrating clips via biportal endoscopic surgery. Global Spine J. 2020;12:452.

10. Hwa Eum J, Hwa Heo D, Son SK, Park CK. Percutaneous biportal endoscopic decompression for lumbar spinal stenosis: a technical note and preliminary clinical results. J Neurosurg Spine. 2016;24(4):602–7.

# Posterolateral Approach for Thoracic Disc Herniation by Unilateral Biportal Endoscopy

Man Kyu Park and Sang-Kyu Son

**Abstract**

The surgery of the thoracic disc herniation (TDH) is technically challenging due to its technical problems, as well as the potential for significant consequences. Therefore, the ideal goal is to obtain adequate decompression without manipulating the spinal cord while avoiding paraspinal muscle/facet injury and consequences. Posterolateral techniques for TDH allow an oblique view of the disc space and avoid thoracic viscera damage problems. However, the traditional posterolateral approach frequently necessitates significant muscle dissection, as well as rib and facet joint excision. The unilateral biportal endoscopy (UBE) technique of TDH with a posterolateral approach has recently offered technically appropriate decompression with minimal muscle injury or facet joint destruction and minimal spinal cord manipulation, has technical advantages, and a low risk of problems and destabilization. This chapter offers the technical aspects of UBE implementation using the posterolateral approach in patients with TDH, as well as specific surgical suggestions to avoid complications.

**Keywords**

Biportal · Endoscopy · Minimally invasive surgery · Thoracic disc herniation · Thoracic spine

## 1 Advantages of this Approach (Introduction)

Thoracic disc herniation (TDH) is an uncommon condition that accounts for approximately 0.15%–4% of all spine discectomy procedures [1, 2]. The surgical approaches for TDH are categorized as posterior, posterolateral, lateral, or anterior transthoracic, thoracoscopic procedures, depending on the location and characteristics of the disc herniation [3–5]. Although anterior or lateral techniques provide the best access to the disc space, they also expose thoracic viscera such the lung, heart, and major arteries [2, 6]. Although posterior approach avoid thoracic viscera injury, there is a high risk of cord injury, paraspinal muscle injury, and bone removal, which can result in postoperative back pain and instability [7]. Many surgeons prefer posterolateral methods for TDH because of these complications. Posterolateral techniques allow an oblique view of the disc space and avoid thoracic viscera damage prob-

**Supplementary Information** The online version contains supplementary material available at https://doi.org/10.1007/978-981-99-1133-2_16.

M. K. Park · S.-K. Son (✉)
Department of Neurosurgery, Good Moonhwa Hospital, Busan, South Korea
e-mail: jihak3@hanmail.net



H. S. Kim et al. (eds.), *Advanced Technique of Endoscopic Cervical and Thoracic Spine Surgery*,
https://doi.org/10.1007/978-981-99-1133-2_16

lems [5]. However, the traditional posterolateral approach frequently necessitates significant muscle dissection as well as rib and facet joint excision [8].

Favorable outcomes and advantages of unilateral biportal endoscopy (UBE) technique have been described for surgery of herniated discs and spinal stenosis in the lumbar spine [9, 10]. The UBE technique of TDH with a posterolateral approach has recently offered technically appropriate decompression with minimal muscle injury or facet joint destruction and minimal spinal cord manipulation, has technical advantages, and a low risk of problems and destabilization.

This chapter covers the technical aspects of UBE implementation using the posterolateral approach in patients with TDH, as well as specific surgical suggestions to avoid complications. Furthermore, we examine the indications for TDH via UBE, and discuss potential problems.

## 2 Indications and Contraindications

Surgical treatment for TDH is recommended if conservative treatment fails or the patient's neurological condition worsens. According to our experience, this technique is suitable for laterally located disc herniation. Conversely, due to limited vision and accessibility, the operation surgery of a centrally located huge substantial calcified herniation is comparatively contraindicated with this technique.

The indications are as follows:

1. Soft or calcified disc herniation
2. Laterally located disc herniation

Contraindications are as follows:

1. Large centrally located calcified disc
2. Instability of the spinal column
3. High-grade deformity

## 3 Anesthesia and Position

After the induction of general endotracheal anesthesia, the patient is positioned prone on a radiolucent table with fluoroscopic guidance. All pressure areas are padded safely and both arms positioned making sure not to overextend at the shoulder beyond 90°. The thoracic cord is vulnerable due to the low canal-to-cord ratio, thoracic kyphosis that pushes the cord anteriorly, and insufficient blood supply in the watershed zone [5]. Therefore, somatosensory and motor-evoked potentials are used to prevent cord injury. The surgeon stands on the ipsilateral side of the pathology of TDH. The endoscopic monitor and fluoroscopy are positioned opposite the surgeon.

## 4 Special Instruments

Most of the equipment used in posterolateral approach for TDH by UBE are comparable to those used in other UBE procedures. This technique requires a diamond drill and a 1 mm Kerrison rongeur. A 0-degree scope is typically utilized, but a 30-degree scope is necessary to approach a centrally located TDH.

## 5 Procedures (Surgical Steps, Videos 1 and 2)

### 5.1 Concept of Posterolateral Approach for TDH by UBE

Traditional posterolateral techniques, such as the costotransversectomy or transpedicular approach, necessitate substantially greater bony excision. Although this method allows for safe TDH access, the amount of bone removed may result in considerable postoperative disability and other problems. Therefore, it is recommended that the posterolateral technique by UBE be used to treat TDH because it is similarly effective and has a

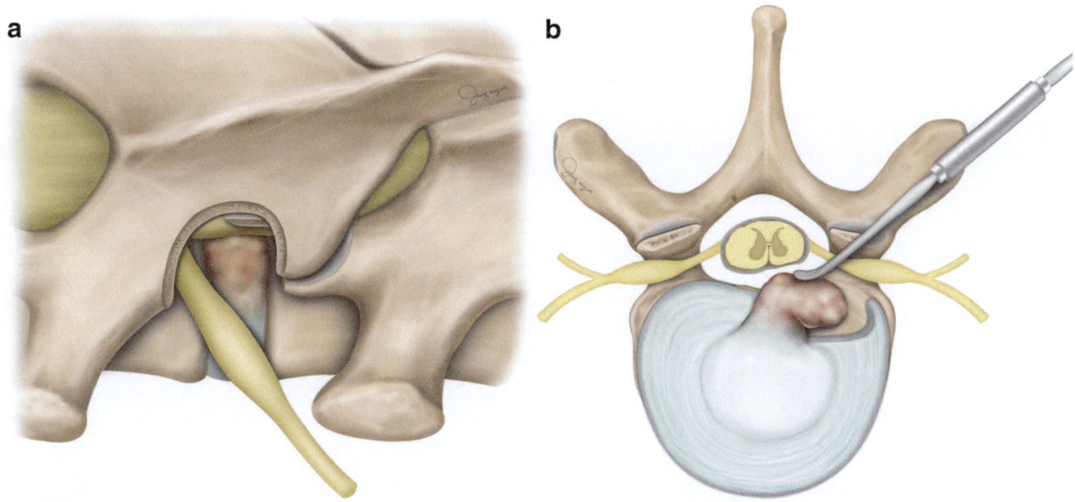


**Fig. 1** Illustration shows posterolateral approach for thoracic disc herniation by unilateral biportal endoscopy. After bone working (**a**). Discectomy (**b**)

lower risk of complications. With the advancement of the endoscope and instruments under endoscopic view, surgeons can more readily reach the disc space with minimal bone removal, if necessary, to reach the centrally located disc (Fig. 1).

## 5.2 Skin Marking and Making Portal

The difficulty of determining the operating level is due to the thoracic spine's unusual architecture. To avoid wrong-level operation, count from an anatomical landmark. The exact surgical level should be determined using lateral and anteroposterior (AP) fluoroscopic guidance.

It is recommended that the scopic portal for endoscopic viewing be utilized with the nondominant hand, whereas the working portal for instrument manipulation be used with the dominant hand. In AP fluoroscopic view, the targeted disc space, transverse process, and facet lateral margin are identified after parallelizing the lower endplate of the upper vertebral body. The lateral aspect of the facet joint, which is located between the upper and lower level pedicles, is the docking point. The two incisions are approximately 3 cm apart, where the center of each incision is located at approximately 3–4 cm lateral to the docking point (Fig. 2a). On preoperative images, an oblique line is drawn from the skin incision to the herniated disc to plan the approach trajectory (Fig. 2b). To have good visualization of the disc space and manipulation of surgical instruments, the required trajectory angle is modified (30–35 degrees to the docking point). The incision's distance from the docking point is determined by the patient's body habitus. A more lateral approach will provide a larger angle of exposure into the ventral dural region in obese patients, enabling a better view toward the centrally located disc.

A series of dilators are inserted through the working portal and docked on the lateral aspect of the facet joint with the aid of fluoroscopy. A scopic portal is then used to insert an endoscopic sheath into the docking point. On the AP and lateral fluoroscopic views, fluoroscopy is used to check the triangular position of the endoscopic sheath and dilator at the docking point (Fig. 2c and d).

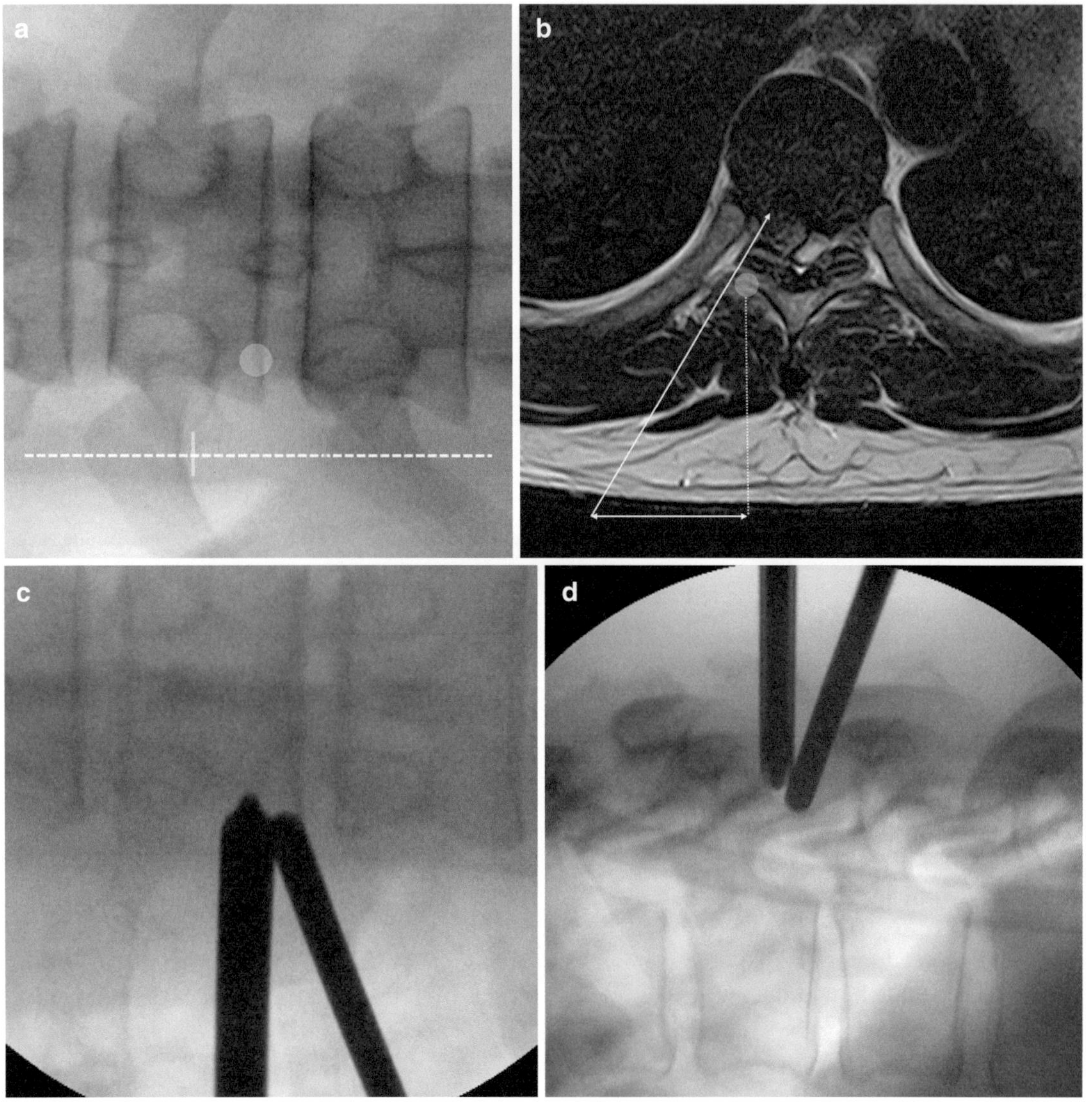


**Fig. 2** Skin incision and docking point on the fluoroscopic anteroposterior view. The docking point (white circle) is the lateral aspect of the facet joint. Two skin incisions (working portal: white line, scopic portal: blue line) are made about 3 cm apart, where the center of each incision is located at approximately 3–4 cm lateral to the docking point (**a**). Determining skin incision and a surgical trajectory using preoperative MRI. The surgical trajectory line is drawn from herniated disc and lateral margin of the facet joint to skin; white circle indication docking point (**b**). Triangulation of the tip of the dilator and the endoscopic sheath above the lateral aspect of the facet joint. AP (**c**) and lateral fluoroscopic images (**d**)

## 5.3 Bone Working

The soft-tissue overlaying the inferior edge of the transverse process and the lateral part of the facet joint is coagulated and removed with a radiofrequency (RF) probe after the endoscope is inserted. The endoscope's range of motion and tilted field of view provide ample working area in all directions, allowing exposure of the inferior edge of the proximal transverse process, lateral margin of the facet joint, and intertransverse membrane (Fig. 3a). After visualizing the lateral portion of

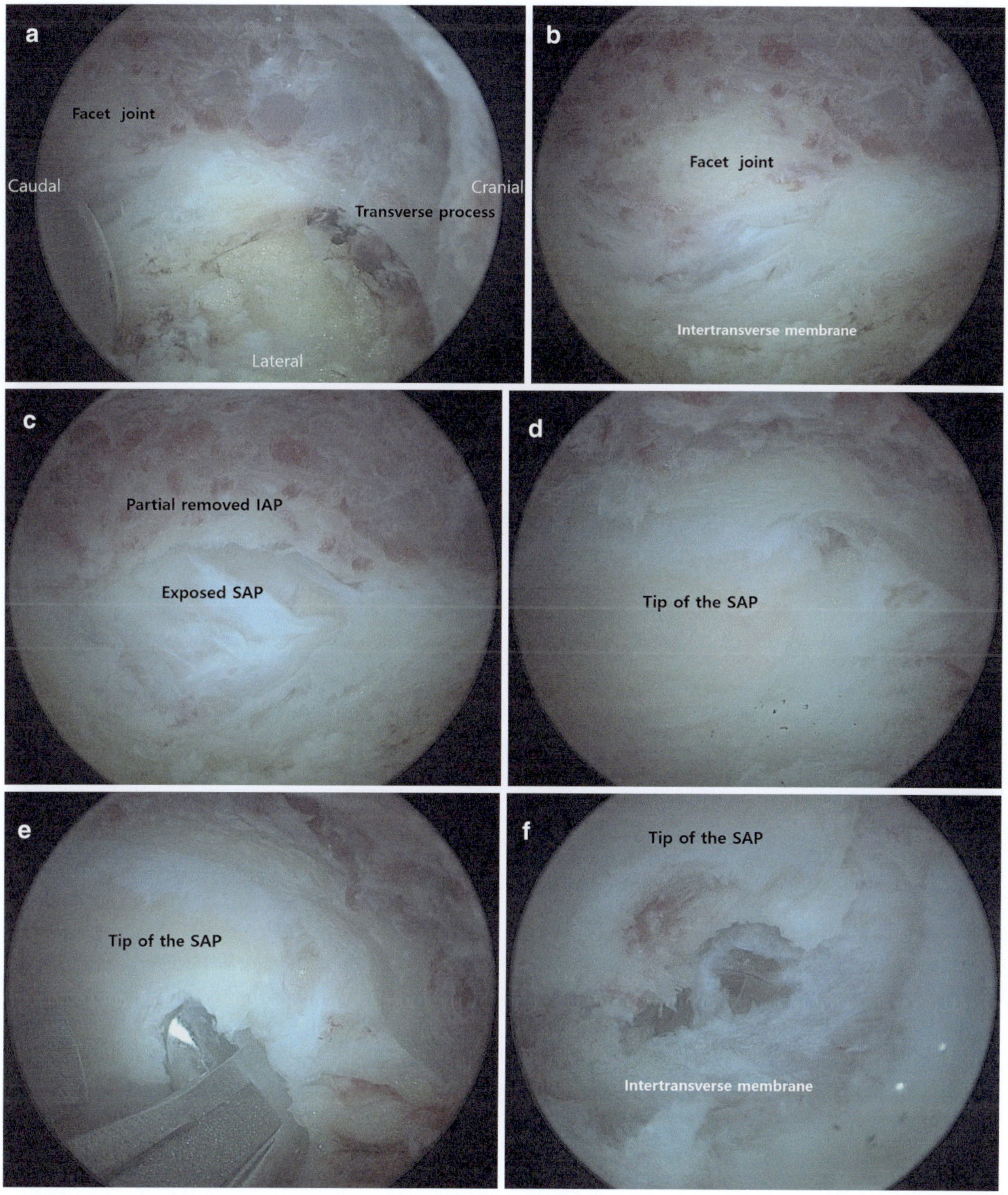


**Fig. 3** Serial sequence endoscopic images of the bone working. The surgical anatomy is first noticed the inferior edge of the proximal transverse process and lateral margin of the facet joint (**a**). A high-speed drill is used to thin the lateral portion of the inferior articular process (IAP) (**b**). The tip of the superior articular process (SAP) is identified when the IAP is partially removed (**c** and **d**). Removal of the tip of the SAP (**e** and **f**). After removal of the tip of the SAP, the disc space and lateral margin of the dural sac is identified (**g**). To access the disc space or disc fragment, the superior aspect of the pedicle can be removed using the drill (**h**). After removing the foraminal ligament, the exiting nerve root (white arrow) and the lateral margin of the dural sac can be identified (**i**). Working within the space defined cranially by the exiting nerve root (white arrow), medially by the lateral margin of the dural sac, and caudally by the superior part of the pedicle, the disk space can be identified (**j**)

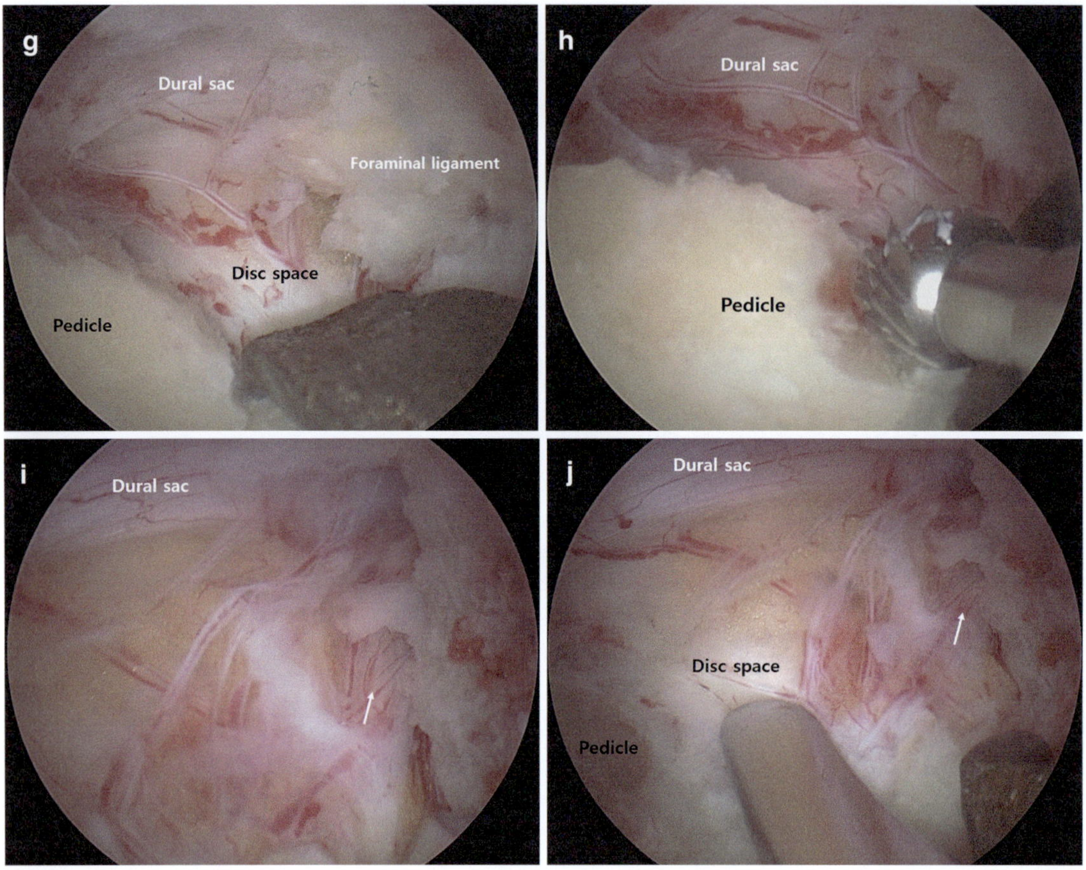


**Fig. 3** (continued)

the facet joint, it is removed to gain access to the disc space. A high-speed drill is used to thin the lateral portion of the inferior articular process (IAP) (Fig. 3b). The tip of the superior articular process (SAP) is identified when the IAP is partially removed using a Kerrison rongeur or osteotome (Fig. 3c and d). Afterward, using Kerrison rongeur, the SAP's tip is removed (Fig. 3e and f). After removal of the tip of the SAP, the disc space and lateral margin of the dural sac is identified (Fig. 3g). The extent of bone removal is determined by endoscope so that only the portion of the facet joint overlying the disc space is removed. The superior portion of the pedicle as well as the lateral aspect of the facet joint had to be removed depending on the disc migration. To access the disc space or disc fragment, the superior aspect of the pedicle can be removed using the drill (Fig. 3h). After removing the foraminal ligament, the exiting nerve root and the lateral margin of the dural sac can be identified (Fig. 3i). Therefore, working within the space defined cranially by the exiting nerve root, medially by the lateral margin of the dural sac, and caudally by the superior part of the pedicle, the disc space can be easily identified and reached under endoscopic guidance (Fig. 1a and 3j).

## 5.4 Discectomy

The optimal view into the ventral space of the dural sac comes from a angling the endoscope (Fig. 4a). A freer elevator is also employed to determine a plane between the ventral region of the dura and the annulus as there is frequent adhesion between the two. A hook-type RF probe is used to incise the annulus once the annulus

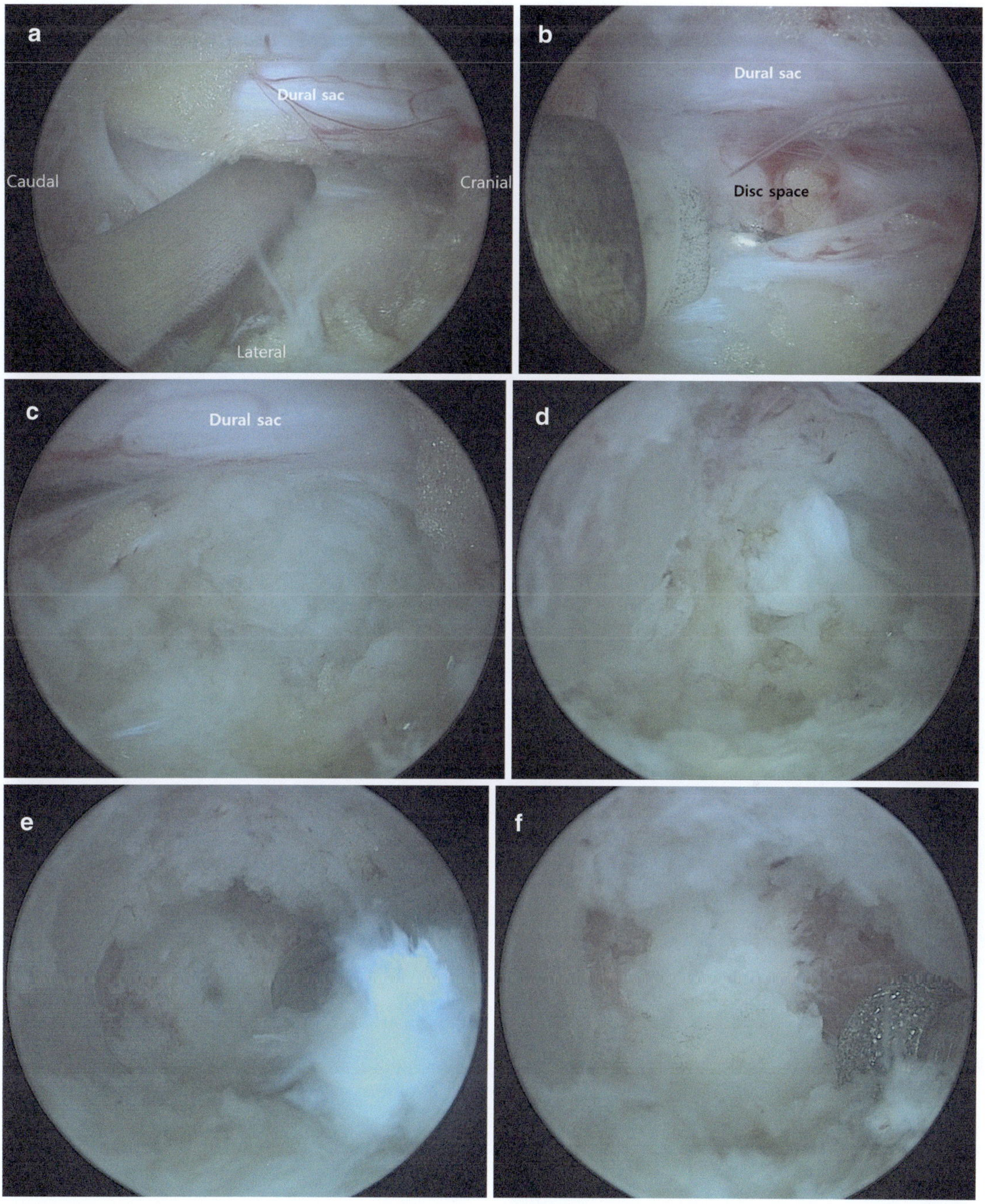


**Fig. 4** Serial sequence endoscopic images of the discectomy. The optimal view into the ventral space of the dural sac comes from a angling the endoscope (**a**). Coagulation of the epidural vessel above annulus (**b**). Annulotomy (**c**). The ruptured disc fragment is removed using a combination of freer elevators (**d**) and pituitary forceps (**e**). Making a space using a diamond drill both in the posterior edge of the endplate and in the vertebral body (**f**). Laterally located disc can be removed under direct visualization (**g**). Push the annulus (white arrow) down into created disc space (asterisk) using curved freer elevator (**h**). Identification of the displaced disc fragment (white arrow) (**i**). The 30 degree of the endoscope allows for direct visualization of the medial side of the disc space (**j**). The area beneath the dura sac is further examined with a freer elevator near the end of the decompression (**k**)

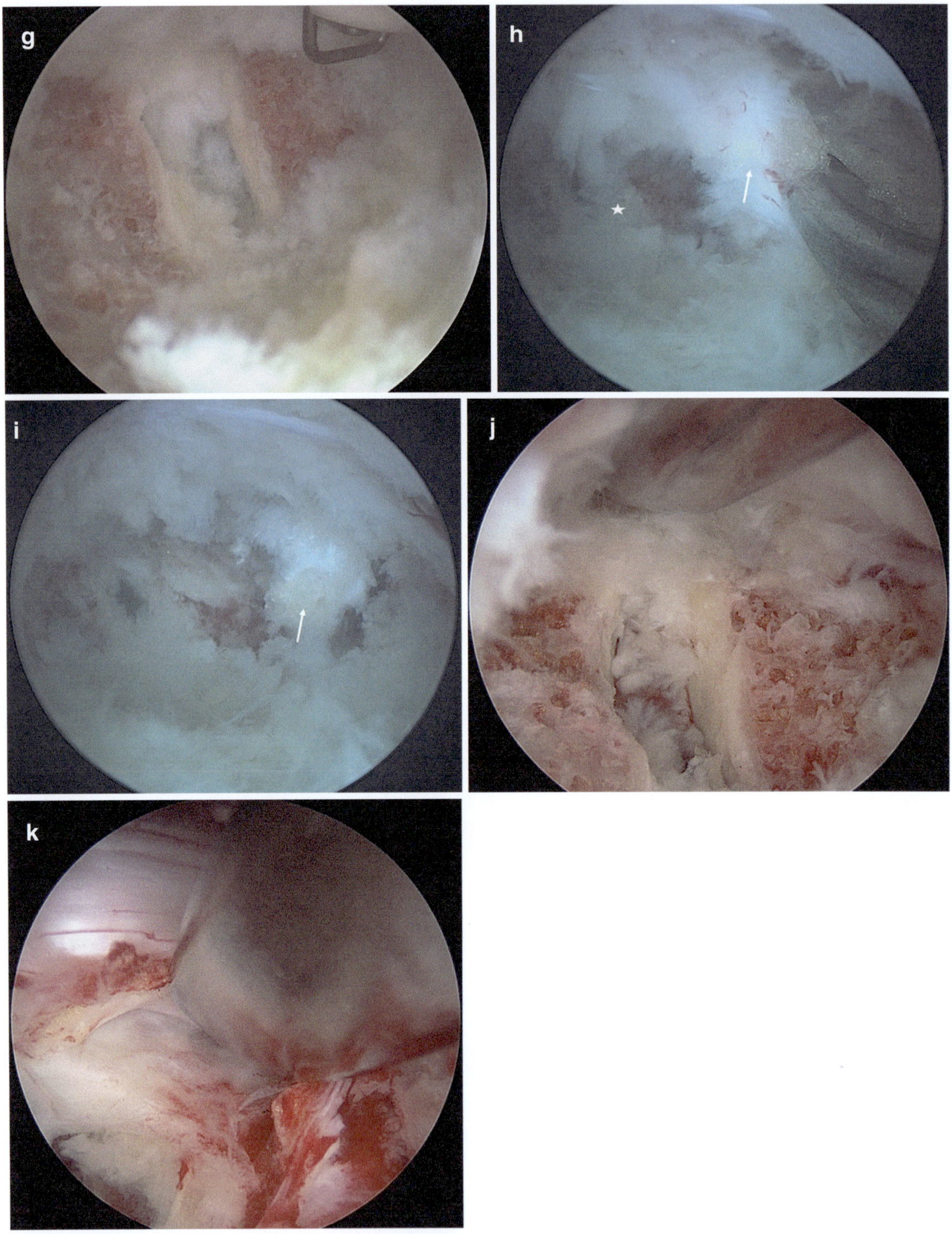


**Fig. 4** (continued)

with epidural vessel has been identified (Fig. 4b and c). The ruptured disc fragment is removed using a combination of freer elevators and pituitary forceps (Fig. 4d and e). If there is centrally located disc or calcified disc, the surgeon should make a space using a diamond drill both in the posterior edge of the endplate and in the vertebral body (Fig. 4f). This technique provides indirect and direct decompression from the ipsilateral to medial side without manipulation of the spinal cord. Using this technique, laterally located disc can be removed under direct visualization (Fig. 4g), whereas centrally located or calcified disc fragments require the use of a curved freer elevator to push the fragment down into the created disc space while avoiding manipulation of the spinal cord (Fig. 1b and 4h). Thereafter, the disc fragment could then be displaced into the disc space and removed using pituitary forceps (Fig. 4i).

Basically, calcified TDH are thick and hard, and removing them is difficult and dangerous. In the case of the calcified TDH, a diamond burr is used to thin out as much as possible the calcified portion. Once thinned out, the remaining calcified disc can be detached from the dura sac using the freer elevator and removed progressively piece by piece using small-sized pituitary forceps. If the dura sac and calcified disc cannot be separated, the calcified portion of the dura is thinned using a diamond drill, leaving a posterior shell. It is known as the floating method that prevent any effort to manipulate the interface between the shell and the ventral dural.

If a 0-degree endoscope cannot visualize the centrally located fragments, a 30-degree scope should be used. The endoscope's 30-degree tilt allows for direct visualization of the medial side of the disc space while avoiding cord manipulation (Fig. 4j). The area beneath the dura sac is further examined with a freer elevator near the end of the decompression to guarantee full decompression, which can be validated using endoscopic guidance (Fig. 4k).

Besides, fusion may or may not be required depending on the amount of facet joint removal required to accomplish complete neural decompression. To give even more segmental stability, percutaneous pedicle screw instrumentation can also be employed.

### 5.5 Postoperative Drain

To prevent postoperative hematoma, a Jackson–Pratt surgical drain (100 cc) is inserted via the working portal after discectomy. Two Jackson–Pratt surgical drains could be implanted if there is considerable bleeding on the operation field.

### 5.6 Postoperative Care

The patient is routinely mobilized without a brace right after surgery. In two days, a postoperative MRI is performed to assess for suspected epidural hematoma and the degree of decompression.

## 6 Illustrated Cases

### 6.1 Case 1: TDH at the T11–T12 Level with Upward Migration

For three months, a 65-year-old man had right-side back pain, lower-extremity paresthesia, and weakness. TDH was found on preoperative MRI at T11–12, and a cranially migrating herniated disc fragment was discovered in the right side of the spinal canal in sagittal/axial view (Fig. 5a–c). From the right side, UBE was used to perform a posterolateral approach at the T11–T12 level. The ruptured disc was removed and the dura sac was decompressed thoroughly. A postoperative MRI confirmed the result after surgery (Fig. 5d–fF). The patient's pain was significantly reduced following surgery. Physical strength in the lower extremities had restored to normal at the 3-month follow-up.

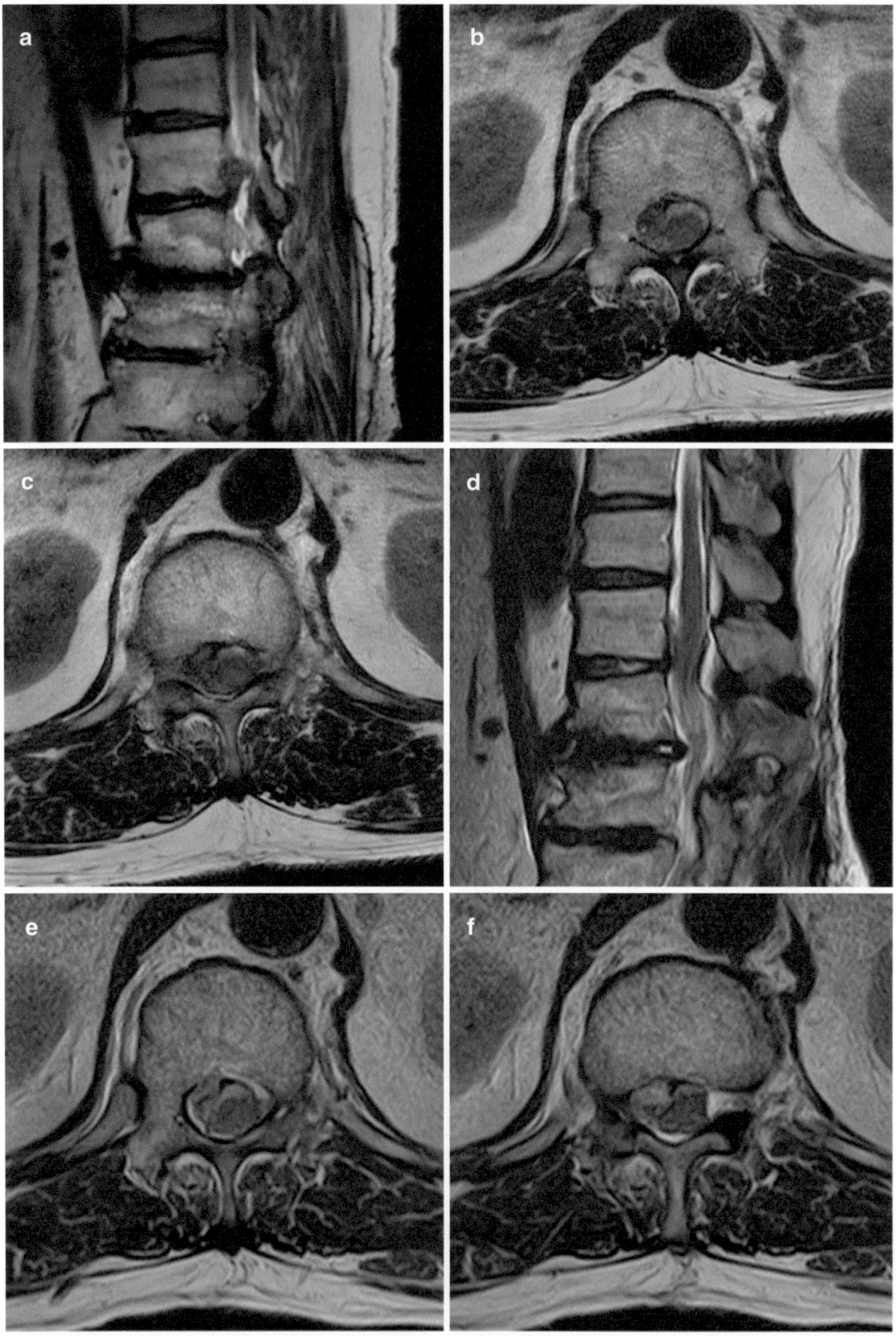


**Fig. 5** Case of a 65-year-old man with thoracic disc herniation at T11–T12 level. Preoperative MR images show upward migrated thoracic disc herniation at T11–12 level (sagittal: **a**, axial: **b** and **c**). Postoperative axial T2-weighted MRI show adequate decompression and no residual disc fragment (sagittal: **d**, axial: **e** and **f**)

### 6.2 Case 2: Myelopathy Due to a TDH at the T8–T9 Level

For 9 months, a 50-year-old woman has been experiencing weakness in both lower extremities. Muscle force loss in the lower limbs was found on the patient's neurological examination, with the loss being more severe on his right lower leg (3/5). Preoperative MRI revealed bilateral paramedian disc herniation (right dominant) at the level of T8–T9, causing spinal cord compression (Fig. 6a and b). UBE used a bilateral posterolateral approach with intraoperative neurophysiological monitoring in this patient. Percutaneous pedicle screw fixation at T8–T9 level was performed to prevent instability in this patient who had bilateral decompression. Postoperative MRI indicated adequate decompression of spinal cord and no evident residual disc herniation at the T8–T9 level (Fig. 6c and d). The patient's muscle force was fully recovered after 3-month follow-up. No evidence of segmental instability was revealed on follow-up radiography.

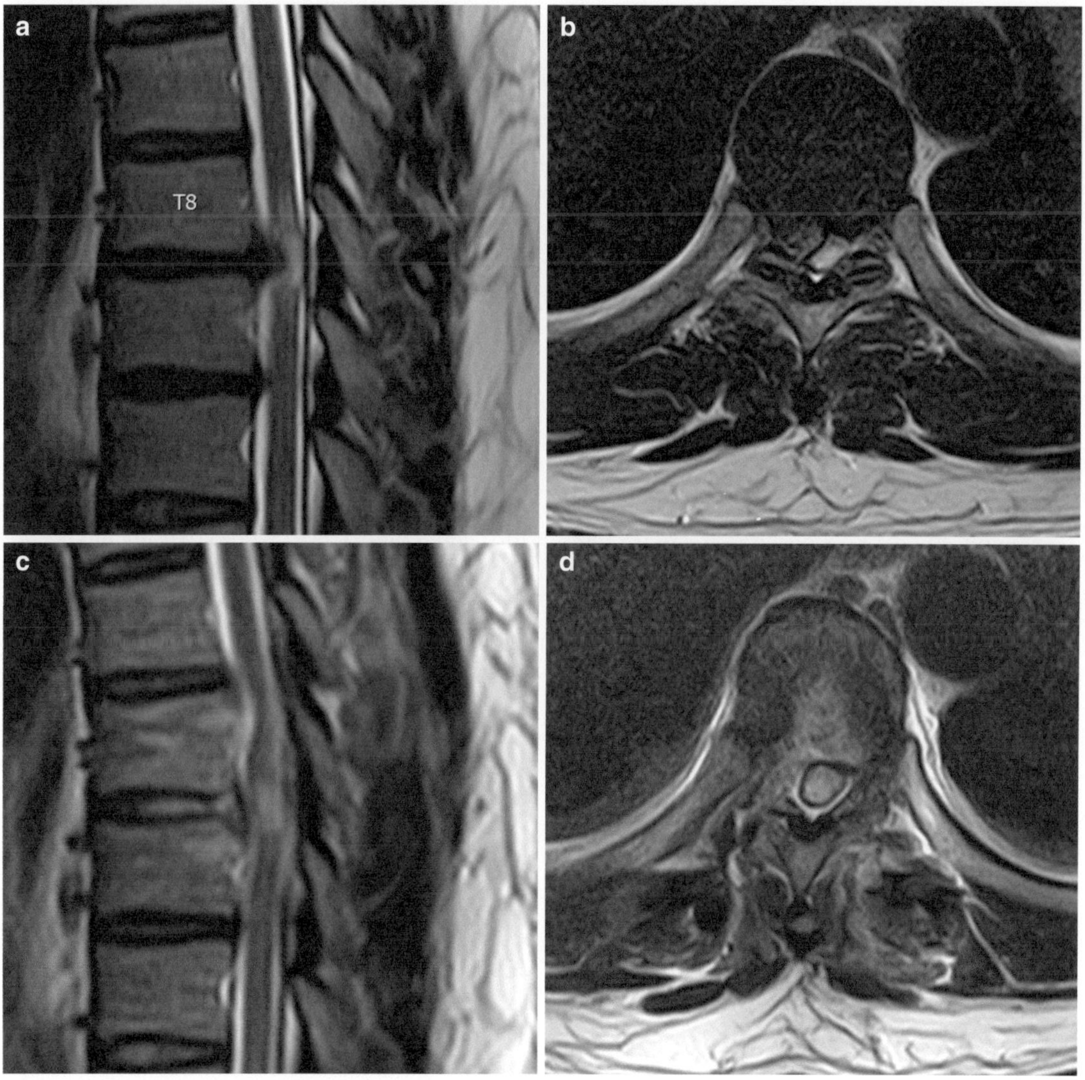


**Fig. 6** Case of a 50-year-old man with thoracic disc herniation at T8–T9 level. Preoperative MRI show bilateral thoracic disc herniation (right dominant), compressing the cord at the T8–T9 level. (MRI sagittal: **a** and axial: **b**). Postoperative axial T2-weighted MRI show well decompression of bilateral TDH (MRI sagittal: **c** and axial: **d**)

## 7 Prevention and Management of Complications

### 7.1 Dural Tear

The adhesion of the disc to the dura sac, which can result in a danger of dura tear, is a specific complication. A small lateral or ventral dura tear can be treated with a fibrin collagen patch (TachoComb) and 5–7 days of bedrest. If the dura tear is large enough that the fibrin collagen patch cannot cover it, the dura defect should be repaired directly with a dural suture. Preoperative CT combined with MRI should be evaluated for the presence of calcification within the disc to prevent this complication. If this is the case, it is suggested that a thinned calcified section be left against the dural sac.

### 7.2 Cord Injury

As the thoracic cord is particularly sensitive to compression, the thoracic decompression should be done carefully to avoid unintended spinal cord compression. Prevention of neurological deterioration is based on some recommendations: (1) using the optimal trajectory that allows excellent disc space exposure with little cord manipulation, (2) using a 30-degree endoscope for more wide vision, (3) using a semi-tubular retractor to ensure continuous fluid output to avoid exaggerated cord pressure, (4) if a centrally located disc or calcified disc is present, the surgeon should create a space between the posterior edge of the endplate and the vertebral body with a diamond drill, and (5) if the calcified disc is difficult to remove due to severe adhesion or dural ossification, it is safe to leave the calcified portion using the floating method.

## 8 Discussion (Surgical Tips and Pitfalls)

Due to the thoracic cord's specific susceptibility to retraction injury, surgery for TDH includes the risk of neurological deterioration. So far, TDH surgery is technically challenging due to its technical problems, as well as the potential for significant consequences. The ideal goal is to obtain adequate decompression without manipulating the spinal cord while avoiding paraspinal muscle/facet injury and consequences.

The posterolateral approach for TDH by UBE has distinct advantages over the conventional approach for TDH: (1) the combination of an angled field of view and freedom of movement allows an adequate working area and minimal manipulation of the spinal cord; (2) the UBE technique under continuous irrigation provides excellent visualization and magnification; (3) the learning curve of this technique did not take a significant time to achieve maximum efficacy compared to other endoscopic techniques; and (4) if the precise route for the endoscope and tools is planned, this surgery can be completed effectively without significant disturbance of the facet joint and musculoligamentous complex.

Only after the surgeon has adequate experience with UBE for lumbar decompression is it advisable to use the posterolateral technique for TDH. Beginner UBE surgeons should avoid patients with large, calcified, centrally located disc due to safety and technical challenges. To avoid difficulties, the surgeon's expertise with thoracic anatomy, as well as their level of comfort and competence with UBE methods, are critical. In addition, for successful surgical and clinical outcomes, physicians must remember the anatomical landmark and the following surgical advice.

1. To have clear sight of the disc space and easy handling of surgical equipment, the required trajectory angle is modified (30–35 degrees to the docking point).
2. Obese patients require a more lateral approach to allow for better vision of the disc area and easier manipulation of surgical instruments.
3. Partial removal of the superior portion of the pedicle may be required in some cases to enable an unobstructed view of the diseased disc and to assist in positioning the scope and instruments deeper and closer to the disc space.

4. The lateral boundary of the dura sac must be identified in order to remove the disc fragment safely and completely.
5. While a centrally located HNP or calcified HNP can be removed under direct view, a space in the disc must first be established, and then a curved freer elevator must be utilized to drive the fragment down into the disc space for removal, avoiding cord manipulation.
6. If removing the calcified disc is difficult due to significant adhesion or dural ossification, the floating approach should be used.
7. A 0-degree endoscope is commonly used. If the centrally located TDH cannot be viewed with a 0-degree endoscope, a 30-degree scope is required.

## References


1. Stillerman CB, Chen TC, Couldwell WT, Zhang W, Weiss MH. Experience in the surgical management of 82 symptomatic herniated thoracic discs and review of the literature. J Neurosurg. 1998;88(4):623–33.
2. Roelz R, Scholz C, Klingler JH, Scheiwe C, Sircar R, Hubbe U. Giant central thoracic disc herniations: surgical outcome in 17 consecutive patients treated by mini-thoracotomy. Eur Spine J. 2016;25(5):1443–51.
3. Sekhar LN, Jannetta PJ. Thoracic disc herniation: operative approaches and results. Neurosurgery. 1983;12(3):303–5.
4. Mulier S, Debois V. Thoracic disc herniations: transthoracic, lateral, or posterolateral approach? A review. Surg Neurol. 1998;49(6):599–606; discussion 8
5. Sharma SB, Kim JS. A review of minimally invasive surgical techniques for the management of thoracic disc herniations. Neurospine. 2019;16(1):24–33.
6. Yoshihara H, Yoneoka D. Comparison of in-hospital morbidity and mortality rates between anterior and nonanterior approach procedures for thoracic disc herniation. Spine (Phila Pa 1976). 2014;39(12):E728–33.
7. Borm W, Bazner U, Konig RW, Kretschmer T, Antoniadis G, Kandenwein J. Surgical treatment of thoracic disc herniations via tailored posterior approaches. Eur Spine J. 2011;20(10):1684–90.
8. Fessler RG, Sturgill M. Review: Complications of surgery for thoracic disc disease. Surg Neurol. 1998;49(6):609–18.
9. Park MK, Son SK, Park WW, Choi SH, Jung DY, Kim DH. Unilateral biportal endoscopy for decompression of extraforaminal stenosis at the lumbosacral junction: surgical techniques and clinical outcomes. Neurospine. 2021;18(4):871–9.
10. Heo DH, Lee DC, Park CK. Comparative analysis of three types of minimally invasive decompressive surgery for lumbar central stenosis: biportal endoscopy, uniportal endoscopy, and microsurgery. Neurosurg Focus. 2019;46(5):E9.